T Cell Biology – From Development to Immunotherapy

Edited by Ling Yin

Published in London, United Kingdom

T Cell Biology - From Development to Immunotherapy
http://dx.doi.org/10.5772/intechopen.1011227
Edited by Ling Yin

Contributors
Adedeji Okikiade, Adán Germán Gallardo Rodríguez, Aldo Mujica Martínez, Christian Omar Ramos Peñafiel, Chunxiao Xue, Claudia Mondragón Albarrán, Cynthia Guadalupe Pelayo Mena, Daniel Moses, Daoyuan Xie, Erika Gómez Zamora, Estibeyesbo Said Plascencia Nieto, Fidelis Nwachukwu, Gabriel Aceves Castillo, Guanting Lu, Huanyuan Wang, Huizhen He, Inaia Phoenix, Jacqueline V. Lara-Espinosa, Jie Zhang, Jing Ni, Jingzhe Ma, Jinping Shu, Ksenia Zornikova, Lianying Wu, Lifang Ma, Ling Yin, María Fernanda Arce-Aceves, Mayra Silva Miranda, Miao He, Mingyue Shang, Moises Leonardo Mendoza Torres, Monica Alethia Cureño Diaz, Okechukwu Nwako, Parv Barot, Qi Qin, Rogelio Hernández-Pando, Sanjay Rathod, Shuai Tan, Shuang Shang, Somia Shehzadi, Vanessa Carregaro, Vasti Lozano-Ordaz, Verónica Fernández Sánchez, Wanling Sun, Wei Wang, Xiaoli Chang, Xiaoyu Li, Yadira Rodríguez- Miguez, Yanet Ventura Enríquez, Yaochi Chen, Yixuan Wang, Yizhang Zhou, Yumeng Li, Yu Tian, Zaid Talal Abdulqader Al-Qadhi, Zhipeng Zhao, Zongqu Sun

First published in London, United Kingdom, 2026 by IntechOpen
IntechOpen is the global imprint of INTECHOPEN LIMITED, registered in England and Wales, registration number: 11086078, 167-169 Great Portland Street, London, W1W 5PF, United Kingdom

For EU product safety concerns: IN TECH d.o.o., Prolaz Marije Krucifikse Kozulić 3, 51000 Rijeka, Croatia, info@intechopen.com or visit our website at intechopen.com.

British Library Cataloguing-in-Publication Data
A catalogue record for this book is available from the British Library

T Cell Biology - From Development to Immunotherapy
Edited by Ling Yin
p. cm.
Print ISBN 978-1-80632-051-6
Online ISBN 978-1-80632-050-9
eBook (PDF) ISBN 978-1-80632-052-3

Meet the editor

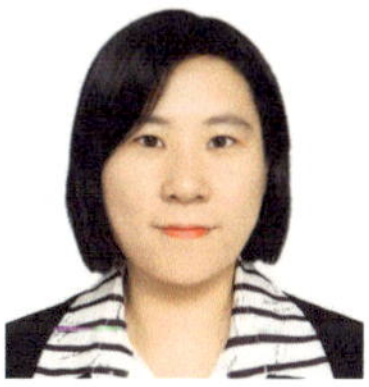

Dr. Ling Yin is a Professor and Dean at the College of Modern Agriculture, Weifang Institute of Technology, China. She received her Ph.D. from South China Agricultural University and completed postdoctoral training at the University of Florida College of Medicine and Fudan University. Her research focuses on gene therapy and cancer immunology, particularly AAV-based therapies and reprogramming the tumor microenvironment. She has published in Gene Therapy, Molecular Therapy, and Drug Discovery Today, serves on multiple editorial boards, and has received the Global Recognition Award and the High-Caliber Talent of Hefei City.

Contents

Preface

T lymphocytes are central to adaptive immunity, orchestrating immune responses against pathogens while maintaining tolerance to self-antigens. This edited volume provides a comprehensive overview of T cell biology, spanning from fundamental developmental mechanisms to cutting-edge therapeutic applications.

The book begins by examining T cell development and differentiation in the thymus, where thymic selection processes shape a functional, self-tolerant T cell repertoire. Subsequent chapters delve into T cell receptor signaling, exploring the molecular architecture of the TCR-CD3 complex, the formation of the immunological synapse, and the intricate signal transduction pathways that govern T cell activation. The volume then surveys the functional specialization of diverse T cell subsets, including helper T cells, cytotoxic T lymphocytes, regulatory T cells, and memory T cells, each playing distinct roles in immune defense and homeostasis.

Moving from basic science to clinical relevance, the book addresses the critical involvement of T cells in human diseases, including autoimmunity, cancer, infectious diseases, and immunodeficiencies. A dedicated section highlights revolutionary T cell engineering approaches, such as CAR-T cell therapies and TCR gene editing, which have transformed cancer immunotherapy. The final chapters showcase emerging technologies reshaping T cell research, including single-cell analysis, spatial transcriptomics, CRISPR screening, and live-cell imaging.

By integrating foundational knowledge with translational applications, this volume serves as an invaluable resource for immunologists, cell biologists, and clinician-scientists. The carefully curated chapters combine rigorous scholarship with accessible explanations, making this book suitable for graduate students, postdoctoral researchers, and established investigators seeking a state-of-the-art synthesis of T cell immunology.

I am grateful to all contributing authors for their outstanding scholarship and to the editorial team at IntechOpen for their professional support throughout the publication process.

Ling Yin
Weill Cornell Medicine,
United States of America

Section 1

T Cell Immunity in Infectious Diseases and Viral Malignancies

Chapter 1

HTLV-1-Driven T-Cell Malignancy: Disruption of T-Cell Development, Immune Function and Opportunities for Therapeutic Innovation

Fidelis Nwachukwu, Daniel Moses, Adedeji Okikiade, Inaia Phoenix and Okechukwu Nwako

Abstract

Human T-cell leukemia virus type 1 (HTLV-1) is a persistent retrovirus that preferentially maintains long-term infection in $CD4^{+}$ T cells and, after decades of latency, causes adult T-cell leukemia/lymphoma (ATLL) in a small subset of carriers. Rather than acute transformation, HTLV-1 drives oncogenesis through chronic immune dysregulation, sustained clonal expansion, and progressive reprogramming of T-cell development and function. This chapter positions HTLV-1 as a model system for dissecting T-cell biology under prolonged oncogenic stress, linking viral persistence, thymic and peripheral fate distortion, immune remodeling, and clonal evolution to delayed and heterogeneous transformation risk. Central to this process are the complementary functions of Tax and HBZ, which maintain proliferative signaling, enforce immune evasion,and stabilize malignant phenotypes. Integrating genomic and epigenomic data, we outline a multistep model of ATLL pathogenesis and connect these dependency networks to mechanism-driven therapies, underscoring the limitations of chemotherapy and the necessity of biomarker-guided, combination treatment strategies.

Keywords: HTLV-1, adult T-cell leukemia/lymphoma, T-cell development, clonal persistence, immune evasion, precision oncology

1. Introduction

Human T-cell leukemia virus type 1 (HTLV-1) is a uniquely instructive pathogen in human immunology and oncology. Unlike acutely transforming oncogenic viruses, HTLV-1 establishes lifelong infection predominantly within CD4+ T lymphocytes and persists through clonal expansion of infected cells rather than sustained productive replication [1–3]. In only a small fraction of infected individuals, this silent, decades-long infection culminates in adult T-cell leukemia/lymphoma (ATLL), an aggressive malignancy characterized by profound immune dysfunction, resistance to conventional therapy, and poor clinical outcomes [4–6].

This prolonged latency and low transformation rate create a paradox that has shaped decades of investigation: HTLV-1 profoundly perturbs T-cell biology in many hosts, yet malignant progression is rare [1, 7]. Globally, an estimated 5–10 million individuals are infected, with marked geographic clustering in southwestern Japan, the Caribbean, parts of South America, and sub-Saharan Africa [8, 9]. Clinical observations from endemic regions consistently demonstrate long-term viral carriage with immune perturbation in the absence of malignancy, emphasizing that ATLL represents the endpoint of a multistep evolutionary process rather than a direct consequence of infection [7, 10].

HTLV-1, therefore, cannot be understood solely as a leukemogenic trigger. Instead, it functions as a chronic biological stressor that incrementally reshapes the T-cell life cycle, altering developmental programming, activation thresholds, immune regulation, and survival signaling over time [1, 11, 12]. Viral gene products, particularly Tax and the HTLV-1 basic leucine zipper factor (HBZ), rewire central signaling networks such as nuclear factor kappa B (NF-κB) and related transcriptional programs, promoting sustained proliferation, immune modulation, and escape from host surveillance [11, 13, 14]. These alterations expand pools of long-lived, developmentally misaligned T cells permissive to secondary genetic and epigenetic events, ultimately stabilizing malignant phenotypes in ATLL [15, 16].

From a translational and precision oncology perspective, ATLL exemplifies a malignancy driven less by early catastrophic genomic instability and more by prolonged immune and signaling dysregulation. Integrated molecular analyses reveal that recurrent genetic and epigenetic alterations in ATLL reinforce virus-induced cellular programs rather than replacing them, underscoring the importance of context-dependent vulnerabilities and pathway dependencies [15–17]. This biology helps explain the limited durability of conventional cytotoxic chemotherapy and highlights the need for biomarker-guided, mechanism-aligned therapeutic strategies [4–6].

In this chapter, HTLV-1 is used as a model system to examine how chronic viral infection disrupts T-cell development, peripheral immune function, and lineage stability, and how these disruptions converge on malignant transformation. We integrate entry and persistence biology, thymic and peripheral fate distortion, immune remodeling, and clonal evolution to motivate mechanism-aligned therapeutic innovation.

2. Why HTLV-1 is a T-cell biology stress test

HTLV-1 is among the most instructive natural models for understanding how chronic viral perturbation reshapes T-cell biology and, in a subset of hosts, culminates in malignant transformation. Unlike acutely transforming oncogenic viruses, HTLV-1 establishes lifelong infection predominantly within CD4+ T lymphocytes and persists primarily through clonal expansion of infected cells rather than sustained productive replication [1–3]. This persistence strategy produces a prolonged latency, often spanning decades between initial infection and the development of ATLL, underscoring that malignant progression is neither inevitable nor immediate [4, 7, 12]. The long latency between infection and malignant transformation reflects progressive immune remodeling and clonal selection within infected T-cell populations, as illustrated in **Figure 1**.

Conceptual schematic illustrating the natural history of HTLV-1 infection. Following the initial infection of CD4+ T cells, the virus persists predominantly through clonal expansion of infected cells rather than sustained productive replication. Over decades, chronic viral pressure reshapes T-cell activation thresholds, immune regulation, and survival signaling, leading to progressive immune remodeling. In a minority of hosts, iterative immune selection and host genomic/epigenomic adaptation culminate in clonal dominance and eventual progression to ATLL.

Globally, HTLV-1 infects an estimated 5–10 million individuals, with pronounced geographic clustering in southwestern Japan, the Caribbean, parts of South America, and sub-Saharan Africa [8, 9]. Despite this substantial burden, ATLL develops in only a minority of infected individuals, revealing a central paradox: HTLV-1 profoundly alters T-cell biology in many hosts, yet only rarely crosses the threshold into overt malignancy [1, 7, 12]. Clinical observations from endemic regions further reinforce this paradox, demonstrating long-term viral carriage with immune perturbation in the absence of malignant transformation [7, 10]. The global distribution, transmission pathways, and relative ATLL risk across endemic regions are summarized in **Table 1**.

This disparity highlights the importance of long-term host-virus interactions, immune selection, and cellular evolution rather than a single oncogenic event [18, 19]. From a translational and precision oncology perspective, HTLV-1 is therefore best understood not simply as a leukemogenic virus but as a chronic biological stressor that incrementally distorts T-cell developmental programs, activation thresholds, and immune regulatory circuits over time [1, 11]. These cumulative perturbations generate cellular states characterized by abnormal persistence, immune evasion, and altered lineage identity, creating fertile ground

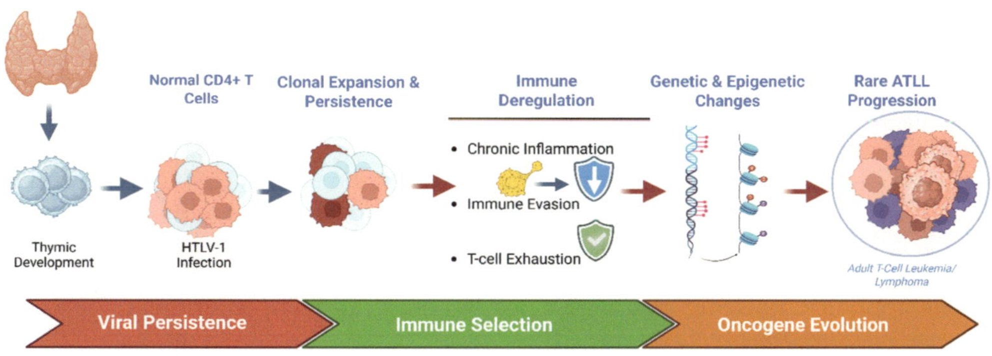

Figure 1.
HTLV-1 as a stress test for T-cell biology.

Region	Estimated prevalence	Predominant transmission routes	ATLL risk
Southwestern Japan	High	Mother-to-child (breastfeeding), sexual	Elevated
Caribbean	High	Sexual, vertical	Elevated
South America	Moderate-high	Sexual, blood exposure	Variable
Sub-Saharan Africa	Moderate	Sexual, vertical	Under-reported
Non-endemic regions	Low	Blood products, migration-associated	Low

Regional clustering reflects differential contributions of breastfeeding-associated vertical transmission, sexual transmission, and blood exposure; ATL risk remains low overall despite endemic prevalence [8, 9].

Table 1.
Global epidemiology and transmission pathways of HTLV-1.

for secondary genetic and epigenetic alterations that ultimately stabilize malignant phenotypes [15, 16, 20, 21]. The rarity of ATLL, despite widespread infection, thus becomes an advantage for biological insight: HTLV-1 exposes how long-term misprogramming of T cells can precede and enable cancer, rather than merely accompany it. Accordingly, this chapter adopts a mechanism-first framework, using HTLV-1 to examine how sustained viral pressure reshapes the T-cell life cycle from developmental programming to peripheral immune function, and how these rewired dependencies inform biomarker-guided and precision therapeutic strategies [5, 6, 22].

3. Cell entry, tropism, and persistence strategy

HTLV-1 can infect multiple immune cell types, including monocytes/macrophages, dendritic cells (DCs), and CD8+ T cells, but it preferentially establishes long-term persistence in CD4+ T cells [23, 24]. Importantly, "cell-free" HTLV-1 is typically poorly infectious; efficient spread is predominantly cell-associated and occurs through structured cell-cell contacts [3]. Dendritic cells are not passive bystanders: HTLV-1 can directly infect DCs, which can then transmit HTLV-1 to CD4+ T cells, and even uninfected DCs can capture virions and transfer them to T cells, supporting early dissemination while limiting exposure to neutralizing antibodies [25, 26].

HTLV-1 entry into CD4+ T cells is mediated by viral envelope interactions with a multicomponent host receptor system that includes the glucose transporter (GLUT1), heparan sulfate proteoglycans (HSPGs), and neuropilin-1 (NRP-1) [27–29]. A coherent entry model involves initial attachment via HSPGs, complexing with NRP-1, and subsequent engagement of GLUT1 to trigger membrane fusion and entry [29, 30]. Differential HSPG expressions on $CD4^+$ T cells have been proposed as one contributor to tropism [26]. NRP-1's capacity to bind VEGF165, and the observation that VEGF165 can inhibit HTLV-1 entry, provide experimental leverage supporting receptor involvement [31].

HTLV-1 spreads predominantly through virological synapses and biofilm-like extracellular assemblies rather than as free virions [32, 33]. Virological synapses help explain preferential CD4+ T-cell infection because HTLV-1 requires sustained cell contact, and CD4+ T cells form stable conjugates via adhesion molecules such as the lymphocyte function-associated antigen-1 (LFA-1) [34]. The coordinated interactions among HSPGs, neuropilin-1, and GLUT1 that facilitate HTLV-1 entry and subsequent cell-to-cell transmission are summarized in **Figure 2**.

Schematic representation of HTLV-1 entry and spread within the host immune compartment. Viral envelope glycoproteins engage a multicomponent receptor system on CD4+ T cells, including HSPGs, NRP-1, and the GLUT1, facilitating membrane fusion and proviral integration. Subsequent viral propagation occurs predominantly through direct cell-to-cell transmission via virological synapses and biofilm-like extracellular assemblies rather than through cell-free virions. Long-term persistence is maintained through clonal expansion of infected T cells, resulting in stable integration-site–defined clones that can persist for decades prior to malignant transformation.

Once integrated, HTLV-1 persistence is achieved primarily through clonal expansion of infected T cells, generating large populations of genetically identical clones with fixed proviral integration sites detectable years before malignancy [1, 18]. Beyond Tax and HBZ, several viral accessory proteins materially support transmission and immune escape. These include p8, which enhances virological synapse formation and promotes the transfer of virions and viral proteins [35]; p12, which can reduce MHC class I surface expression and decrease CD8+ T-cell killing [36]; and p30, which functions as a post-transcriptional negative regulator of viral replication and promotes latency by constraining viral gene expression, including Tax-dependent programs [37].

A defining feature of HTLV-1 persistence is asymmetric viral gene expression over time. The viral transactivator Tax is a strong early driver of transcriptional activation, proliferation, and inflammatory signaling, most notably via NF-κB. However, it is highly immunogenic, and sustained expression renders infected cells vulnerable to cytotoxic T-lymphocyte-mediated clearance [11, 13, 38]. In contrast, HBZ is more consistently expressed at low levels and is considerably less immunogenic, supporting infected-cell survival and immune modulation while evading immune detection [11, 14, 39]. The complementary functional roles of Tax and HBZ in viral persistence and oncogenic conditioning are summarized in **Table 2**.

This division of labor allows HTLV-1 to balance proliferative drive with immune invisibility, enabling lifelong persistence and creating the biological substrate for clonal selection and malignant evolution [1, 18].

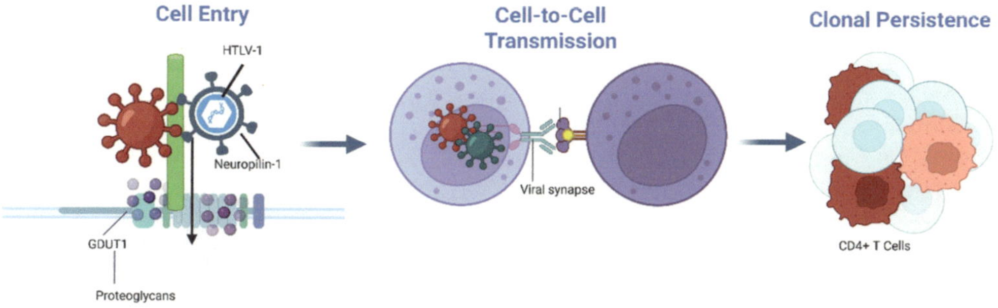

Figure 2.
Cell entry, cell-to-cell transmission, and clonal persistence of HTLV-1 in CD4+ T-cells.

Feature	Tax	HBZ	Functional consequence
Expression pattern	Intermittent, often silenced	Persistent, low-level	Immune selection favors HBZ
Immunogenicity	High	Low	Enables immune evasion
NF-κB activation	Strong	Indirect/modulatory	Sustained survival signaling
Proliferation	Potent driver	Maintenance	Clonal expansion
Immune regulation	Pro-inflammatory	Regulatory/exhaustion-like	Impaired surveillance
Role in ATLL	Early expansion	Later persistence	Malignant fixation

Tax primarily amplifies activation and proliferation with high immune visibility, whereas HBZ supports persistence, immune modulation, and malignant maintenance with lower immunogenicity [11, 13, 14].

Table 2.
Comparative roles of tax and HBZ in HTLV-1–driven T-cell reprogramming.

4. Interference with T-cell development and lineage programming

Although HTLV-1 infection is most readily detected in peripheral blood, accumulating evidence supports the concept that viral perturbation extends upstream into programs governing T-cell identity, lineage commitment, and fate stability. HTLV-1 can infect hematopoietic progenitors and multiple thymocyte stages, including double-negative (DN), double-positive (DP), and single-positive (SP) subsets, supporting the plausibility of early developmental perturbation [40]. Experimental work in a humanized $Rag2^{-}/^{-}\gamma c^{-}/^{-}$ mouse model demonstrated that HTLV-1 infection of immature thymocytes accelerated maturation and was associated with the accumulation of activated SP CD4+ and CD8+ T cells [40]. Mechanistically, Tax suppresses transcription of the pre-T-cell receptor α chain (pTα), potentially compromising β-selection and increasing apoptosis risk [41]. A coherent compensatory model is that Tax-driven NF-κB activation provides survival signals that partially substitute for pre-TCR-mediated cues, enabling thymocytes to bypass normal constraints while retaining proliferative capacity [13, 41].

Clinical observations in HTLV-1-associated myelopathy (HAM) provide additional support for lineage distortion under chronic viral pressure. Reports describe expanded CD4+/CD8+ populations and the emergence of DP T cells with elevated Tax expression, mixed helper/cytotoxic phenotypes, and inflammatory cytokine profiles consistent with altered differentiation and tissue-homing behavior [42]. These developmental distortions in thymic selection and peripheral signaling pathways are conceptually illustrated in **Figure 3**.

Conceptual schematic illustrating how chronic HTLV-1 infection perturbs thymic and peripheral T-cell fate decisions. Viral gene products, particularly Tax and HBZ, alter basal signaling thresholds within developing thymocytes and mature CD4+ T cells through sustained activation of pathways such as nuclear factor kappa B (NF-κB) and Janus kinase/signal transducer and activator of transcription (JAK/STAT). These signaling shifts bias survival independently of canonical selection checkpoints (β-selection, positive and negative selection), promoting the expansion of developmentally misaligned T-cell populations that retain proliferative and activation capacity. Over time, this chronic distortion of

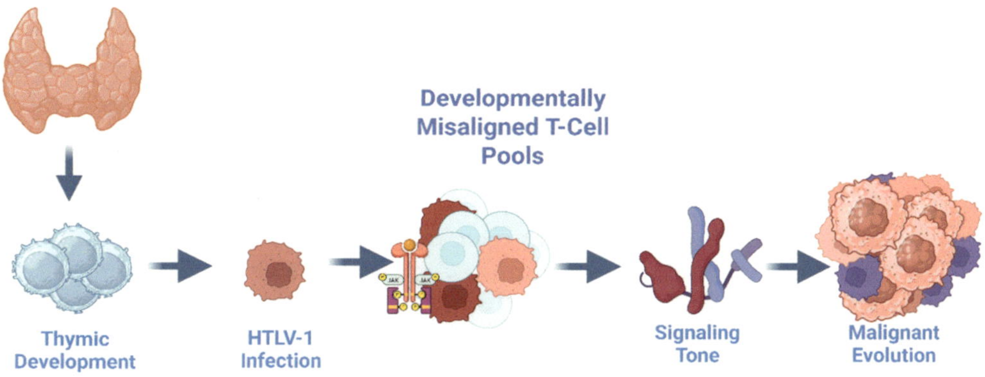

Figure 3.
Disruption of T-cell development and lineage programming by HTLV-1.

lineage fidelity generates long-lived, activation-biased T-cell pools that are permissive to secondary genetic and epigenetic events, facilitating clonal evolution and eventual malignant transformation.

Crucially, these alterations do not imply wholesale failure of T-cell development. Rather, HTLV-1 induces a subtle but chronic distortion of lineage fidelity, expanding pools of long-lived, activation-biased T cells that deviate from canonical differentiation trajectories while retaining survival and self-renewal capacity [1, 11]. Over decades, such cells accumulate secondary genetic and epigenetic alterations that stabilize aberrant signaling states and reduce reliance on viral transactivation [15–17, 21]. Large-scale genomic and epigenomic analyses provide compelling support for this model: recurrent alterations converge on pathways already stressed by HTLV-1 infection, including T-cell receptor signaling, NF-κB regulation, transcriptional control, and chromatin remodeling [15, 16, 20]. Rather than introducing entirely new oncogenic programs, these changes reinforce and lock in virus-induced cellular states, converting chronic dysregulation into fixed malignant identity [15, 16].

5. Functional rewiring of T-cells in HTLV-1 infection

Tax and HBZ are critical for viral gene expression and contribute directly to cellular transformation [11, 43]. Tax is an early, highly immunogenic driver of transformation through transcriptional activation, proliferation, and DNA damage, and is often downregulated after transformation is established [13, 44]. Tax engages host pathways, particularly NF-κB, promoting chronic T-cell activation and growth factor-independent proliferation [13]. Tax also inhibits DNA repair pathways, increasing mutational burden and genetic instability [45, 46]. Because Tax is a major target of cytotoxic T-cell responses, immune selection favors reduced Tax expression in later disease stages [1, 38].

HBZ is consistently expressed in ATLL and contributes to proliferation, apoptosis resistance, autophagy regulation, and immune evasion [14, 39, 47]. HBZ can suppress apoptosis through its effects on transcriptional regulators and survival pathways and may inhibit autophagy via mTOR pathway involvement [47–49]. HBZ supports immune escape by dampening antiviral and inflammatory pathways, shifting T-cell function toward regulatory phenotypes, and maintaining latency while minimizing immune recognition [14, 50, 51]. HBZ also suppresses Tax-mediated transcription from the 5' long terminal repeat (LTR) and contributes to reduced viral protein expression, supporting immune invisibility [51, 52]. This functional division of labor between early Tax activity and sustained HBZ expression is summarized schematically in **Figure 4**.

The resulting immune environment is characterized by chronic immune activation coupled with ineffective antitumor immunity, which are features consistent with immune dysfunction and exhaustion-like states broadly described in chronic immune stimulation settings [53]. This immune rewiring helps explain why ATLL behaves differently from other aggressive lymphomas: the disease is not merely resistant to immune clearance; it emerges and persists within an immune landscape shaped by long-term viral modulation [4–6].

Side-by-side model summarizing how HTLV-1 balances proliferative drive with immune invisibility through differential viral gene expression. Tax functions predominantly as an early, high-amplitude transactivator that promotes transcriptional activation, proliferation, and pro-inflammatory signaling (including strong NF-κB pathway engagement), but it is highly immunogenic and therefore subject to strong cytotoxic T-cell-mediated negative selection. In contrast, HBZ is typically expressed more persistently at low levels, supports infected-cell survival and immune modulation, and contributes to immune evasion by dampening

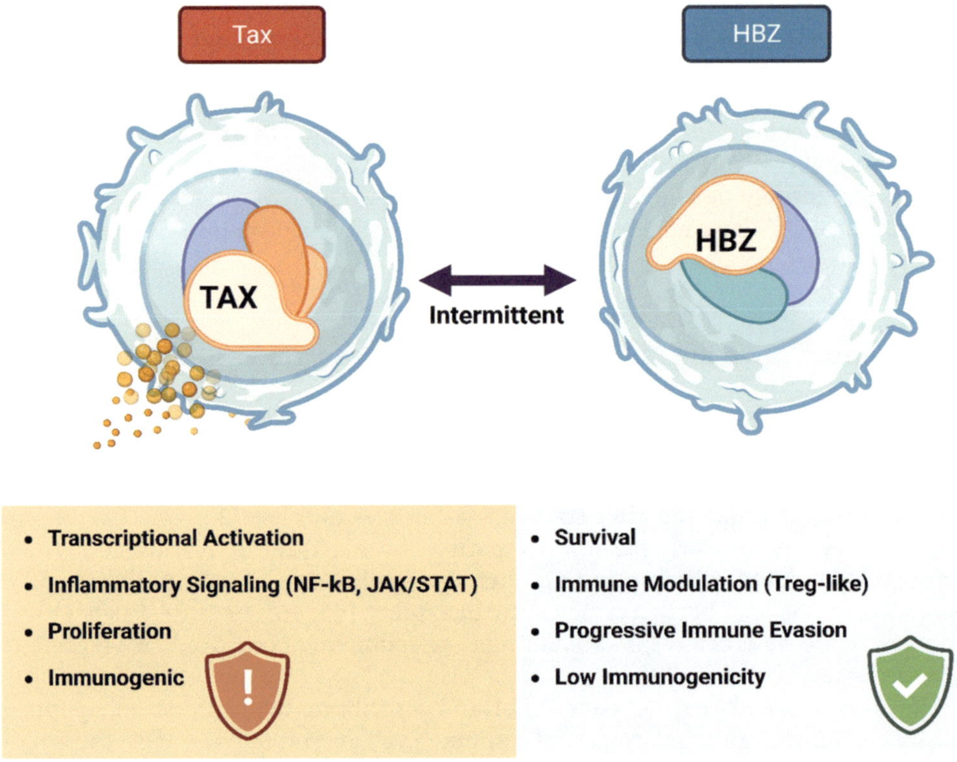

Figure 4.
Functional division of labor between Tax and HBZ in HTLV-1-infected T cells.

inflammatory and antiviral signaling and maintaining low antigen visibility. Together, intermittent Tax activity and sustained HBZ expression enable lifelong persistence and progressively condition infected clones for clonal dominance and malignant fixation.

6. From viral rewiring to ATLL: A multistep model of T-cell oncogenesis

ATLL represents the endpoint of a prolonged, multistep evolutionary process shaped by persistent viral pressure, immune selection, and progressive stabilization of host genomic and epigenomic alterations [1, 18]. Early HTLV-1 infection establishes a polyclonal reservoir of infected CD4+ T cells defined by unique proviral integration sites; over time, immune selection, particularly cytotoxic T-lymphocyte pressure against highly immunogenic proteins such as Tax, edits this reservoir, enriching clones that reduce immune visibility while retaining proliferative and survival advantages [1, 38]. This yields oligoclonal and eventually monoclonal dominance, often detectable years before clinical malignancy [1]. The evolutionary trajectory from polyclonal infection to clonal dominance and malignant fixation is illustrated in **Figure 5**.

As clonal dominance is established, secondary host genetic and epigenetic alterations accumulate, converging on pathways already stressed by chronic viral signaling. Integrated molecular analyses identify recurrent alterations affecting proximal T-cell receptor signaling, NF-κB regulation, transcriptional control, and chromatin modifiers, supporting the model that transformation reinforces virus-biased programs rather than replacing them [15, 17]. Epigenomic studies demonstrate polycomb-dependent remodeling and DNA methylation changes that lock in survival and immune-evasive transcriptional states [16, 21]. Polycomb-mediated loss of miR-31 has been shown to activate NIK-dependent NF-κB signaling in ATLL, illustrating how epigenetic dysregulation can directly reinforce survival pathways central to HTLV-1-conditioned biology [20]. Consistent with immune selection, advanced ATLL often exhibits reduced or absent Tax expression despite clear viral origin, reflecting progressive uncoupling of malignant maintenance from viral transactivation [1, 15].

Viewed through this lens, ATLL is best understood as an evolutionary endpoint shaped by iterative selection rather than abrupt transformation, in which viral persistence, immune pressure, and host genomic/epigenomic adaptation act sequentially and synergistically [18]. This framework explains prolonged latency, biological heterogeneity, and therapeutic resistance, and motivates biomarker-guided,

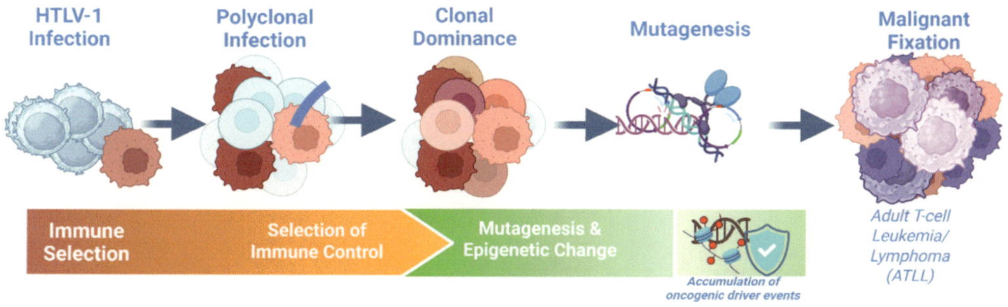

Figure 5.
Multistep model of ATLL oncogenesis from HTLV-1 infection to malignant fixation.

Altered pathway	Representative alterations (examples)	Functional impact	Translational relevance
T-cell receptor (TCR)/proximal signaling	Activating alterations in PLCG1, VAV1, CARD11	Lower activation threshold; sustained signaling	Pathway-dependency stratification; targeted inhibition concepts [15, 17]
NF-κB regulation and survival signaling	Loss of TNFAIP3 (A20) and other lesions converging on NF-κB	Anti-apoptotic tone; survival advantage	Explains chemo resistance; motivates combinatorial targeting [15, 17]
Transcriptional control/lineage stability	Recurrent transcriptional program disruption reported in integrated analyses.	Malignant identity fixation; lineage rigidity	Supports epigenetic and immune combinations; predicts limited reversibility [15, 16]
Epigenetic regulation (Polycomb/methylation)	Polycomb-dependent remodeling; aberrant methylation programs; miRNA network disruption, including miR-31 loss.	Transcriptional fixation; persistent immune-evasive states; NIK-dependent NF-κB activation.	Rationale for epigenetic therapeutics: biomarker development in methylation/miRNA signatures [16, 20, 21]
Cell-cycle control/genomic stability	Recurrent disruption of checkpoints and proliferative enforcement.	Clonal dominance and progression	Risk modeling and progression biomarkers [15, 18]

Recurrent ATLL alterations reinforce virus-stressed pathways (activation/survival and transcriptional control) and stabilize immune-evasive phenotypes, contributing to therapeutic resistance and supporting biomarker-guided, mechanism-aligned treatment design.

Table 3.
Recurrent genetic and epigenetic alterations in ATLL and their functional impact.

mechanism-aligned intervention [4–6, 22]. Integrated genomic and epigenomic studies indicate that recurrent ATLL lesions do not create an entirely new biology; rather, they reinforce virus-conditioned signaling and transcriptional states, locking in survival advantage, immune evasion, and clonal dominance (**Table 3**).

Multistep timeline illustrating how ATLL emerges through decades of constrained clonal evolution under persistent viral pressure. Early infection establishes a polyclonal reservoir of infected CD4+ T cells, each defined by a distinct proviral integration site. Over time, immune selection, particularly cytotoxic T-cell pressure against immunogenic viral programs such as Tax, progressively edits this reservoir, enriching clones that reduce immune visibility while retaining proliferative and survival advantages, resulting in oligoclonal and eventually clonal dominance. As dominant clones persist, recurrent host genetic and epigenetic alterations accumulate and converge on pathways already stressed by HTLV-1–conditioned signaling (e.g., TCR/proximal signaling, NF-κB regulation, transcriptional control, chromatin remodeling), stabilizing survival and immune-evasive states and culminating in malignant fixation as ATLL. The model also captures progressive uncoupling of tumor maintenance from overt viral transactivation (often reduced Tax expression) as host-encoded programs become entrenched.

7. Animal models and *in vivo* validation

Mechanistic claims in HTLV-1 biology and ATLL evolution are strongest when supported by complementary *in vivo* platforms that parse persistence, immune remodeling, and transformation-linked phenotypes. In rabbit infection models (New Zealand White), HTLV-1 transmission and persistence are robustly studied in an *in vivo* infection setting, where infection is primarily cell-associated (whole blood/washed cells transmit infection, whereas cell-free plasma is ineffective) and where CD4 predominance emerges over time through post-infection clonal selection rather than strict entry tropism. These models are also uniquely suited for testing molecular clones and gene-function requirements *in vivo*, including determinants of viral persistence such as HBZ [54].

In parallel, transgenic mouse systems provide targeted validation of viral programs: Tax models capture high-amplitude inflammatory/survival signaling and oncogenic stress, whereas HBZ transgenic mice support a persistence-first framework in which chronic HBZ expression promotes immune remodeling, including Treg-skewing and effector/memory $CD4^+$ expansion, as well as lymphoproliferative disease over time [55].

For therapeutic evaluation, immunodeficient xenograft models (ATL cell lines or primary ATL cells) offer tractable tumor-control and pharmacodynamic readouts for pathway-directed interventions (e.g., NF-κB and proteostasis dependence), while humanized mouse platforms enable partial validation in a human-cell developmental context and have been used to model ATL-like outgrowth from infected human hematopoietic progenitors. Importantly, immune-evasion conclusions should be framed most strongly in humanized systems rather than immunodeficient xenografts [54].

Together, these models provide a pragmatic translational bridge between Tax/HBZ-driven molecular circuitry and in vivo therapeutic stress-testing [54, 55].

8. Therapeutic innovation mapped to rewired T-cell nodes

Therapeutic failure in ATLL is biologically driven: cytotoxic chemotherapy can reduce bulk disease but does not dismantle the core dependencies created by chronic HTLV-1 pressure (survival signaling, epigenetic fixation, and immune dysfunction), allowing residual clones to persist and re-expand. Therefore, therapy must move beyond class-level concepts toward agent-level, dependency-matched interventions with explicitly reported trial outcomes. For immune-phenotype targeting, CCR4 is commonly expressed in ATLL, and the anti-CCR4 monoclonal antibody mogamulizumab has shown measurable activity, for example, ORR 11% vs. 0% when added to chemotherapy in a randomized program and ORR ~50% in phase II relapsed ATLL, supporting sequencing strategies when CCR4 expression is confirmed [56]. For survival-axis disruption, proteasome inhibition with bortezomib has been evaluated in phase II relapsed/refractory ATLL with ORR 6.7% and median progression-free survival (PFS) of 38 days, highlighting limited single-agent durability and the rationale for combinations [57]. For transcriptional rigidity, HDAC inhibition (e.g., romidepsin) yields ORR ~25%–38% in broader mature T-cell lymphoma cohorts but remains best positioned in ATLL as a sensitizing state-modifier rather than curative monotherapy [58]. Together, these examples reinforce the central translational principle of ATLL management: durable control requires sequencing and combination strategies engineered around dependency networks, not isolated node inhibition. A mechanism-aligned framework linking these biological dependencies to representative therapeutic strategies is illustrated in **Figure 6**.

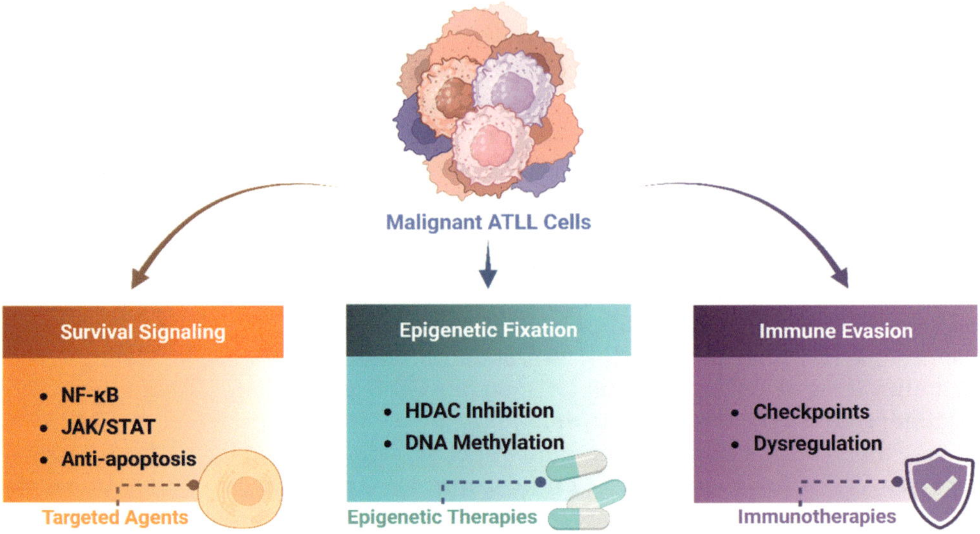

Figure 6.
Therapeutic targeting of rewired T-cell dependencies in ATLL.

From a mechanism-first perspective, three interdependent biological axes dominate ATLL maintenance: survival signaling, epigenetic fixation, and immune dysregulation. Persistent activation of survival pathways, particularly NF-κB and related networks, creates a strong anti-apoptotic tone that confers resistance to cytotoxic stress [11, 13]. Targeted agents aimed at these pathways are conceptually attractive but are often limited by pathway redundancy and adaptive escape, supporting rational combination strategies rather than isolated node targeting [5, 6].

Epigenetic fixation is a second major barrier. ATLL exhibits polycomb-dependent remodeling and aberrant methylation programs that lock malignant cells into rigid transcriptional states [16, 21]. Epigenetic therapies (e.g., HDAC and DNA methyltransferase (DNMT) inhibitors) can relax transcriptional constraints and restore partial flexibility, but their impact is often constrained by toxicity, incomplete reprogramming, and persistence of immune dysfunction, supporting their use as sensitizers within multimodal regimens rather than definitive monotherapies [5, 6].

Immune dysregulation is both a driver of disease and a therapeutic hazard. ATLL arises in a context of chronic immune activation coupled with ineffective antitumor immunity, shaped by decades of viral immune modulation [1, 14]. While checkpoint blockade has transformed other cancers, immune checkpoint modulation can be hazardous in dysregulated immune contexts, highlighting that immune state is itself a biomarker and that immunotherapy must be guided by mechanistic understanding and careful selection [5, 6, 55].

The most rational therapeutic strategies are, therefore, combinatorial and sequential, integrating agents that attenuate survival signaling, relax epigenetic constraints, and restore effective immune surveillance. Such approaches require biomarker-guided frameworks accounting for clonal architecture, immune competence, and pathway dependency, rather than uniform regimens borrowed from other lymphoid malignancies [4, 6, 22]. Selected therapeutic agents mapped to major biological dependency nodes in ATLL are summarized in **Table 4**.

Mechanism-aligned framework mapping core biological dependencies in ATLL to representative therapeutic classes. Chronic HTLV-1–conditioned survival signaling, particularly NF-κB–biased anti-apoptotic tone, is targeted by proteasome inhibition (e.g., bortezomib) to disrupt constitutive survival pathways. Epigenetic fixation

Dependency node	Agent (example)	Target/Mechanism	Clinical evidence	Practical limitation
Immune phenotype and trafficking	Mogamulizumab	Anti-CCR4 monoclonal antibody (antibody-dependent cellular cytotoxicity [ADCC] against $CCR4^{+}$ malignant T cells)	Randomized trial (mogamulizumab + chemotherapy vs. chemotherapy): ORR 11% vs. 0% (best overall response reported as 28% vs. 8% in some summaries of the same program). Phase II relapsed ATLL: ORR ~50% with median PFS on the order of months.	Immune toxicity risk; requires CCR4 assessment; access constraints [56].
NF-κB-biased survival signaling	Bortezomib	Proteasome inhibition → indirect suppression of NF-κB survival tone	Phase II relapsed/refractory ATLL: ORR 6.7%; median PFS 38 days (limited single-agent activity and durability).	Limited single-agent durability; cytopenias/neuropathy; regimen compatibility [57].
Epigenetic fixation/transcriptional rigidity	Romidepsin (HDAC inhibitor class)	HDAC inhibition → chromatin modulation and transcriptional reprogramming	In mature T-cell lymphoma cohorts (peripheral T-cell lymphoma/cutaneous T-cell lymphoma (PTCL/CTCL)), ORR is typically ~25%–38% in pivotal studies; ATLL-specific benefit is less well-defined and often pursued as a combination sensitizer rather than definitive monotherapy.	Toxicity (cytopenias, infections, ECG/QT considerations); incomplete reprogramming; relapses without a combinatorial strategy [58].
Curative-intent consolidation	Allogeneic hematopoietic stem cell transplantation (HSCT)	Graft-versus-tumor effect	Across transplant series, long-term overall survival (OS) is commonly ~30%–40% in selected eligible patients, with substantial transplant-related mortality.	Limited eligibility; high-resource dependence; donor access barriers.

Where trial-level effect sizes are cited, report outcomes explicitly (e.g., ORR, CR rate, PFS/OS, toxicity signals) from the primary clinical trial manuscripts to avoid overgeneralization and ensure reproducibility of claims.

Table 4.
Selected clinical agents mapped to rewired T-cell biology in ATLL.

and transcriptional rigidity, driven by polycomb remodeling and aberrant methylation programs, are addressed using histone deacetylase (HDAC) inhibitors (e.g., romidepsin) as state-modifying agents that partially restore transcriptional flexibility. Immune-phenotype targeting exploits CCR4 expression on ATLL cells using anti-CCR4 monoclonal antibodies (e.g., mogamulizumab) to enhance immune-mediated clearance. The model emphasizes pathway redundancy, adaptive resistance, and immune context as major barriers to durable control, supporting combination and sequencing strategies rather than single-node inhibition.

Mechanism-aligned therapy in ATLL benefits from matching interventions to dominant dependencies. CCR4-directed therapy (mogamulizumab) operationalizes phenotype targeting in CCR4+ disease and is best positioned within sequencing strategies rather than as an isolated maneuver. Proteasome inhibition (bortezomib) supports survival-node disruption consistent with NF-κB–biased anti-apoptotic tone but typically requires combination approaches to prevent adaptive escape. Epigenetic state modifiers (e.g., HDAC inhibition) are most rational as sensitizers that relax transcriptional rigidity and enhance vulnerability to immune-mediated or cytotoxic clearance. For eligible patients, allogeneic transplantation remains the principal curative-intent option, emphasizing that durable control requires both biological alignment and realistic pathway-to-access planning.

9. Clinical reality check: Why chemotherapy fails and sequencing matters

Despite advances in supportive care and transplantation strategies, outcomes for aggressive ATLL remain poor, particularly outside specialized centers [4, 6]. Conventional chemotherapy frequently induces transient cytoreduction but fails to achieve durable remission, reflecting biological resistance rather than therapeutic insufficiency [4, 5]. ATLL cells are preconditioned for survival through chronic anti-apoptotic signaling, transcriptional inflexibility, and immune escape, allowing residual disease to persist and re-expand after treatment [11, 15, 16].

Treatment sequencing is therefore critical. Interventions that modulate immune function or epigenetic state may need to precede or accompany cytotoxic therapy to meaningfully alter disease trajectory [6]. Allogeneic stem cell transplantation remains a potentially curative option for a subset of patients, but its applicability is limited by age, comorbidities, and access to specialized care [6].

Global implementation constraints further complicate management. In many HTLV-1-endemic regions, limited access to diagnostic infrastructure, targeted agents, and transplantation magnifies disease burden and delays intervention [8, 9]. This reality supports context-appropriate translational strategies that balance biological insight with feasibility [10].

10. Public health and resource-adapted strategies in endemic settings

Because HTLV-1 transmission is sustained through breastfeeding-associated vertical transmission, sexual transmission, and blood exposure, prevention and early identification are essential complements to therapeutic innovation. Priority strategies include strengthening blood-product screening, targeted antenatal testing where feasible, counseling on breastfeeding alternatives when maternal HTLV-1 infection is identified, and building surveillance in endemic and migration-linked regions. In resource-limited settings, pragmatic treatment algorithms should emphasize (i) early recognition and confirmation of HTLV-1 infection, (ii) rapid clinical subtyping and tempo assessment of ATLL, (iii) infection prevention and supportive care, and (iv) referral pathways for patients likely to benefit from targeted agents or transplantation. This approach ties mechanistic insight to feasible implementation and reduces delays that amplify morbidity in endemic regions.

11. Future directions: What HTLV-1 and ATLL teach us about T-cell immunology

Beyond its clinical significance, HTLV-1-driven ATLL offers enduring lessons for immunology and cancer biology. It demonstrates that T-cell identity is plastic and vulnerable to chronic perturbation, that immune escape can be achieved through functional remodeling rather than antigen loss alone, and that malignancy can emerge from prolonged dysregulation without early catastrophic genomic events [1, 18, 19]. From a translational perspective, ATLL underscores the need for mechanism-aligned biomarkers capturing immune competence, pathway dependency, epigenetic state, and clonal architecture [15, 16, 22]. Future advances will depend on integrating viral biology, host immune context, and clonal evolution into unified treatment frameworks rather than extrapolating directly from other lymphoid malignancies [5, 6].

List of abbreviations

HTLV-1	human T-cell leukemia virus type 1
ATLL	adult T-cell leukemia/lymphoma
ADCC	antibody-dependent cellular cytotoxicity
DCs	dendritic cells
HSPGs	heparan sulfate proteoglycans
NRP-1	neuropilin-1
GLUT1	glucose transporter 1
VEGF165	vascular endothelial growth factor 165
LFA-1	lymphocyte function-associated antigen-1
MHC	major histocompatibility complex
LTR	long terminal repeat
TCR	T-cell receptor
NF-κB	nuclear factor kappa B
JAK/STAT	Janus kinase/signal transducer and activator of transcription
DN	double negative
DP	double positive
SP	single positive
HAM	HTLV-1-associated myelopathy
PTCL	peripheral T-cell lymphoma
CTCL	cutaneous T-cell lymphoma
HSCT	hematopoietic stem cell transplantation
ORR	overall response rate

CR	complete response
PFS	progression-free survival
OS	overall survival
mTOR	mechanistic target of rapamycin
DNMT	DNA methyltransferase

Artificial intelligence use disclosure

The authors acknowledge the use of ChatGPT (OpenAI) for language polishing of the manuscript. All scientific interpretations, clinical statements, and reference selections were performed and verified by the authors.

Acknowledgments

The authors thank colleagues and collaborators who provided intellectual input and constructive feedback during the preparation of this chapter. The publication of this work was supported by professional development funds from Roseman University College of Medicine, Nevada, USA.

Conflict of Interest

The authors declare no conflict of interest.

Author details

Fidelis Nwachukwu[1*], Daniel Moses[2], Adedeji Okikiade[3], Inaia Phoenix[1] and Okechukwu Nwako[4]

1 Foundational Sciences, Roseman University College of Medicine, Las Vegas, Nevada, USA

2 Clinical Sciences, Roseman University College of Medicine, Las Vegas, Nevada, USA

3 Clinical Sciences, California Northstate University, Elk Grove, California, USA

4 Internal Medicine, Federal University of Technology, Owerri, Imo State, Nigeria

*Address all correspondence to: fnwachukwu@roseman.edu; ayofidel@gmail.com

References

[1] Bangham CRM, Matsuoka M. Human T-cell leukaemia virus type 1: Parasitism and pathogenesis. Philosophical Transactions of the Royal Society B: Biological Sciences. 2017;**372**(1732):20160272. DOI: 10.1098/rstb.2016.0272

[2] Matsuoka M, Jeang KT. Human T-cell leukaemia virus type 1 (HTLV-1) infectivity and cellular transformation. Nature Reviews Cancer. 2007;**7**(4):270–280. DOI: 10.1038/nrc2111

[3] Mazurov D, Ilinskaya A, Heidecker G, Lloyd P, Derse D. Quantitative comparison of HTLV-1 and HIV-1 cell-to-cell infection with new replication dependent vectors. PLoS Pathogens. 2010;**6**(2):e1000788. DOI: 10.1371/journal.ppat.1000788

[4] Ishitsuka K, Tamura K. Human T-cell leukaemia virus type I and adult T-cell leukaemia–lymphoma. The Lancet Oncology. 2014;**15**(11):e517–e526. DOI: 10.1016/S1470-2045(14)70202-5

[5] Hermine O, Ramos JC, Tobinai K. A review of new findings in adult T-cell leukemia-lymphoma: A focus on current and emerging treatment strategies. Advances in Therapy. 2018;**35**(2):135–152. DOI: 10.1007/s12325-018-0658-4

[6] Cook LB, Fuji S, Hermine O, et al. Revised adult T-cell leukemia–lymphoma international consensus meeting report. Journal of Clinical Oncology. 2019;**37**(8):677–687. DOI: 10.1200/JCO.18.00501

[7] Bangham CR. HTLV-1 infections. Journal of Clinical Pathology. 2000;**53**(8):581–586. DOI: 10.1136/jcp.53.8.581

[8] Gessain A, Cassar O. Epidemiological aspects and world distribution of HTLV-1 infection. Frontiers in Microbiology. 2012;**3**:388. DOI: 10.3389/fmicb.2012.00388

[9] Proietti FA, Carneiro-Proietti ABF, Catalan-Soares BC, Murphy EL. Global epidemiology of HTLV-I infection and associated diseases. Oncogene. 2005;**24**(39):6058–6068. DOI: 10.1038/sj.onc.1208968

[10] Nwachukwu F, Browne R, Barnard T, Snagg N. Human T-cell lymphotropic virus (HTLV-1) and adult T-cell leukaemia/lymphoma (ATL): Case report and literature review. West Indian Medical Journal. 2022;**69**(7):530–534. DOI: 10.7727/wimj.2016.163

[11] Giam CZ, Semmes OJ. HTLV-1 infection and adult T-Cell leukemia/lymphoma-a tale of two proteins: Tax and HBZ. Viruses. 2016;**8**(6):161. DOI: 10.3390/v8060161

[12] Yasunaga J, Matsuoka M. Human T-cell leukemia virus type I induces adult T-cell leukemia: From clinical aspects to molecular mechanisms. Cancer Control. 2007;**14**(2):133–140. DOI: 10.1177/107327480701400206

[13] Mohanty S, Harhaj EW. Mechanisms of Oncogenesis by HTLV-1 Tax. Pathogens. 2020;**9**(7):543. DOI: 10.3390/pathogens9070543

[14] Zhao T. The Role of HBZ in HTLV-1-Induced Oncogenesis. Viruses. 2016;**8**(2):34. DOI: 10.3390/v8020034

[15] Kataoka K, Nagata Y, Kitanaka A, et al. Integrated molecular analysis of adult T-cell leukemia/lymphoma.

Nature Genetics. 2015;**47**(11):1304–1315. DOI: 10.1038/ng.3415

[16] Fujikawa D, Nakagawa S, Hori M, et al. Polycomb-dependent epigenetic landscape in adult T-cell leukemia. Blood. 2016;**127**(14):1790–1802. DOI: 10.1182/blood-2015-08-662593

[17] Kogure Y, Kataoka K. Genetic alterations in adult T-cell leukemia/lymphoma. Cancer Science. 2017;**108**(9):1719–1725. DOI: 10.1111/cas.13303

[18] Greaves M, Maley CC. Clonal evolution in cancer. Nature. 2012;**481**(7381):306–313. DOI: 10.1038/nature10762

[19] Hanahan D, Weinberg RA. Hallmarks of cancer: The next generation. Cell. 2011;**144**(5):646–674. DOI: 10.1016/j.cell.2011.02.013

[20] Yamagishi M, Nakano K, Miyake A, et al. Polycomb-mediated loss of miR-31 activates NIK-dependent NF-κB pathway in adult T cell leukemia and other cancers. Cancer Cell. 2012;**21**(1):121–135. DOI: 10.1016/j.ccr.2011.12.015

[21] Feinberg AP, Koldobskiy MA, Göndör A. Epigenetic modulators, modifiers and mediators in cancer aetiology and progression. Nature Reviews Genetics. 2016;**17**(5):284–299. DOI: 10.1038/nrg.2016.13

[22] Garraway LA, Verweij J, Ballman KV. Precision oncology: An overview. Journal of Clinical Oncology. 2013;**31**(15):1803–1805. DOI: 10.1200/JCO.2013.49.4799

[23] Franchini G, Mann DL, Popovic M, Zicht RR, Gallo RC, Wong-Staal F. HTLV-I infection of T and B cells of a patient with adult T-cell leukemia-lymphoma (ATLL) and transmission of HTLV-I from B cells to normal T cells. Leukemia Research. 1985;**9**(11):1305–1314. DOI: 10.1016/0145-2126(85)90116-x

[24] de Castro-amarante MF, Pise-Masison CA, McKinnon K, et al. Human T Cell leukemia virus type 1 infection of the three monocyte subsets contributes to viral burden in humans. Journal of Virology. 2015;**90**(5):2195–2207. DOI: 10.1128/JVI.02735-15

[25] Macatonia SE, Cruickshank JK, Rudge P, Knight SC. Dendritic cells from patients with tropical spastic paraparesis are infected with HTLV-1 and stimulate autologous lymphocyte proliferation. AIDS Research and Human Retroviruses. 1992;**8**(9):1699–1706. DOI: 10.1089/aid.1992.8.1699

[26] Jones KS, Petrow-Sadowski C, Huang YK, Bertolette DC, Ruscetti FW. Cell-free HTLV-1 infects dendritic cells leading to transmission and transformation of CD4(+) T cells. Nature Medicine. 2008;**14**(4):429–436. DOI: 10.1038/nm1745

[27] Manel N, Kim FJ, Kinet S, Taylor N, Sitbon M, Battini JL. The ubiquitous glucose transporter GLUT-1 is a receptor for HTLV. Cell. 2003;**115**(4):449–459. DOI: 10.1016/s0092-8674(03)00881-x

[28] Jones KS, Petrow-Sadowski C, Bertolette DC, Huang Y, Ruscetti FW. Heparan sulfate proteoglycans mediate attachment and entry of human T-Cell leukemia virus Type 1 virions into CD4 + T Cells. Journal of Virology. 2005;**79**(20):12692–12702. DOI: 10.1128/JVI.79.20.12692-12702.2005

[29] Ghez D, Lepelletier Y, Lambert S, et al. Neuropilin-1 is involved in human

T-cell lymphotropic virus type 1 entry. Journal of Virology. 2006;**80**(14):6844–6854. DOI: 10.1128/JVI.02719-05

[30] Jones KS, Lambert S, Bouttier M, et al. Molecular aspects of HTLV-1 entry: Functional domains of the HTLV-1 surface subunit (SU) and their relationships to the entry receptors. Viruses. 2011;**3**(6):794–810. DOI: 10.3390/v3060794

[31] Lambert S, Bouttier M, Vassy R, et al. HTLV-1 uses HSPG and neuropilin-1 for entry by molecular mimicry of VEGF165. Blood. 2009;**113**(21):5176–5185. DOI: 10.1182/blood-2008-04-150342

[32] Igakura T, Stinchcombe JC, Goon PK, et al. Spread of HTLV-I between lymphocytes by virus-induced polarization of the cytoskeleton. Science. 2003;**299**(5613):1713–1716. DOI: 10.1126/science.1080115

[33] Pais-Correia AM, Sachse M, Guadagnini S, et al. Biofilm-like extracellular viral assemblies mediate HTLV-1 cell-to-cell transmission at virological synapses. Nature Medicine. 2010;**16**(1):83–89. DOI: 10.1038/nm.2065

[34] Gross C, Thoma-Kress AK. Molecular Mechanisms of HTLV-1 Cell-to-Cell Transmission. Viruses. 2016;**8**(3):74. DOI: 10.3390/v8030074

[35] Van Prooyen N, Gold H, Andresen V, et al. Human T-cell leukemia virus type 1 p8 protein increases cellular conduits and virus transmission. Proceedings of the National Academy of Sciences of the United States of America. 2010;**107**(48):20738–20743. DOI: 10.1073/pnas.1009635107

[36] Silverman LR, Phipps AJ, Montgomery A, Ratner L, Lairmore MD. Human T-Cell lymphotropic virus type 1 open reading frame II-encoded p30 ii is required for in vivo replication: Evidence of in vivo reversion. Journal of Virology. 2004;**78**(8):3837–3845. DOI: 10.1128/jvi.78.8.3837-3845.2004

[37] Nicot C, Dundr M, Johnson JM, et al. HTLV-1-encoded p30II is a post-transcriptional negative regulator of viral replication. Nature Medicine. 2004;**10**(2):197–201. DOI: 10.1038/nm984

[38] Kannagi M, Harada S, Maruyama I, et al. Predominant recognition of human T cell leukemia virus type I (HTLV-I) pX gene products by human CD8+ cytotoxic T cells directed against HTLV-I-infected cells. International Immunology. 1991;**3**(8):761–767. DOI: 10.1093/intimm/3.8.761

[39] Satou Y, Yasunaga J, Yoshida M, Matsuoka M. HTLV-I basic leucine zipper factor gene mRNA supports proliferation of adult T cell leukemia cells. Proceedings of the National Academy of Sciences of the United States of America. 2006;**103**(3):720–725. DOI: 10.1073/pnas.0507631103

[40] Villaudy J, Wencker M, Gadot N, et al. HTLV-1 propels thymic human T cell development in "human immune system" Rag2^{-}/$^{-}$ gamma c^{-}/$^{-}$ mice. PLoS Pathogens. 2011;7(9):e1002231. DOI: 10.1371/journal.ppat.1002231

[41] Wencker M, Sausse C, Derse D, Gazzolo L, Duc Dodon M. Human T-cell leukemia virus type 1 Tax protein down-regulates pre-T-cell receptor alpha gene transcription in human immature thymocytes. Journal of

Virology. 2007;**81**(1):301–308. DOI: 10.1128/JVI.00766-06

[42] Maher AK, Aristodemou A, Giang N, et al. HTLV-1 induces an inflammatory CD4+CD8+ T cell population in HTLV-1-associated myelopathy. JCI Insight. 2024;**9**(1): e173738. DOI: 10.1172/jci.insight.173738

[43] Green PL, Chen IS. Regulation of human T cell leukemia virus expression 1. The FASEB Journal. 1990;**4**(2):169–175. DOI: 10.1096/fasebj.4.2.2404818

[44] Bangham CRM. HTLV-1 persistence and the oncogenesis of adult T-cell leukemia/lymphoma. Blood. 2023;**141**(19):2299–2306. DOI: 10.1182/blood.2022019332

[45] Jeang KT, Giam CZ, Majone F, Aboud M. Life, death, and tax: Role of HTLV-I oncoprotein in genetic instability and cellular transformation. Journal of Biological Chemistry. 2004;**279**(31):31991–31994. DOI: 10.1074/jbc.R400009200

[46] Hollingworth R, Grand RJ. Modulation of DNA damage and repair pathways by human tumour viruses. Viruses. 2015;**7**(5):2542–2591. DOI: 10.3390/v7052542

[47] Ma G, Yasunaga J, Matsuoka M. Multifaceted functions and roles of HBZ in HTLV-1 pathogenesis. Retrovirology. 2016;**13**:16. DOI: 10.1186/s12977-016-0249-x

[48] Tanaka-Nakanishi A, Yasunaga J, Takai K, Matsuoka M. HTLV-1 bZIP factor suppresses apoptosis by attenuating the function of FoxO3a and altering its localization. Cancer Research. 2014;**74**(1):188–200. DOI: 10.1158/0008-5472.CAN-13-0436

[49] Kim YC, Guan KL. mTOR: A pharmacologic target for autophagy regulation. Journal of Clinical Investigation. 2015;**125**(1):25–32. DOI: 10.1172/JCI73939

[50] Zhao T, Satou Y, Sugata K, et al. HTLV-1 bZIP factor enhances TGF-β signaling through p300 coactivator. Blood. 2011;**118**(7):1865–1876. DOI: 10.1182/blood-2010-12-326199

[51] Philip S, Zahoor MA, Zhi H, Ho YK, Giam CZ. Regulation of human T-lymphotropic virus type I latency and reactivation by HBZ and Rex. PLoS Pathogens. 2014;**10**(4):e1004040. DOI: 10.1371/journal.ppat.1004040

[52] Gaudray G, Gachon F, Basbous J, Biard-Piechaczyk M, Devaux C, Mesnard JM. The complementary strand of the human T-cell leukemia virus type 1 RNA genome encodes a bZIP transcription factor that down-regulates viral transcription. Journal of Virology. 2002;**76**(24):12813–12822. DOI: 10.1128/jvi.76.24.12813-12822.2002

[53] Wherry EJ, Kurachi M. Molecular and cellular insights into T cell exhaustion. Nature Reviews Immunology. 2015;**15**(8):486–499. DOI: 10.1038/nri3862

[54] Panfil AR, Al-Saleem JJ, Green PL. Animal Models Utilized in HTLV-1 Research. Virology: Research and Treatment. 2013;**4**:49–59. DOI: 10.4137/VRT.S12140

[55] Nakajima S, Okuma K. Mouse Models for HTLV-1 Infection and Adult T Cell Leukemia. International Journal of Molecular Sciences. 2023;**24**(14):11737. DOI: 10.3390/ijms241411737

[56] Phillips AA, Fields PA, Hermine O, et al. Mogamulizumab versus

investigator's choice of chemotherapy regimen in relapsed/refractory adult T-cell leukemia/lymphoma. Haematologica. 2019;**104**(5):993–1003. DOI: 10.3324/haematol.2018.205096

[57] Ishitsuka K, Utsunomiya A, Katsuya H, et al. A phase II study of bortezomib in patients with relapsed or refractory aggressive adult T-cell leukemia/lymphoma. Cancer Science. 2015;**106**(9):1219–1223. DOI: 10.1111/cas.12735

[58] Barbarotta L, Hurley K. Romidepsin for the treatment of Peripheral T-Cell Lymphoma. Journal of the Advanced Practitioner in Oncology. 2015;**6**(1):22–36

Chapter 2

Perspective Chapter: A New Immune Perspective Related to Platelet–T-Cell Crosstalk

Shuai Tan, Huizhen He, Mingyue Shang, Yumeng Li, Xiaoli Chang, Yaochi Chen, Jingzhe Ma, Yixuan Wang, Jing Ni, Chunxiao Xue, Zongqu Sun, Yizhang Zhou, Xiaoyu Li, Huanyuan Wang, Qi Qin, Wei Wang and Wanling Sun

Abstract

Platelets are increasingly recognized as immune modulators that influence T-cell activation and metabolism through direct interactions and mediator release. This review focuses on platelet–T-cell crosstalk in aplastic anemia (AA) and hematological disorders. Platelet factor 4/C-X-C motif chemokine ligand 4 (CXCL4) and transforming growth factor-beta (TGF-β) serve as central mediators. PF4 binds T-cell CXCR3 to activate the Akt-PGC1α-TFAM axis, reprogramming mitochondrial metabolism and promoting T Helper 1 (Th1) polarization while restraining T Helper 17 (Th17) responses. TGF-β exerts context-dependent effects – inducing regulatory T-cells (Tregs) under homeostasis but driving Th17 differentiation in inflammatory conditions like AA. In hematological malignancies, this crosstalk extends to tumor metabolic reprogramming and immunosuppression via microparticles. Emerging evidence also implicates platelet–T-cell interactions in neurological disorders, including myasthenia gravis and ischemic stroke. Understanding this axis offers therapeutic opportunities, including thrombopoietin receptor agonists (e.g., eltrombopag) that modulate platelet production and immunity, and strategies targeting PF4/CXCR3 or TGF-β signaling to restore immune homeostasis.

Keywords: platelet, T-cell, PF4/CXCL4, TGF-β, crosstalk

1. Introduction

Aplastic anemia (AA) is a severe bone marrow failure (BMF) syndrome characterized by peripheral pancytopenia and marrow hypocellularity [1, 2], primarily driven by T-cell-mediated immune destruction of hematopoietic stem cells (HSC) [3]. Although timely intervention with intensive immunosuppressive therapy (IST) or hematopoietic stem cell transplantation (HSCT) is critical for survival, approximately one-third of patients fail to achieve long-term survival. Notably, adding eltrombopag (EPAG), a thrombopoietin receptor agonist (TPO-RA), to IST enhances hematologic response rates [4]. The immune crosstalk between platelets and T-cells is a significant recent discovery in acquired AA pathophysiology (**Figure 1**).

In AA, activated platelets release soluble mediators such as platelet factor 4 (PF4/CXCL4), which bind to chemokine receptors CXCR3/CXCR5 on T-cells. This interaction activates the Akt–PGC1α–TFAM signaling axis, reprogramming mitochondrial energy metabolism and altering reactive oxygen species (ROS) and ATP (Adenosine triphosphate) production. Such metabolic reprogramming drives aberrant T-cell activation and differentiation, promoting proinflammatory $CD4^+$ T-cell subsets (Th1, Th17) while potentially suppressing Tregs, and enhancing $CD8^+$ cytotoxic T-cell effector functions [5–7], including perforin/granzyme release and secretion of inflammatory cytokines such as IFN-γ [8] and TNF-α. Targeting this platelet–T-cell interaction, for instance, by inhibiting PF4 signaling or its downstream metabolic pathways, may offer a novel immunomodulatory strategy for AA [9].

Moreover, platelet–T-cell interactions form a critical immune-thrombotic axis with multifaceted roles in disease pathogenesis. In autoimmune disorders, activated platelets, via P-selectin, bind Tregs, disrupting their suppressive function and promoting autoantibody production in systemic lupus erythematosus (SLE) and lupus nephritis [10]. P-selectin-PSGL1 interactions also activate autoreactive $CD4^+$ T cells, fueling kidney damage. In multiple sclerosis (MS), platelet–T cell engagement drives neuroinflammation via CD40 ligand (CD40L)-mediated T-cell migration across the blood–brain barrier (BBB) [11]. In rheumatoid arthritis (RA), platelets can suppress T-cell proliferation and proinflammatory cytokine secretion while enhancing antiinflammatory interleukin-10 (IL-10) production [12].

In cardiovascular disease, platelet–T-cell crosstalk drives atherosclerosis and acute coronary syndromes. Activated platelets release microvesicles (pMVs) carrying CD40L and regulated upon activation, normal T-Cell expressed and secreted (RANTES), recruiting T-cells to plaques and promoting destabilization [13]. Platelets also directly activate T-cells via P-selectin, enhancing endothelial adhesion and forming a vicious cycle where T-cell-derived interleukin-1 Beta (IL-1β) further potentiates platelet activation and thrombosis [14]. $CD8^+$ T-cells further modulate plaque stability by hydrolyzing prothrombotic nucleotides via CD39 [15]. Elevated pMVs perpetuate synovial inflammation in RA and correlate with thrombotic risk in antiphospholipid syndrome [13].

In infectious diseases, platelets shape T-cell responses through direct and indirect mechanisms. Upon activation, they release a multitude of soluble mediators – such as sCD84, CD40L, TGF-β, and PF4 – which can directly suppress T-cell proliferation or modulate their function [16]. More importantly, platelets significantly impair dendritic cell (DC) function by suppressing proinflammatory cytokine production (tumor necrosis factor-alpha (TNF-α), IL-12, IL-6), consequently weakening Th1 differentiation and cellular immune responses against pathogens [17]. Conversely, in the context of certain viral infections, such as HIV, platelets can form complexes with CD8 + T-cells, prompting their functional exhaustion and cell death [18].

This interaction is especially pronounced in hematologic diseases. In immune thrombocytopenia (ITP), pathogenesis stems from collective T-cell subset dysfunction: pathogenic Th1, Th17, T Helper 22 (Th22), and T follicular helper (Tfh) cells are overactivated, while Tregs and CD8 + Tregs are insufficient, leading to

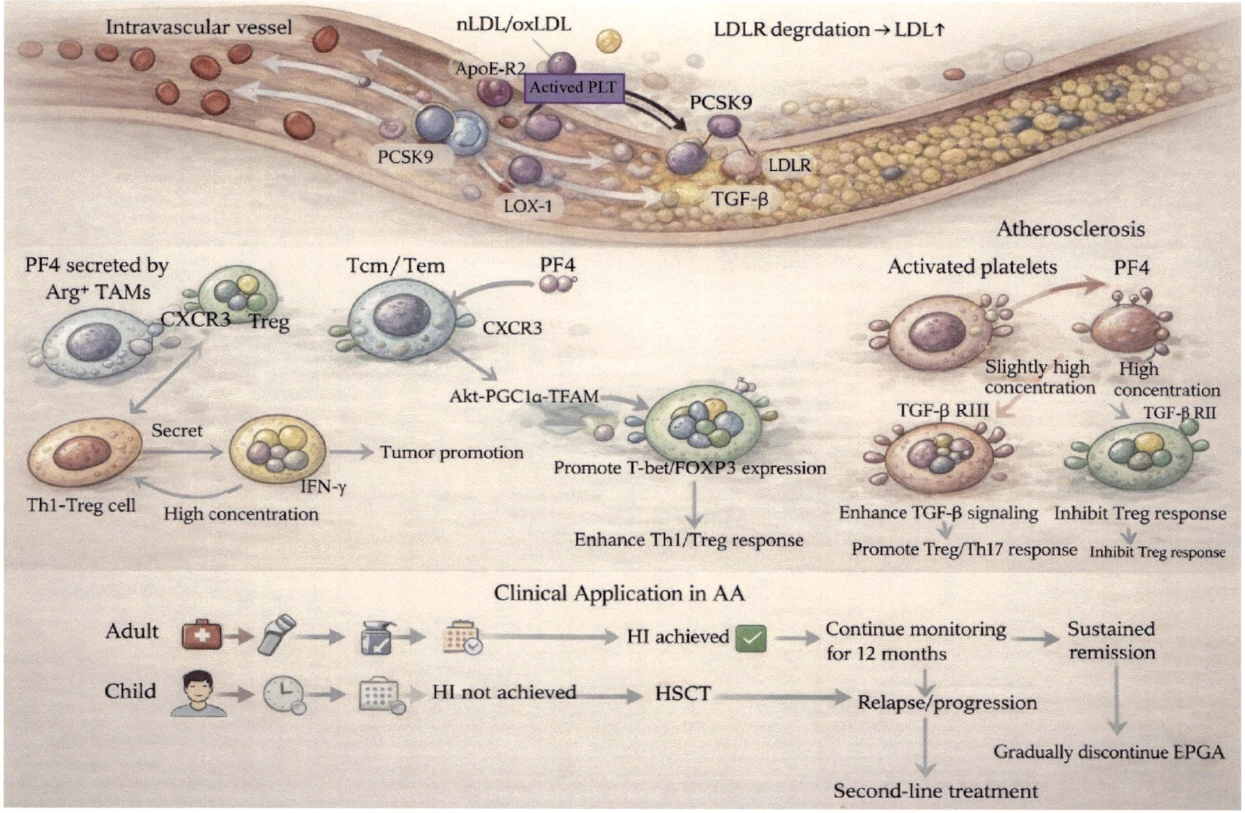

Figure 1.
The platelet factor 4 (PF4) signaling axis linking lipid metabolism, immune dysregulation, and clinical strategy in aplastic anemia. This schematic illustrates the multifaceted role of PF4, bridging metabolic cues and immune pathology in aplastic anemia (AA). The upper cascade shows how oxidized LDL (oxLDL) activates platelets (PLT) via surface receptors to secrete PF4, which then acts as a central mediator. PF4 engages cells like Treg via CXCR3, modulating mitochondrial biogenesis (TFAM) and TGF-β signaling (Smad2/3) to influence immune suppression and Th1-Treg polarization. The lower panel outlines the integrated clinical management strategy for AA, detailing the initiation, maintenance, and assessment points for eltrombopag (EPAG) combined with immunosuppressive therapy (IST) in both adult and pediatric patients.

a coordinated autoimmune attack on platelets [19]. Furthermore, low-dose decitabine has been shown to correct the Treg cell deficiency and counteract the hyperactivation of effector T-cells (such as Th1 and Th17) in ITP. It restores immune tolerance by rebalancing the Treg/Teff equilibrium and suppressing the signal transducer and activator of transcription 3 (STAT3) signaling pathway [20].

In conclusion, the interaction between platelets and T-cells has significant implications in various pathological contexts, including autoimmune diseases, hematological malignancies, infections, and central nervous system (CNS) disorders. In this chapter, we synthesize mechanistic and clinical evidence to propose a conceptual framework wherein platelets act as context-dependent regulators of T-cell fate.

2. Platelet–T-cell crosstalk in AA and BMF

2.1 TPO-RA EPAG with AA patients

TPO-RAs exert therapeutic effects by functioning as exogenous agonists of the myeloproliferative leukemia protein (c-MPL) receptor, mimicking its native ligand, thrombopoietin. This binding activates the Janus kinase 2 (JAK2)/signal transducer and activator of transcription 5 (STAT5), phosphatidylinositol 3-kinase (PI3K)/AKT, and mitogen-activated protein kinase (MAPK) pathways, which collectively promote megakaryocytic differentiation, cytoplasmic maturation, and subsequent platelet shedding into the bloodstream. Additionally, c-MPL expression has been documented on hematopoietic stem and progenitor cells (HSPCs). Activation of c-MPL signaling by TPO-RAs may help counteract the loss of HSPCs that underlies BMF in AA [21]. The therapeutic efficacy of the use of TPO-RAs in AA extends beyond increasing platelet counts, positioning them as pivotal regulators of the hyperactive bone marrow immune microenvironment. This immunomodulatory mechanism is primarily mediated by TPO-RA-augmented platelets through soluble mediators (most notably PF4/CXCL4 and TGF-β) and via direcT-cell–cell contact [22]. The efficacy of the combination therapy may be explained by a temporally and hierarchically coordinated mechanism: TPO-RAs exert their hematopoiesis-sustaining effects across the hematopoietic hierarchy, from stem cells to progenitor cells. This establishes a functional bridge, providing a critical window during which IST can effectively curb the immune-mediated attack on the hematopoietic compartment. Conceptually, IST dampens immune attack, whereas TPO-RAs support hematopoietic recovery. This paradigm is supported by responses to EPAG even in refractory severe aplastic anemia (SAA) [23].

In previously untreated SAA patients, prospective studies demonstrate that IST (antithymocyte globulin (ATG) plus cyclosporine) combined with eltrombopag achieves a higher hematologic response rate than IST monotherapy [24]. This notion has likewise been substantiated by evidence from randomized controlled trials [23]. However, a significant limitation in the current evidence base is the lack of standardization in EPAG administration across pivotal trials. Critical parameters, specifically the optimal time to initiate EPAG after ATG and the ideal maintenance duration, vary considerably and remain unresolved. Pediatric practice remains more uncertain because evidence regarding the incremental benefit of adding EPAG to IST in children is less consistent than in adults [25].

Our recently published meta-analysis, pooling 21 studies (n = 2,239), found that EPAG plus immunosuppression increased overall and complete response rates at 3 and 6 months, though differences were not statistically evident at 12 months. For adult patients, we recommend incorporating EPAG within 7 days of initiating IST and maintaining it for 3 months; if not started within this timeframe, continuation for 6 months is advised. For children, maintenance therapy for at least 6 months is recommended, though pediatric regimens remain heterogeneous. Notably, extending EPAG therapy beyond 12 months does not yield significantly improved outcomes compared with IST alone [26].

2.2 Platelet–T-cell crosstalk

As previously mentioned, platelets are increasingly recognized as active immunomodulators that shape T-cell responses through both soluble mediators and contact-dependent mechanisms. Platelets contain two types of granules, with α-granules harboring hemostatic factors alongside key immune mediators, including CD40L, P-selectin (CD62P), PF4/CXCL4, C–C motif chemokine ligand 5 (CCL5), and TGF-β (**Figure 1**) [11].

Among these, PF4 plays a particularly prominent role in the regulation of T-cell-mediated immune responses. Specifically, PF4 has been shown to limit Th17 differentiation within the tumor microenvironment [27] and induce apoptosis in myeloma models by inhibiting the IL6-STAT3 signaling pathway [28], suggesting a potential tumor-suppressive function. Furthermore, it has been reported to promote Th1 differentiation, potentially through the regulation of STAT1- and STAT3-dependent signaling pathways, while simultaneously enhancing the chemotaxis, activation, and effector functions of $CD8^+$ cytotoxic T lymphocytes. In contrast, PF4 appears to restrain Th2- and Th17-associated immune responses, thereby contributing to a shift toward a type 1-dominant immune profile. These regulatory effects are further reinforced by PF4 cooperation with other platelet-derived mediators, including CCL5 and TGF-β, which together fine-tune $CD4^+$ T-cell responses [22]. In parallel, direct platelet–T-cell interactions mediated by CD40L promote T-cell activation and proliferation and modulate $CD8^+$ T-cell responses [29], while P-selectin/PSGL-1 signaling attenuates Treg suppressive function [30]. Emerging evidence also suggests that platelet-derived mitochondria can regulate $CD4^+$ T-cell activity through the CXCR4/stromal cell-derived factor 1 (SDF-1) axis [31].

TGF-β is a key immunoregulatory mediator linking platelet activation to adaptive immune modulation. Stored within platelet α-granules alongside PF4/CXCL4 and other bioactive mediators, TGF-β is released upon platelet activation to coordinate thrombosis, inflammation, and immunity. As platelets constitute the predominant circulating source of TGF-β, this cytokine serves as a reliable marker of in vivo platelet activation [32].

TGF-β represents a central immunoregulatory mediator linking platelet activation to adaptive immune modulation. Platelets constitute the predominant circulating source of TGF-β, rendering this cytokine a reliable marker of in vivo platelet activation [32]. In T-cell differentiation, TGF-β promotes Treg generation, maintaining immune tolerance while suppressing $CD8^+$ T-cell overactivation. However, in the presence of proinflammatory cytokines such as interleukin-6 (IL-6), TGF-β can drive Th17 differentiation, highlighting its context-dependent and dual-edged role in immune regulation – an aspect particularly relevant in BMF syndromes. Beyond T-cell differentiation, platelet-derived TGF-β exerts broad immunosuppressive functions by directly impairing effector lymphocyte activity and compromising natural killer (NK) cell cytolytic function [32].

Platelet–T-cell crosstalk also involves the active blockade of apoptotic programs. Platelets induce the overexpression of cyclooxygenase-2 (COX-2) in tumor cells through GPVI receptors. COX-2-derived prostaglandin E2 (PGE2) triggers the downregulation of the proapoptotic protein p21 and the upregulation of cyclin B1, effectively bypassing p53-mediated cell cycle arrest [33]. This antiapoptotic signaling allows tumor cells to persist despite the presence of cytotoxic T-cells or chemotherapy.

Collectively, these findings highlight the complex interplay between platelets and immune cells. However, several of the described mechanisms are based on inferences from the existing literature and still require further validation.

3. Platelet–T-cell crosstalk in other hematological malignancies

The acute myeloid leukemia (AML) microenvironment is characterized by an increase in Tregs and a decrease in helper T-cells [27]. T-cell exhaustion is further exacerbated by an expansion of CD8 + populations expressing PD-1 [34]. Platelet-induced AKT signaling contributes to the phenotypic shift of CD8 + early memory T-cells toward senescence, significantly enhancing resistance to induction chemotherapy [35].

Multiple myeloma (MM) cells utilize sialyl Lewis a/x to bind platelet P-selectin, forming a physical "cloak" [36]. This shield not only suppresses NK cell cytotoxicity but also impedes the formation of stable immune synapses between T-cells and myeloma clones, thereby facilitating immune escape.

In diffuse large B-cell lymphoma (DLBCL), TGF-β activates cancer-associated fibroblasts (CAFs) to construct physical barriers, directly suppressing CD8 + T-cell function and inducing exhaustion [37]. The loss of TGF-β-mediated growth inhibition is a fundamental step in lymphomagenesis [38].

Given the current paucity of direct experimental evidence, the precise mechanisms governing platelet–T-cell interactions in hematological malignancies remain incompletely defined. Consequently, much of our current understanding is extrapolated from related disease contexts or inferred from indirect observations, underscoring the need for dedicated mechanistic studies to validate these postulated pathways.

4. Platelet–T-cell crosstalk in the CNS

The CNS also harbors specialized T-cells termed tissue-resident memory T-cells (TRM cells), typically generated following CNS infections. These cells persist in tissues after infection resolution, enabling faster and more robust responses to reinfection by the same pathogen. Unlike other T-cells in the blood, TRM cells do not circulate in peripheral blood but reside in target tissues. They rely on specific surface molecules (CD49, CD69, and CD103) for stable tissue residency [39, 40].

Traditionally, the CNS has been considered an immune-privileged site, primarily due to its isolation by the BBB. Under healthy conditions, the BBB remains intact and is maintained by endothelial cells, the basement membrane, pericytes, and astrocytic endfeet. In the vascular lumen, platelets circulate in a resting state, sustaining vascular integrity but not triggering immune activation. A limited number of T-cells are present in the circulation; besides, T-cell immune surveillance is restricted to CNS interface regions. Within the CNS, microglia remain in a resting, ramified state, and neurons preserve normal function [42-44, 41–43] **(Figure 2a)**. Early pathological activation: under injury or inflammatory conditions, the permeability of the BBB increases. This is accompanied by endothelial disruption and swelling or retraction of astrocytic endfeet. Platelets are rapidly activated, followed by pseudopod-forming morphological changes and the release of granules or soluble mediators, like ATP, which activate endothelial P2Y2 receptors, increasing the permeability of the BBB [33]. Activated platelets promote T-cell adhesion to the endothelium, inducing T-cell recruitment and extravasation across the compromised BBB. Meanwhile, infiltrating T-cells and platelet-derived signals induce early microglial activation, leading to neuroinflammatory responses [44, 45] **(Figure 2b)**.

MS has long been regarded as an autoimmune attack on the CNS mediated by T-cells. However, recent studies indicate that synergistic effects between platelets and T-cells play a crucial role in the pathogenesis of MS. Platelets initiate immune responses, driving peripheral immune activation and CNS neuroinflammation through interactions with T-cells. In MS and its animal model (experimental autoimmune encephalomyelitis [EAE]), platelets are among the earliest activated cells. They initiate and shape the initial immune response through multiple pathways [46]. First, activated platelets release large quantities of extracellular vesicles (EVs). These EVs serve as critical signaling carriers, rich in proteins, lipids, and microRNAs, which can be internalized by immune cells to broadly regulate immune cell function and inflammatory responses [47]. Second, platelets are a key source of bioactive lipids such as prostaglandins and platelet-activating factor (PAF). These lipids play a crucial role in CNS immunity, directly modulating T-cell activation and differentiation pathways [48]. Platelets and their secreted bioactive substances create a proinflammatory microenvironment in the periphery, promoting T-cell differentiation toward pathogenic Th1 and Th17 subtypes, thereby laying the groundwork for CNS invasion [49]. Furthermore, activated platelets rapidly adhere to the surface of inflammation-activated cerebral vascular endothelial cells, leading to high expression of platelet adhesion molecules such as P-selectin. This further induces endothelial cells to express molecules like vascular cell adhesion molecule-1 (VCAM-1) [46]. This process enables T-cells expressing very late antigen-4 (VLA-4) to firmly adhere to the vascular wall and successfully traverse the BBB into the brain parenchyma and spinal cord [49]. Within the CNS, Th1 cells activate macrophages/microglia by secreting interferon-gamma (IFN-γ), while Th17 cells release cytokines like IL-17, directly damaging oligodendrocytes and compromising BBB integrity, leading to demyelination and axonal injury [49]. Concurrently, platelets activate microglia and astrocytes by releasing proinflammatory factors like ROS and nitric oxide (NO), driving their polarization toward harmful phenotypes [46]. Neuroantigens and inflammatory signals released by T-cells continuously activate platelets and innate immune

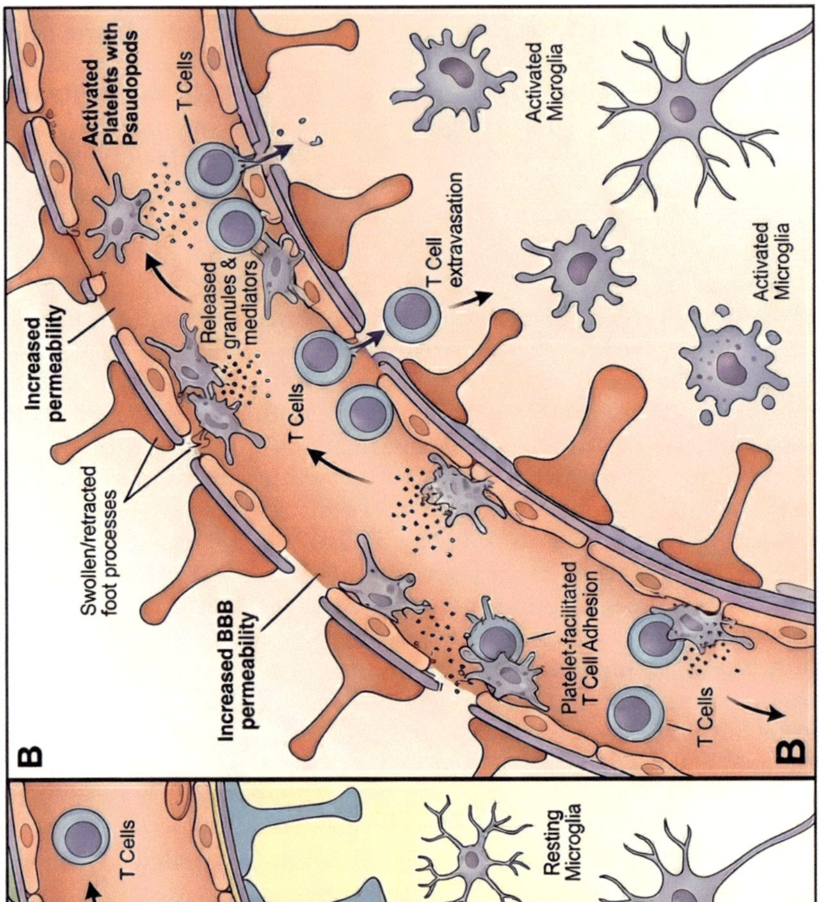

Figure 2.
Platelet and T-cell dynamics at the CNS interface: from physiological homeostasis to pathological activation. (a) Physiological homeostasis. (b) Early pathological activation.

cells, further recruiting additional T-cells and exacerbating inflammation and pathology.

5. Discussion and prospect

Therefore, PF4 may be an important potential new target in tumor immunotherapy. Platelets, traditionally recognized for their roles in hemostasis and thrombosis, are now acknowledged as key immune modulators. Accumulating evidence indicates that platelets dynamically influence T-cell activation, differentiation, metabolism, and trafficking through direct cellular interactions and the release of bioactive mediators [50].

Previous studies suggest that platelets regulate different T-cell subsets in multiple aspects. PF4 primarily released by platelets, is an essential mediator for CD4 + central and effector memory T-cell responses. It acts via the CXCR3 receptor to activate the Akt-PGC1α-TFAM pathway, promoting mitochondrial biosynthesis and enhancing Th1 and Treg cell activation [5, 6]. PF4 also facilitates Treg polarization toward a Th1-Treg phenotype within the tumor microenvironment and has been associated with poor prognosis when highly expressed in tumor-associated macrophages (TAMs) [51]. This regulation is time and concentration-dependent and synergizes with TGFβ to modulate T-cell subsets via distinct receptor-binding modes [5, 6]. Functional platelet–T-cell interactions, crucial for optimal immune modulation, require direct cell–cell contact and platelet-derived PF4, as evidenced by spleen-specific Treg/Th17 impairment upon contact blockade and restoration by PF4-reconstitution [22].

AA is a T-cell-mediated autoimmune disorder of the hematopoietic system, characterized by severe depletion of HSPCs, leading to pancytopenia [52]. Overactivated T-cells in AA directly induce HSPC apoptosis via FAS/Fas ligand (FASL), TNF-related apoptosis-inducing ligand (TRAIL)/death receptor (DR), and other DR pathways, and promote inflammatory homing through CCL5–CCR5 while secreting IFN-γ, TNF-α, and other proinflammatory cytokines, ultimately leading to bone marrow aplasia and hematopoietic failure [9]. Early AA is dominated by Th1 responses, while later stages involve Th17 and effector memory $CD8^+$ T-cells [53]. Megakaryocytes may also acquire immune properties and present antigens via major histocompatibility complex Class II (MHC II), further impairing (HSC function [54].

Key cytokines such as PF4 and TGF-β play central roles in immune dysregulation, HSPC damage, and BMF. Bone marrow macrophages, particularly the M1 subtype, drive T-cell activation through the TNF-α/TNF-α receptor pathway, further exacerbating HSPC injury. Beyond their hemostatic function, platelets also participate in T-cell immunoregulation via mechanisms such as the Akt-PGC1α-TFAM pathway or PF4-mediated activity [55]. Through cellular metabolic processes, PF4 mediates $CD4^+$ memory T-cell responses and functions as a crucial chemokine and platelet activation signal. By binding to CXCR3, PF4 decreases PGC1α phosphorylation and inhibits Akt activity, increasing TFAM production and PGC1α function to support mitochondrial biogenesis and increase Th1 and Treg responses. T-box transcription factor (T-bet) and Forkhead Box P3 (FoxP3) expression are further upregulated, and $CD4^+$ T effector responses are strengthened by increased mitochondrial mass, which also increases oxygen consumption and ATP/ROS generation [6]. However, PF4 also exhibits dual pathological potential: on one hand, it may exert immunomodulatory effects by promoting Treg differentiation and function, aiding in the restoration of immune tolerance; on the other hand, in the inflammatory milieu of AA, PF4-driven mitochondrial biogenesis is more likely to provide sustained energy and biosynthetic support to already activated autoreactive Th1 cells, enhancing their proliferation, survival, and production of effector cytokines such as IFN-γ, thereby intensifying immune attacks on HSPCs.

Moreover, platelets are the largest reservoir of circulating TGF-β [56]. In healthy states, TGF-β1 released from activated platelets maintains immune homeostasis through the canonical SMAD family member 2/3 (Smad2/3) signaling pathway, promoting Treg differentiation and suppressing effector T-cell function [57, 58]. However, within the disrupted bone marrow microenvironment of AA, the overall immunosuppressive network is compromised, potentially overwhelming the homeostatic function of TGF-β1. Its capacity to promote Th17 differentiation may instead exacerbate inflammatory responses in the presence of proinflammatory cytokines such as IL-6 and IL-21. Notably, plasma TGF-β1 levels are significantly elevated in responders to TPO-RA therapy [59]. Therefore, a crucial therapeutic strategy to restore immunological tolerance and rectify aberrant T-cell activation in AA is to increase functional platelets (and TGF-β1) via TPO-RAs in conjunction with antiinflammatory tactics.

This study explores the role of platelets as immune coordinators in AA. Through the secretion of PF4 and TGF-β, platelets interact with T-cells and macrophages, influencing immune polarization and promoting IFN-γ and TNF-α production, thereby exacerbating immune-mediated HSPC injury.

These findings offer a new perspective for understanding the immunopathology of AA, highlighting the significance of platelet–T-cell interactions in disease progression. They also suggest potential directions for therapeutic development. Targeting platelet-mediated immune regulation – for instance, by using TPO-RAs such as EPAG to simultaneously increase platelet counts and correct immune imbalances, or by developing interventions focused on specific pathways such as PF4/CXCR3 – may represent promising strategies for improving patient outcomes. Further investigation into the platelet-driven immune regulatory network is essential for achieving a comprehensive understanding of AA pathogenesis and for advancing combined immunotherapeutic approaches. Currently, research on the crosstalk between T-cells and platelets in hematological malignancies remains limited, and the underlying mechanism has not yet been fully elucidated. Therefore, given the limited evidence currently available, the mechanisms underlying platelet–T-cell crosstalk can only be inferred from existing studies.

Not only can platelets interact with T-cells, but their by-products, platelet-derived microparticles (PMPs), can also interact with T-cells. PMPs are ultramicro membranous vesicles shed from the serous membranes of platelets, containing high levels of phosphatidylserine and comprising lipids, proteins, messenger RNAs (mRNAs), microRNAs (miRNAs), and even DNA, which play an important role in cancer progression, thrombosis, cell–cell communication, inflammation, etc. [55]. PMPs participate in immune modulation by interacting with Tregs, including inhibiting Treg proliferation, mainly through CXCR3 [53]. A previous study has demonstrated platelet activation in AML and low-stage B-cell lymphoma (BCL). Moreover, a recent study has found that platelets can bind to lymphocytes in AML and BCL patients, and this interaction is associated with altered immune responses.

However, the patterns of platelet activation in AML and BCL are not the same. In AML patients, the expression of CD61 and CD42b was significantly decreased compared with controls, while CD61 PMP levels were markedly increased, indicating intravascular activation of platelets. Meanwhile, leukemia cells can also stimulate platelet activation [55]. In low-stage BCL patients, increased platelet counts and activation were observed, accompanied by upregulation of T-cell markers. In contrast, these markers were reduced in high-stage BCL patients. These findings suggest that T-cell function is modulated by platelet status and dynamically regulated during BCL progression [56].

In MPN (Myeloproliferative Neoplasms)patients, increased frequencies of PLT–CD8 T-cell aggregates have been observed in both peripheral blood and bone marrow. Common driver mutations in MPN, including JAK2, calreticulin (CALR), and MPL, are associated with the formation of these aggregates. The extent of platelet binding varies among different mutations: triple-negative patients show lower PLT binding, whereas MPL-mutated cases exhibit higher levels. JAK2-mutated patients display lower levels of PLT–CD8 aggregates than CALR-mutated patients, and platelet counts correlate with PLT binding in JAK2-mutated but not CALR-mutated MPN. These findings suggest that enhanced PLT–T-cell interaction depends not only on JAK–STAT activation but also on thrombopoietin receptor–related pathways [57]. In MPN, platelet activation leads to increased release of PF4 and CCL5; meanwhile, IL-1β may also be produced by activated platelets. These factors can promote immune cell chemotaxis toward platelets, suggesting that they may enhance platelet–immune cell interactions [58]. Generally, PLT binding to memory and antigen-specific $CD8^{+}$T-cells is associated with reduced proliferation and cytokine production. Platelet–T-cell crosstalk may therefore contribute to immune suppression through platelet-derived TGF-β and P-selectin/PSGL-1 interactions, impairing antitumor T-cell function [57].

Currently, there are no direct mechanistic studies that have clearly demonstrated the interaction between platelets and T-cells in myelodysplastic syndromes (MDS) and MM. In MDS, platelet activation appears to be impaired, as reflected by altered CD63 expression and reduced CD154 and Toll-like receptor 4 (TLR4) levels, suggesting dysregulated platelet-mediated immune function [59]. Although direct platelet–T-cell interactions were not examined, these changes may influence immune crosstalk. In MM, a low platelet-to-lymphocyte ratio (PLR) has been identified as an independent predictor of poor overall survival. However, this association is based on cell counts and does not provide direct evidence of platelet–T-cell interaction [60]. Taken together, while current evidence allows for reasonable inference, direct functional experiments are needed to validate platelet–T-cell interactions in hematological malignancies.

Platelet–T-cell crosstalk occurs not only in hematological diseases but also in neurological disorders. In myasthenia gravis (MG), dysregulated platelet activation is associated with disease severity. Activated platelets promote $CD4^{+}$ T-cell proliferation, skew responses toward a Th1 phenotype, and inhibit Treg differentiation, mainly through RANTES-mediated signaling [61]. Ischemic stroke, caused by a sudden disruption of blood flow to the brain, is a leading cause of death and exerts a heavy burden on both patients and public health systems. In ischemic stroke, platelet–T-cell crosstalk exhibits a dynamic, stage-dependent pattern. During the hyperacute phase, Tregs interact with platelets in the vasculature, inducing thrombosis, microvasculature dysfunction, and facilitating initial T-cell migration into the ischemic brain via platelet-derived factors such as CD84. In the acute phase, this interaction enhances T-cell infiltration and proinflammatory cytokine production, thereby exacerbating tissue injury [43].

In addition, high-sensitivity multiplex proteomics and immunoassay technologies play a crucial role in identifying biomarkers for CNS diseases. For instance, in cognitive impairment disorders, these ultra-sensitive detection techniques can accurately capture trace amounts of potential biomarkers related to platelet–T-cell crosstalk (such as specific subtypes of EVs and soluble P-selectin) from plasma or cerebrospinal fluid (CSF) at the very early stages of cognitive decline. This provides key targets and technical support for noninvasive early screening and precise intervention in CNS diseases.

Author contributions

The authors contributed to the study conception and design: S. Tan, Q. Qin, W. Wang, and W.L. Sun. S. Tan, H.Z. He, M.Y. Shang, Y.M. Li, X.L. Chang, Y.C. Chen, J. Ni, J.Z. Ma, Y.X. Wang, C.X. Xue, Z.Q. Sun, Y.Z. Zhou, X.Y. Li, H.Y. Wang, Q. Qin, W. Wang, and W.L. Sun performed the literature review, interpreted the data, and wrote the manuscript. S. Tan, H.Z. He, M.Y. Shang, and Y.M. Li interpreted the data, wrote the manuscript, and revised the manuscript. S. Tan, Q. Qin, W. Wang, and W.L. Sun designed the study, interpreted the data, and organized the research. All authors provided critical feedback during manuscript preparation and approved the final version for publication.

Acknowledgments

The study was supported by grants from the National Natural Science Foundation of China (NSFC) (project no. 82300161); Beijing High Innovation Program·Spring Bud Project (project no. 2-1-008-0262); Xuanwu Hospital Talent Convergence Program (project no. HZ2025ZCYX003); Beijing Future Talent Training Program in the Medical-Engineering Field (project no. MBRC0012025063); the Natural Science Foundation of Beijing Municipality (project no. Z200022); National Key R&D Program of China (project no. 2025YFE0206600); Capital's Funds for Health Improvement and Research (project no. 2024-2-1032); Beijing Nova Program (project no. 20240484566); Beijing Natural Science Foundation (project no. L251023); Xuanwu Hospital Talent Convergence Program (project no. HZ2025PYYX005); Beijing High-level Overseas Returnee Talent Funding Project (project no. 2-2-008-0243); Capital Medical University Science and Innovation Elite Plan Project (project no. 2024KCJY0405); the "National Natural Science Foundation of Youth Cultivation Project" of "Xuanwu Hospital, Capital Medical University, Beijing, China" (project no. QNPY2022014); and the "Person of Outstanding Ability Training Program" of "Xuanwu Hospital, Capital Medical University, Beijing, China" (project no. YC20220127). All authors provided critical feedback during manuscript preparation and approved the final version for publication. Last but not least, many thanks to our friend ***Dr. Mohamed Elsherif Badr (Chinese Institutes for***

Medical Research (CIMR), Beijing) for the help. These illustrations were conceived and designed by the author, with initial concept images generated by Google Gemini AI, followed by optimization and final design using Figuredraw and PowerPoint.

The authors acknowledge the use of DeepSeek for language polishing, which enhances the clarity and readability of their manuscript.

Conflict of Interest

The authors state that they have no conflicts of interest.

Acronyms and abbreviations

AA	Aplastic anemia
PF4	Platelet factor 4
CXCL4	C-X-C motif chemokine ligand 4
TGF-β	Transforming growth factor-beta
CXCR3	C-X-C motif chemokine receptor 3
Th1	T helper 1
Th17	T helper 17
Treg	Regulatory T-cell
IFN-γ	Interferon-gamma
TNF-α	Tumor necrosis factor-alpha
IST	Immunosuppressive therapy
HSCT	Hematopoietic stem cell transplantation
EPAG	Eltrombopag
TPO-RA	Thrombopoietin receptor agonist
ROS	Reactive oxygen species
Akt	Akt/PKB(Akt/Protein Kinase B)
PGC1α	Peroxisome proliferator-activated receptor gamma coactivator 1-alpha
TFAM	Mitochondrial transcription factor A
SLE	Systemic lupus erythematosus
PSGL-1	P-selectin glycoprotein ligand 1
RA	Rheumatoid arthritis
pMVs	Platelet-derived microvesicles
CD40L	CD40 ligand
RANTES	Regulated upon activation, normal T-cell expressed and secreted
IL-1β	Interleukin-1 beta
ITP	Immune thrombocytopenia
Tfh	T follicular helper cells
STAT3	Signal transducer and activator of transcription 3
BMF	Bone marrow failure
c-MPL	Myeloproliferative leukemia protein
JAK2	Janus kinase 2
STAT5	Signal transducer and activator of transcription 5
PI3K	Phosphatidylinositol 3-Kinase

MAPK	Mitogen-activated protein kinase
HSPCs	Hematopoietic stem and progenitor cells
ATG	Antithymocyte globulin
SAA	Severe aplastic anemia
CsA	Cyclosporine
CCL5	C-C motif chemokine ligand 5
SDF-1	Stromal cell-derived factor 1
NK	Natural killer
Smad2/3	Smad family member 2/3
AML	Acute MYELOID LEUKEMIA
PD-1	Programmed cell death protein 1
MM	Multiple myeloma
DLBCL	Diffuse large B-cell lymphoma
CAFs	Cancer-associated fibroblasts
COX-2	Cyclooxygenase-2
CNS	Central nervous system
TRM	Tissue-resident memory T-cells
BBB	Blood–brain barrier
MS	Multiple sclerosis
EAE	Experimental autoimmune encephalomyelitis
EVs	Extracellular vesicles
PAF	Platelet-activating factor
VCAM-1	Vascular cell adhesion molecule-1
VLA-4	Very late antigen-4
NO	Nitric oxide
T-bet	T-box transcription factor
FoxP3	Forkhead box P3
TAMs	Tumor-associated macrophages
FASL	Fas ligand
TRAIL	TNF-related apoptosis-inducing ligand
DR	Death receptor
MHC II	Major histocompatibility complex class II
Th22	T helper 22
MDS	Myelodysplastic syndromes
TLR4	Toll-like receptor 4
PLR	Platelet-to-lymphocyte ratio
MG	Myasthenia gravis
CSF	Cerebrospinal fluid
CALR	Calreticulin
JAK	Janus kinase
HSC	Hematopoietic stem cell
OXPHOS	Oxidative phosphorylation

Author details

Shuai Tan[1,2,3†], *Huizhen He[1,2,3†], Mingyue Shang[1,2,3†], Yumeng Li[1,2,3†], Xiaoli Chang[1,2,3], Yaochi Chen[1,2,3], Jingzhe Ma[1,2,3], Yixuan Wang[4], Jing Ni[1,2,3], Chunxiao Xue[1,2,3], Zongqu Sun[1,2,3], Yizhang Zhou[1,2,3,5], Xiaoyu Li[1,2,3,5], Huanyuan Wang[1,2,3], Qi Qin[4*], Wei Wang[6,7*] and Wanling Sun[1,2,3*]

1 Department of Hematology, Xuanwu Hospital, Capital Medical University, Beijing, China

2 Comprehensive Center for Neuro-oncology, Xuanwu Hospital, Capital Medical University, Beijing, China

3 National Center for Neurological Disorders, Beijing, China

4 Department of Neurology and Innovation Center for Neurological Disorders, Xuanwu Hospital, Capital Medical University, National Center for Neurological Disorders, Beijing, China

5 Department of Hematology, Xiong'an Xuanwu Hospital, Hebei, China

6 National Institute of Biological Sciences, Beijing, China

7 Tsinghua Institute of Multidisciplinary Biomedical Research, Tsinghua University, Beijing, China

† These authors contributed equally

*Address all correspondence to: tanshuai@xwhosp.org; qinqibao@126.com; wangwei@nibs.ac.cn; wanlingsun@xwhosp.org

References

[1] Thaiss CA, Tian Y, Winer DA, et al. Aging and immunity. Immunity. 2025;**58**(11):2609–2612. DOI: 10.1016/j.immuni.2025.10.019

[2] Masopust D, Awasthi A, Bosselut R, et al. Guidelines for T cell nomenclature. Nature Reviews Immunology. 2025:10–1038. DOI: 10.1038/S41577-025-01238-2

[3] Brodsky RA, Jones RJ. Aplastic anaemia. The Lancet. 2005;**365**(9471):1647–1656. DOI: 10.1016/S0140-6736(05)66515-4

[4] Goronkova O, Novichkova G, Salimova T, et al. Efficacy of combined immunosuppression with or without eltrombopag in children with newly diagnosed aplastic anemia. Blood Advances. 2023;**7**(6):953–962. DOI: 10.1182/bloodadvances.2021006716

[5] Tan S, Zhang J, Sun Y, et al. Platelets enhance CD4+ central memory T cell responses via platelet factor 4-dependent mitochondrial biogenesis and cell proliferation. Platelets. 2022;**33**(3):360–370. DOI: 10.1080/09537104.2021.1936479

[6] Tan S, Li S, Min Y, et al. Platelet factor 4 enhances CD4(+) T effector memory cell responses via Akt-PGC1α-TFAM signaling-mediated mitochondrial biogenesis. Journal of Thrombosis and Haemostasis. 2020;**18**(10):2685–2700. DOI: 10.1111/jth.15005

[7] Huang G, Zhang Y, Wei X, et al. CD8(+)GITR(+) T cells may negatively regulate T cell overactivation in aplastic anemia. Immunological Investigations. 2021;**50**(4):406–415. DOI: 10.1080/08820139.2020.1770785

[8] Alvarado LJ, Huntsman HD, Cheng H, et al. Eltrombopag maintains human hematopoietic stem and progenitor cells under inflammatory conditions mediated by IFN-γ. Blood. 2019;**133**(19):2043–2055. DOI: 10.1182/blood-2018-11-884486

[9] Tan S, He H, Li Y, et al. Platelets as a potential new immune coordinator in T cell-mediated aplastic anemia. Frontiers in Oncology. 2025;**15**:1568169

[10] Maugeri N, Manfredi AA. Platelets as drivers of immunothrombosis in rheumatic diseases. Nature Reviews Rheumatology. 2025;**21**(8):478–493. DOI: 10.1038/s41584-025-01276-z

[11] Scherlinger M, Richez C, Tsokos GC, et al. The role of platelets in immune-mediated inflammatory diseases. Nature Reviews Immunology. 2023;**23**(8):495–510. DOI: 10.1038/s41577-023-00834-4

[12] Chellamuthu G, Muthu S, Khanna M, et al. "Platelet-rich plasma holds promise in management of rheumatoid arthritis"-systematic review. Rheumatology International. 2021;**41**(11):1895–1903. DOI: 10.1007/s00296-021-04849-9

[13] Badimon L, Suades R, Fuentes E, et al. Role of platelet-derived microvesicles as crosstalk mediators in atherothrombosis and future pharmacology targets: A link between inflammation, atherosclerosis, and thrombosis. Frontiers in Pharmacology. 2016;7:293

[14] Pedicino D, Giglio AF, Ruggio A, et al. Inflammasome, T lymphocytes and innate-adaptive immunity

crosstalk: Role in cardiovascular disease and therapeutic perspectives. Thrombosis and Haemostasis. 2018;**118**(8):1352–1369. DOI: 10.1055/S-0038-1666860

[15] Schäfer S, Zernecke A. CD8(+) T cells in atherosclerosis. Cells. 2020;**10**(1):37. DOI: 10.3390/cells10010037

[16] Schuhmann MK, Stoll G, Bieber M, et al. CD84 links T cell and platelet activity in cerebral thrombo-inflammation in acute stroke. Circulation Research. 2020;**127**(8):1023–1035. DOI: 10.1161/circresaha.120.316655

[17] Saris A, Steuten J, Schrijver DP, et al. Inhibition of dendritic cell activation and modulation of T cell polarization by the platelet secretome. Frontiers in Immunology. 2021;**12**:631285

[18] Wu F, Li Y, Jiang N, et al. Increased platelet-CD8+ T-cell aggregates displaying high activation, exhaustion, and tendency to death correlate with disease progression in people with HIV-1. Journal of Leukocyte Biology. 2024;**116**(1):166–176. DOI: 10.1093/jleuko/qiae048

[19] Bu S, Liu M, Yang L, et al. The function of T cells in immune thrombocytopenia. Frontiers in Immunology. 2025;**16**:1499014

[20] Han P, Hou Y, Zhao Y, et al. Low-dose decitabine modulates T-cell homeostasis and restores immune tolerance in immune thrombocytopenia. Blood. 2021;**138**(8):674–688. DOI: 10.1182/blood.2020008477

[21] Olnes MJ, Scheinberg P, Calvo KR, et al. Eltrombopag and improved hematopoiesis in refractory aplastic anemia. The New England Journal of Medicine. 2012;**367**(1):11–19. DOI: 10.1056/NEJMoa1200931

[22] Min Y, Hao L, Liu X, et al. Platelets fine-tune effector responses of naïve CD4(+) T cells via platelet factor 4-regulated transforming growth factor β signaling. Cellular and Molecular Life Sciences. 2022;**79**(5):247. DOI: 10.1007/s00018-022-04279-1

[23] Peffault De Latour R, Kulasekararaj A, Iacobelli S, et al. Eltrombopag added to immunosuppression in severe aplastic anemia. The New England Journal of Medicine. 2022;**386**(1):11–23. DOI: 10.1056/NEJMoa2109965

[24] Townsley DM, Scheinberg P, Winkler T, et al. Eltrombopag added to standard immunosuppression for aplastic anemia. The New England Journal of Medicine. 2017;**376**(16):1540–1550. DOI: 10.1056/NEJMoa1613878

[25] Groarke EM, Patel BA, Gutierrez-Rodrigues F, et al. Eltrombopag added to immunosuppression for children with treatment-naïve severe aplastic anaemia. British Journal of Haematology. 2021;**192**(3):605–614. DOI: 10.1111/bjh.17232

[26] Tan S, He H, Ni J, et al. Meta-analysis evaluating the efficacy and safety of various Bruton tyrosine kinase (BTK) inhibitors for central nervous system lymphoma: Novel covalent BTK inhibitors, except for ibrutinib, also demonstrate good efficacy in the treatment of primary central nervous system lymphoma. Cancer. 2025;**131**(18):e70083. DOI: 10.1002/cncr.70083

[27] Tian T, Yu S, Liu L, et al. The profile of T helper subsets in bone marrow microenvironment is distinct for different stages of acute myeloid leukemia patients and chemotherapy partly ameliorates these variations. PLoS One. 2015;**10**(7):e0131761. DOI: 10.1371/journal.pone.0131761

[28] Kulkarni A, Bazou D, Santos-Martinez MJ. Bleeding and thrombosis in multiple myeloma: Platelets as key players during cell interactions and potential use as drug delivery systems. International Journal of Molecular Sciences. 2023;**24**(21):15855. DOI: 10.3390/ijms242115855

[29] Aloui C, Prigent A, Sut C, et al. The signaling role of CD40 ligand in platelet biology and in platelet component transfusion. International Journal of Molecular Sciences. 2014;**15**(12):22342–22364. DOI: 10.3390/ijms151222342

[30] Scherlinger M, Guillotin V, Douchet I, et al. Selectins impair regulatory T cell function and contribute to systemic lupus erythematosus pathogenesis. Science Translational Medicine. 2021;**13**(600):eabi4994. DOI: 10.1126/scitranslmed.abi4994

[31] Yu H, Hu W, Song X, et al. Immune MODULATION OF PLATELET-DERIVED MITOCHONDRIA ON MEMORY CD4(+) T cells in humans. International Journal of Molecular Sciences. 2020;**21**(17):6295. DOI: 10.3390/ijms21176295

[32] Tan S, Sun Y, Sheng Z, et al. Platelet-specific TGFβ deficiency aggravates atherosclerosis, vascular inflammation, and hypercholesterolemia in mice. Thrombosis and Haemostasis. 2025. DOI: 10.1055/a-2694-1383

[33] Schlesinger M. Role of platelets and platelet receptors in cancer metastasis. Journal of Hematology & Oncology. 2018;**11**(1):125. DOI: 10.1186/s13045-018-0669-2

[34] Tan J, Chen S, Lu Y, et al. Higher PD-1 expression concurrent with exhausted CD8+ T cells in patients with de novo acute myeloid leukemia. Chinese Journal of Cancer Research. 2017;**29**(5):463–470. DOI: 10.21147/j.issn.1000-9604.2017.05.11

[35] Mazziotta F, Biavati L, Rimando J, et al. CD8+ T-cell differentiation and dysfunction inform treatment response in acute myeloid leukemia. Blood. 2024;**144**(11):1168–1182. DOI: 10.1182/blood.2023021680

[36] Natoni A, Cerreto M, De Propris MS, et al. Sialofucosylation enables platelet binding to myeloma cells via P-selectin and suppresses NK cell-mediated cytotoxicity. Cancers. 2023;**15**(7):2154. DOI: 10.3390/cancers15072154

[37] Apollonio B, Spada F, Petrov N, et al. Tumor-activated lymph node fibroblasts suppress T cell function in diffuse large B cell lymphoma. The Journal of Clinical Investigation. 2023;**133**(13):e166070. DOI: 10.1172/JCI166070

[38] Clozel T, Yang S, Elstrom RL, et al. Mechanism-based epigenetic chemosensitization therapy of diffuse large B-cell lymphoma. Cancer Discovery. 2013;**3**(9):1002–1019. DOI: 10.1158/2159-8290.cd-13-0117

[39] Ok AK, Farber DL, Zou W. Tissue-resident memory T cells in tumor immunity and immunotherapy. The Journal of Experimental Medicine.

2021;**218**(4):e20201605. DOI: 10.1084/jem.20201605

[40] Wang X, Tian Z, Peng H. Tissue-resident memory-like ILCs: Innate counterparts of T(RM) cells. Protein & Cell. 2020;**11**(2):85–96. DOI: 10.1007/s13238-019-0647-7

[41] Rego S, Sanchez G, Da Mesquita S. Current views on meningeal lymphatics and immunity in aging and Alzheimer's disease. Molecular Neurodegeneration. 2023;**18**(1):55. DOI: 10.1186/s13024-023-00645-0

[42] Ruiz-Fernández I, Sánchez-Díaz R, Ortega-Sollero E, et al. Update on the role of T cells in cognitive impairment. British Journal of Pharmacology. 2024;**181**(6):799–815. DOI: 10.1111/bph.16214

[43] Zhang D, Ren J, Luo Y, et al. T cell response in ischemic stroke: From mechanisms to translational insights. Frontiers in Immunology. 2021;**12**:707972

[44] Wang CS, Kavalali ET, Monteggia LM. BDNF signaling in context: From synaptic regulation to psychiatric disorders. Cell. 2022;**185**(1):62–76. DOI: 10.1016/j.cell.2021.12.003

[45] Shi L, Sun Z, Su W, et al. Treg cell-derived osteopontin promotes microglia-mediated white matter repair after ischemic stroke. Immunity. 2021;**54**(7):1527–1542. DOI: 10.1016/j.immuni.2021.04.022

[46] Orian JM, D'Souza CS, Kocovski P, et al. Platelets in multiple sclerosis: Early and central mediators of inflammation and neurodegeneration and attractive targets for molecular imaging and site-directed therapy. Frontiers in Immunology. 2021;**12**:620963

[47] Chapman LM, Aggrey AA, Field DJ, et al. Platelets present antigen in the context of MHC class I. Journal of Immunology (Baltimore, Md.: 1950). 2012;**189**(2):916–923. DOI: 10.4049/jimmunol.1200580

[48] Kihara Y. Systematic understanding of bioactive lipids in neuro-immune interactions: Lessons from an animal model of multiple sclerosis. Advances in Experimental Medicine and Biology. 2019;**1161**:133–148. DOI: 10.1007/978-3-030-21735-8_13

[49] Angelini G, Bani A, Constantin G, et al. The interplay between T helper cells and brain barriers in the pathogenesis of multiple sclerosis. Frontiers in Cellular Neuroscience. 2023;**17**:1101379

[50] Tian Y, Zong Y, Pang Y, et al. Platelets and diseases: Signal transduction and advances in targeted therapy. Signal Transduction and Targeted Therapy. 2025;**10**(1):159. DOI: 10.1038/s41392-025-02198-8

[51] Kuratani A, Okamoto M, Kishida K, et al. Platelet factor 4-induced TH1-Treg polarization suppresses antitumor immunity. Science. 2024;**386**(6724):eadn8608. DOI: 10.1126/science.adn8608

[52] Feng X, Scheinberg P, Samsel L, et al. Decreased plasma cytokines are associated with low platelet counts in aplastic anemia and immune thrombocytopenic purpura. Journal of Thrombosis and Haemostasis. 2012;**10**(8):1616–1623. DOI: 10.1111/j.1538-7836.2012.04757.x

[53] Contursi A, Tacconelli S, Di Berardino S, et al. Platelets as crucial players in the dynamic interplay of inflammation, immunity, and cancer: Unveiling new strategies for cancer prevention. Frontiers in Pharmacology. 2024;**15**:1520488

[54] Zhu C, Lian Y, Wang C, et al. Single-cell transcriptomics dissects hematopoietic cell destruction and T-cell engagement in aplastic anemia. Blood. 2021;**138**(1):23–33. DOI: 10.1182/blood.2020008966

[55] Guo J, Cui B, Zheng J, et al. Platelet-derived microparticles and their cargos: The past, present and future. Asian Journal of Pharmaceutical Sciences. 2024;**19**(2):100907. DOI: 10.1016/j.ajps.2024.100907

[56] Dinkla S, van Cranenbroek B, van der Heijden WA, et al. Platelet microparticles inhibit IL-17 production by regulatory T cells through P-selectin. Blood. 2016;**127**(16):1976–1986. DOI: 10.1182/blood-2015-04-640300

[57] Carnaz Simões AM, Holmström MO, Aehnlich P, et al. Patients with myeloproliferative neoplasms harbor high frequencies of CD8 T cell-platelet aggregates associated with T cell suppression. Frontiers in Immunology. 2022;**13**:866610

[58] Marin Oyarzún CP, Heller PG. Platelets as mediators of thromboinflammation in chronic myeloproliferative neoplasms. Frontiers in Immunology. 2019;**10**:1373. DOI: 10.3389/fimmu.2019.01373

[59] Liu J, Niu H, Yue L, et al. Abnormal platelet phenotypes in patients with myelodysplastic syndromes. International Journal of Laboratory Hematology. 2020;**42**(4):371–379. DOI: 10.1111/ijlh.13191

[60] Zhang Q, Wang Y, Shi W, et al. The prognostic value of the platelet-to-lymphocyte ratio in multiple myeloma patients treated with a bortezomib-based regimen. Scientific Reports. 2025;**15**(1):1819. DOI: 10.1038/s41598-024-84343-x

[61] Wen Q, Zhang S, Wang Y, et al. Platelet activation plays a pro-inflammatory role in myasthenia gravis. Nature Communications. 2025;**16**(1):8779. DOI: 10.1038/s41467-025-63750-2

[62] Burnouf T, Walker TL. The multifaceted role of platelets in mediating brain function. Blood. 2022;**140**(8):815–827. DOI: 10.1182/blood.2022015970

Chapter 3

T Lymphocytes in Pulmonary Tuberculosis: Immunity, Immunopathology and Therapeutic Potential

Jacqueline V. Lara-Espinosa, Mayra Silva Miranda, María Fernanda Arce-Aceves, Vasti Lozano-Ordaz, Yadira Rodríguez- Miguez and Rogelio Hernández-Pando

Abstract

Tuberculosis (TB), caused primarily by *Mycobacterium tuberculosis* (*Mtb*), remains a major global health challenge and the leading cause of death worldwide from a single infectious agent. In developed countries, TB is a prototypical re-emerging infectious disease, while in developing nations, it is a devastating health issue. In humans and mice, cell-mediated immunity, driven by T lymphocytes, plays a crucial role in coordinating and regulating the immune response to eliminate *Mtb*. Significant evidence indicates that $CD4^+$ T helper lymphocytes (Th-1 cells) and Th-17 cells are vital to the protective immune response against *Mtb*. $CD4^+$ Th-1 cells activate macrophages, enhancing their ability to eliminate mycobacteria. They also recruit additional immune cells to infection and inflammation sites and promote the cytotoxicity of $CD8^+$ T lymphocytes, which are essential for killing infected cells through apoptosis. Indeed, the immune response to *Mtb* involves a carefully balanced interaction between protective inflammation and tissue-damaging pathology. Therefore, the involvement of anti-inflammatory cells, such as Th-2 lymphocytes and T regulatory cells, is also critical in modulating and controlling inflammation that can cause tissue damage. In this chapter, the roles of various T-lymphocyte subtypes in the immune response to *Mtb* are discussed, along with the different T-cell immune evasion strategies *Mtb* employs to prevent clearance. Additionally, novel immunotherapeutic approaches aimed at enhancing protective T-cell activity or suppressing harmful T-cell effects are explored, providing potential methods to facilitate pathogen eradication and reduce the lengthy chemotherapy required for this significant infectious disease.

Keywords: tuberculosis, T-lymphocytes, immunotherapy, evasion, Immunoregulation

1. Introduction

Tuberculosis (TB) is a lung infection caused by bacteria of the Mycobacterium tuberculosis Complex (MTBC), particularly *Mycobacterium tuberculosis* (*Mtb*) and *M. africanum* [1]. According to the World Health Organization (WHO), TB remains the principal cause of death due to an infectious agent [2]. In 2024, there were 10.7 million new cases of TB reported worldwide and 1.23 million deaths [2]. Although the lungs are the primary site of infection, the bacteria can disseminate via the bloodstream or lymphatic system, leading to extrapulmonary manifestations of TB [3]. After infection with *Mtb*, it is estimated that only 5% of people will develop active TB, while 95% will eliminate the bacteria or control the infection. The outcome of *Mtb* infection is closely related to the strength of the host's immune system and to components inherent to mycobacteria [4].

The innate immune response, particularly macrophages, is essential for controlling *Mtb*. Cell-mediated immunity, driven by T lymphocytes, coordinates and regulates host defenses against *Mtb*. Substantial evidence demonstrates that cluster of differentiation 4 ($CD4^+$) T helper type 1 (Th-1) cells, simultaneously with T helper type 17 (Th-17) cells, are critical components of the protective immune response. Th-1 cells promote macrophage activation, thereby enhancing intracellular mycobacterial killing and facilitating the recruitment of additional immune cells to sites of infection and inflammation. Moreover, Th-1-derived signals support the cytotoxic function of cluster of differentiation 8 ($CD8^+$) T lymphocytes, which contribute to host defense by inducing apoptosis in infected cells. Therefore, TB is not only an infectious disease but also an immune-mediated disease.

The human *Mtb* is an exceptionally successful pathogen that has evolved multiple effective mechanisms to evade the host immune response. These mechanisms include surviving and replicating within macrophages, blocking phagosome–lysosome fusion, limiting phagosomal acidification, expressing virulence factors, resisting reactive oxygen species (ROS), suppressing protective cytokines such as interleukin (IL)-12 and tumor necrosis factor (TNF)-α, evading antigen presentation, and inhibiting apoptosis. In addition, *Mtb* dampens the host-protective T helper 1 (Th-1) immune response while promoting T helper type 2 (Th-2)-type cytokines, which are anti-inflammatory and favor its persistence [5]. *Mtb*'s capacity to modulate the host's immune response has enabled it to be a successful human pathogen [6].

This chapter examines the functional roles of the major T-lymphocyte subsets involved in the immune response to *Mtb*, as well as the diverse immune evasion strategies the bacterium employs to subvert T-cell-mediated clearance. In addition, emerging host-directed and immunotherapeutic strategies aimed at enhancing protective T-cell responses or attenuating deleterious immune mechanisms are discussed, highlighting their potential to improve pathogen elimination and shorten the prolonged chemotherapy currently required for effective TB treatment.

2. Mycobacterium tuberculosis

Mtb is a member of the MTBC, comprising 10 human-adapted and nine animal-adapted lineages that share more than 99.9% sequence identity over homologous regions, yet are associated with distinct global distributions and host tropisms [6].

DOI: http://dx.doi.org/10.5772/intechopen.1015455

Mtb is the primary causative agent of TB in humans. It is a slow-growing, obligate-aerobic, facultatively intracellular bacterium that infects phagocytic cells, including macrophages and neutrophils. *Mtb* is neither Gram-positive nor Gram-negative and is acid-fast, identifiable by Ziehl-Neelsen staining [7]. Approximately 10% of its genome comprises genes from the Proline-Glutamic Acid (PE) and Proline-Proline-Glutamic Acid (PPE) families, which encode antigens involved in immune evasion and immunopathogenesis [7]. *Mtb* has a highly specialized cell envelope composed of three layers: the plasma membrane, the cell wall core, and an outer membrane. Nearly 60% of its biomass consists of complex lipids, conferring marked hydrophobicity. The plasma membrane provides structural integrity and is surrounded by a densely cross-linked peptidoglycan layer covalently linked to arabinogalactan, which contributes to cell wall thickness and barrier function. Terminal arabinogalactan residues are esterified with mycolic acids, the dominant cell wall components, forming a hydrophobic outer shell that restricts antibiotic penetration and protects against oxidative stress and complement-mediated damage. The outer membrane is enriched in mycolic acids and complex glycolipids, including trehalose monomycolate, trehalose dimycolate (TDM), phosphatidylinositol mannosides, lipomannan, lipoarabinomannan (LAM), phthiocerol dimycocerosates, and sulfolipids. This structure confers on *Mtb* resistance to desiccation, disinfectants, antibiotics, and oxidative stress [8] (**Figure 1**).

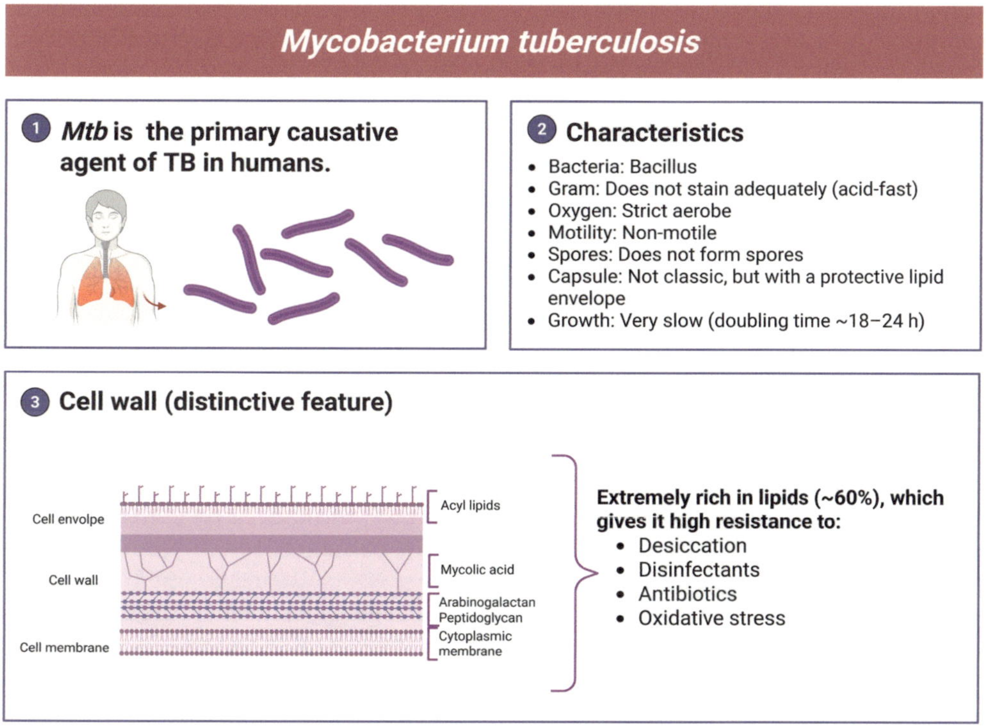

Figure 1.
General characteristics and cell wall structure of Mtb. Mtb, *the primary causative agent of TB, is a non-motile, strictly aerobic, acid-fast bacillus with slow growth. Its cell envelope is lipid-rich (~60%) and composed of a cytoplasmic membrane, peptidoglycan–arabinogalactan complex, and an outer layer of mycolic acids and acyl lipids. This structure provides resistance to desiccation, disinfectants, antibiotics, and oxidative stress, promoting persistence and pathogenicity. Created in BioRender. Barrios, J. (2026) https://biorender.com/p81rqi9.*

3. Pulmonary TB

Pulmonary TB is a chronic infectious disease caused by *Mtb* and other bacteria of the MTBC. Its pathophysiology is shaped by complex interactions between the bacillus and the host immune system, reflecting prolonged coevolution [9, 10]. Infection begins with the inhalation of aerosols containing viable bacilli, which reach the pulmonary alveoli and are phagocytosed mainly by alveolar macrophages and dendritic cells. However, the pathogen employs multiple evasion mechanisms, including inhibition of phagosome-lysosome fusion, resistance to oxidative stress, and modulation of inflammatory pathways, thereby allowing it to survive and replicate within cells. The innate immune response recruits neutrophils, natural killer cells (NK cells), and monocytes, and releases cytokines and factors, such as vascular endothelial growth factor (VEGF), that promote inflammation, angiogenesis, and tissue remodeling. Later, adaptive immunity, driven by interferon gamma (IFN-γ) and tumor necrosis factor-α (TNF-α), produced by $CD4^+$ Th-1 lymphocytes, activates macrophages and induces granuloma formation. Granulomas are dynamic structures designed to contain bacterial spread but can also serve as niches for persistence and latency [11]. Clinically, the disease may manifest as primary TB, common in immunocompromised individuals, or as a latent infection, which remains symptomless for years. Reactivation results in secondary TB, characterized by systemic symptoms such as fever, night sweats, weight loss, and loss of appetite, along with respiratory symptoms like chronic cough, hemoptysis, and chest pain in pulmonary cases. Additionally, hematogenous spread can cause extrapulmonary TB, affecting lymph nodes, the genitourinary system, bones, the central nervous system, or leading to miliary TB [12]. Overall, the balance between immune containment, chronic inflammation, and tissue damage influences disease progression, contagiousness, and the wide range of TB symptoms (**Figure 2**).

4. Immune response against *mycobacterium tuberculosis*

The human immune system is complex, with both the innate and adaptive responses working together to control pathogens and develop immunological memory [13]. As we mentioned, *Mtb* is an intracellular bacterium; these pathogens can establish persistent, lifelong infections, evade host immune surveillance, and cause disease by replicating within host cells [14].

The immune response to *Mtb* in pulmonary TB results from complex, dynamic interactions between innate and adaptive immunity, influenced by genetic and environmental factors from both the host and the pathogen. Initially, innate cells such as macrophages, dendritic cells, neutrophils, NK cells, and innate lymphoid cells (ILCs) recognize the bacillus through pattern recognition receptors and activate microbicidal, inflammatory, and regulatory mechanisms that determine early control or progression of the infection [15]. Later, adaptive immunity, driven by $CD4^+$ Th-1, Th-17, and Th-22 lymphocytes, along with $CD8^+$ lymphocytes and B cells, strengthens macrophage activation, IFN-γ production, and granuloma formation, which are key structures that contain bacterial spread. However, *Mtb* can alter this response toward Th-2 and regulatory profiles, promoting an alternatively activated macrophage (M2) phenotype, chronic inflammation, tissue damage, and bacterial persistence [16]. Therefore, the balance between protective and harmful

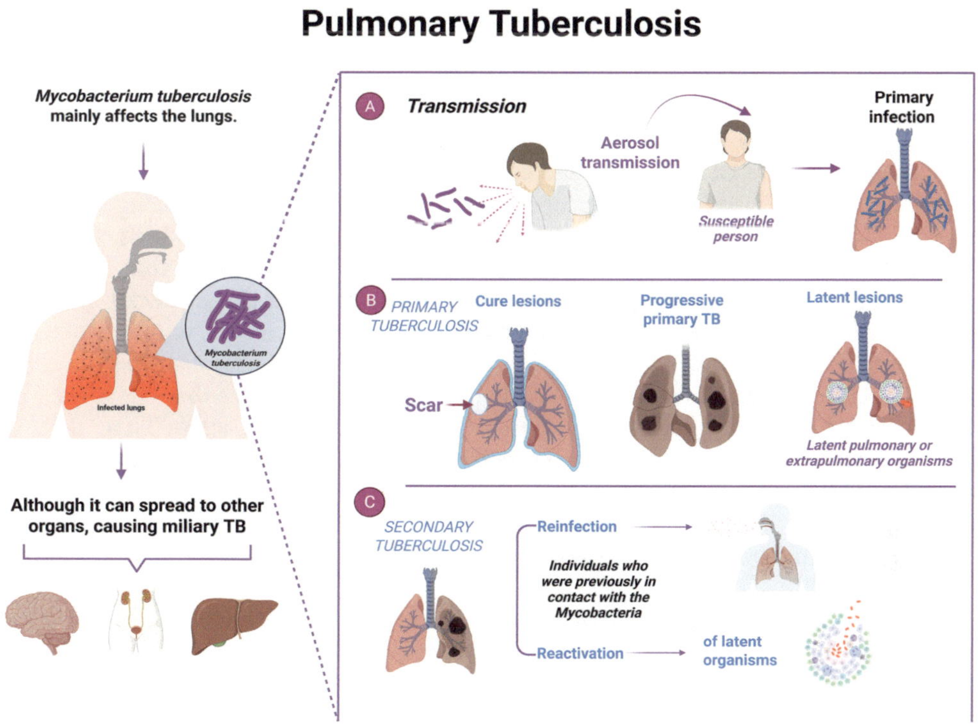

Figure 2.
Pathogenesis and clinical outcomes of pulmonary TB. (a) Mtb *is transmitted via inhaled aerosol droplets, establishing primary lung infection. (b) Primary TB may resolve with fibrosis, progress to active disease, or persist as latent infection. (c) Latent bacilli can later reactivate or reinfect, particularly during immune compromise, and may disseminate hematogenously, causing extrapulmonary or miliary TB. Created in BioRender. Barrios, J. (2026) https://biorender.com/etvrei8.*

responses shapes the clinical spectrum of the disease and fosters growing interest in host-directed therapies aimed at reducing inflammation and lung damage.

5. Protective T cell responses in pulmonary TB

In TB, T lymphocytes play a central role in protective immunity against *Mtb*, coordinating the cellular response necessary to contain the intracellular infection. In particular, $CD4^+$ Th1 T lymphocytes form the main axis of protection by producing cytokines such as IFN-γ and TNF-α, which activate infected macrophages and enhance their microbicidal mechanisms, including the production of reactive nitrogen and oxygen species. This activation promotes the formation and maintenance of granulomas, organized immune structures that limit bacterial dissemination. Furthermore, $CD8^+$ T lymphocytes contribute to infection control by lysing infected cells and releasing proinflammatory cytokines, facilitating the elimination of the bacillus from its intracellular niches. The coordinated interaction between $CD4^+$ Th1 T lymphocytes, $CD8^+$ T lymphocytes, and macrophages determines a balance between bacterial control and tissue damage, which is essential to contain the infection and prevent progression to active disease.

5.1 CD4⁺ T cells as key regulators of the immune response to *Mtb*

CD4⁺ T cells are T cells that express the CD4 receptor. These cells recognize antigens that are presented on the surface of host cells by MHC class II molecules. CD4⁺ T cells are essential for mounting a controlled and effective immune response to pathogens. Naïve CD4⁺ T cells become activated after engaging with the antigen-MHC complex [17]. When an appropriately activated antigen-presenting cell recognizes a specific antigen, naïve CD4⁺ T cells undergo multiple rounds of division and can differentiate into various effector T helper (Th) cell subsets that coordinate different protective immune responses. The development of these specialized effector T cells is regulated by distinct sets of transcription factors, whose expression is influenced by multiple signals, especially soluble factors that act on responding CD4⁺ T cells during activation. CD4⁺ T helper (Th) subsets have distinct roles: Th-1 cells are vital for macrophage activation via IFN-γ and TNF-α, while Th-17 cells promote neutrophil recruitment and secrete cytokines such as IL-17 [18]. The next section will describe the function of each subset in TB.

5.1.1 Th1-mediated immunity and macrophage activation in the control of Mtb

Antigen presentation via major histocompatibility complex (MHC) class II molecules leads to the differentiation of Th-1 cells, which secrete pro-inflammatory cytokines such as IFN-γ and TNF, thereby helping to restrict mycobacterial growth [19].

TB is an intracellular infection in which cellular immunity determines the clinical outcome. In this context, Th-1 cells represent the functional axis of the protective response, not only due to their direct effector capacity but also because of their role in organizing the pulmonary inflammatory microenvironment. Differentiation toward the Th-1 phenotype is driven by IL-12, produced by macrophages, NK cells, and dendritic cells upon recognition of mycobacterial patterns, which activates the signal transducer and activator of transcription 4 (STAT4) and the transcription factor T-bet, leading to sustained IFN-γ production [20–22]. This polarization is not an incidental phenomenon but an indispensable requirement for establishing an effective antimicrobial response.

Th-1-derived IFN-γ is the main activator of infected macrophages, promoting the expression of major histocompatibility complex class II molecules, increasing TNF-α production, and favoring the induction of the inducible nitric oxide synthase enzyme (iNOS), thereby generating reactive nitrogen species [23]. This classically activated macrophage phenotype (M1) optimizes the macrophage's microbicidal capacity and limits intracellular replication of *Mtb*. The non-redundant relevance of this pathway is evident in murine models deficient in IFN-γ or its receptor, which develop progressive and disseminated disease [24], as well as in patients with defects in the IL-12/IFN-γ axis, who exhibit increased susceptibility to mycobacteria.

Beyond macrophage activation, Th-1 cells play a structural role in organizing and maintaining the tuberculous granuloma, a dynamic immunological cellular complex that serves to contain the bacilli and restrict their dissemination. TNF-α, induced and sustained in part by Th-1 signals, is essential for initiating and preserving granuloma integrity; its pharmacological neutralization is associated with granuloma breakdown and reactivation of latent TB [25]. Thus, the Th-1 response not only contains the bacilli and restricts antimicrobial functions but also coordinates interactions among macrophages, lymphocytes, and other immune populations within the lung.

Although Th-1 predominance correlates with bacterial control, its overactivation can contribute to immunopathology, leading to tissue necrosis, pulmonary cavitation, and functional impairment [26]. Furthermore, the efficacy of the Th-1 response depends on its proper integration with other immune axes, such as the balance with Th-17 responses, which facilitate cell recruitment, and the containment of Th-2 or regulatory profiles that could attenuate protective immunity [20]. Therefore, we cannot reduce the role of Th-1 lymphocytes in TB to the simple production of IFN-γ but must conceive of it as a central regulatory system that integrates inflammatory signals, tissue structure, and bacterial control.

Taken together, experimental and clinical evidence position the IL-12/IFN-γ/Th-1 axis as the core of protective immunity against *Mtb*, but also as a component whose magnitude and duration must be modulated (**Figure 3**) [27]. The outcome of the infection (controlled latency, active progression, or severe lung damage) depends on the quality, intensity, and regulation of the Th-1 response, making this axis a strategic target for both vaccine design and the development of host-directed therapies [28].

5.1.2 Th17 immunity at the interface of granuloma formation and host protection

Coordinated adaptive immune responses are necessary to control *Mtb* infection. As commented before, Th-1 cells are traditionally known to produce interferon-γ (IFN-γ), which triggers macrophage bactericidal activity [20, 29]. However, increasing evidence indicates that Th-17 cells and the cytokine IL-17A play a crucial role in determining protective immunity, granuloma dynamics, and vaccine-induced responses during TB [30].

The signal transducer and activator of transcription 3 (STAT3) and the retinoic acid receptor-related orphan receptor gamma t (RORγt) transcriptional programs drive Th-17 differentiation [31]. The C–C chemokine receptor type 6 (CCR6) is a marker of a unique subset of $CD4^+$ T lymphocytes that produce IL-17A, IL-17 F, IL-21, and granulocyte-macrophage colony-stimulating factor (GM-CSF). Their differentiation from naïve $CD4^+$ cells requires cytokines, including IL-6, IL-1β, transforming growth factor beta (TGF-β), and, particularly, IL-23, which maintain lineage integrity and effector function [32, 33]. These cytokine environments engage Th-17 cells.

Th-17 cells facilitate trafficking to mucosal tissues, including the lung [34, 35]. Indeed, Th-17 cells are key modulators of mucosal immunity and host defense against *Mtb*. These lymphocytes promote early protective responses by recruiting neutrophils, establishing chemokine gradients, and supporting granuloma organization [36–40]. During *Mtb* infection, antigen-specific $IL\text{-}17A^+$ $CD4^+$ T cells are primarily found in pulmonary compartments rather than peripheral blood, indicating tissue-restricted immune responses that shape granuloma architecture [34, 40].

Mtb-specific $IL\text{-}17A^+$ and $IFN\text{-}\gamma^+/IL\text{-}17A^+$ double-positive $CD4^+$ T cells have been detected in bronchoalveolar lavage fluid in non-human primate models of latent TB infection, suggesting a coordinated recruitment of Th-1 and Th-17 cells during subclinical infection. This balanced cellular response between Th-1 and Th-17 correlates with sustained bacterial containment, enhanced effector cell recruitment, and suppression of bacillary replication [34, 35].

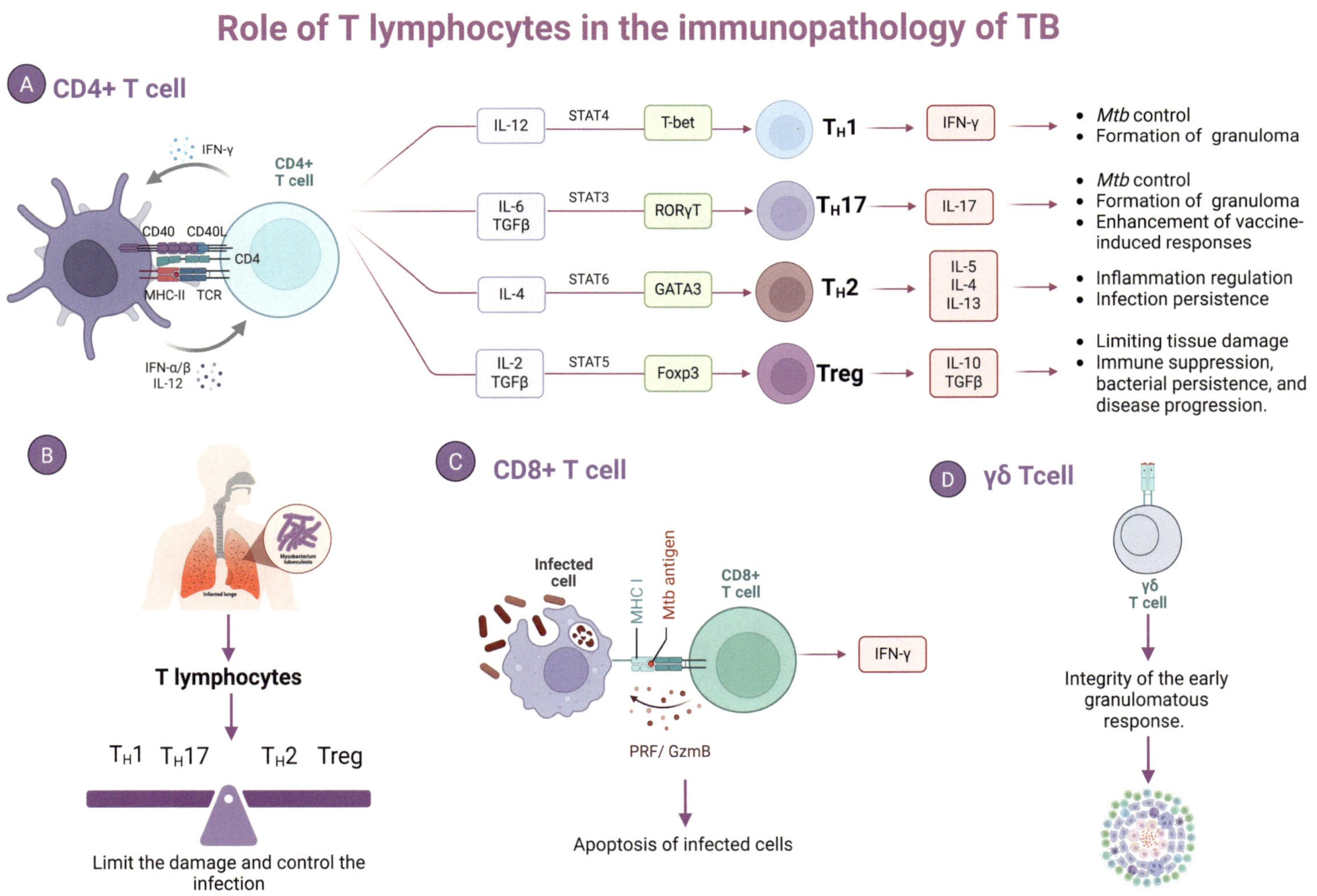

Figure 3.
Role of T lymphocytes in TB immunopathology. (a) CD4⁺ T cells differentiate into subsets that shape TB outcomes: th1 cells produce IFN-γ, activating macrophages and promoting granuloma formation; Th17 cells secrete IL-17, supporting granulomas and vaccine responses; Th2 cells (IL-4, IL-5, IL-13) regulate inflammation but may impair Th1 responses and favor fibrosis; Treg cells (IL-10, TGF-β) limit tissue damage yet can enhance immune suppression. (b) Disease outcome depends on the balance among these subsets. (c) CD8⁺ T cells recognize Mtb *antigens on MHC I, produce IFN-γ, and induce apoptosis via perforin and granzyme B. (d) γδ T cells contribute to early defense and granuloma maintenance. Created*

Th-17 cells promote an early wave of neutrophils and stimulate epithelial and stromal cells to release signals, such as C–X–C motif chemokine ligand 1 (CXCL1), C–X–C motif chemokine ligand 8 (CXCL8), and C–C motif chemokine ligand 20 (CCL20), which enhance the migration of immune cells to the infected lung tissue [35, 41]. During an *Mtb* challenge, the ability of Th-17 cells to remember and respond effectively is mediated by signals from IL-23 and by their precise cellular placement, which is guided by chemokine receptors such as C–X–C chemokine receptor type 5 (CXCR5), positioning Th-17 cells close to macrophages and B-cell follicles to boost their ability to optimize antimicrobial activity and eliminate infections [42].

The balance between Th-1 and Th-17 immunity is crucial. Excessive amounts of IL-17A can cause exaggerated inflammation mediated by neutrophils, which is associated with tissue damage and disease progression to active TB. In contrast, insufficient Th-17 activity may reflect an impaired immune system's ability to eliminate or reduce the *Mtb* bacterial burden [43, 44]. Regulatory systems that control programmed cell death protein 1 (PD-1)/programmed death-ligand 1 (PD-L1) interactions and modulate IL-23 receptor signaling can affect Th-17 cell function and might determine clinical outcomes [45]. When the immune system is dysregulated, especially during viral coinfections such as SARS-CoV-2, it can disrupt the balance of certain immune cells, thereby affecting Th-17 homeostasis and potentially TB susceptibility and disease severity [46]. These interactions underscore the complexity of the immune networks that govern TB pathogenesis.

Th-17 cells play a significant role in the development of TB vaccines. Evidence suggests that vaccines that elicit long-lasting Th-17 memory, boost early chemokine production, and accelerate the arrival of Th-1 cells after *Mtb* exposure in experimental models [47]. These teamwork-like responses improve early bacterial control, supporting the idea that a balanced Th-1-Th-17 immune response might be more effective than Th-1-focused strategies alone. Moreover, the way antigens are recognized appears to affect Th-17 cell development, which could help in developing better vaccines and provide insights for rational vaccine design [42, 48, 49].

In conclusion, Th-17 lymphocytes are essential for the protective immune response to TB but can also contribute to tissue damage. Th-17 cells contribute substantially to host defense against *Mtb* through cytokine-mediated recruitment of innate and adaptive effectors, maintenance of granuloma structure, and enhancement of vaccine-induced responses (**Figure 3**). However, both excessive or deficient Th-17 lymphocyte activity can compromise the disease outcome. Future research should define the immunological thresholds that distinguish protective from pathological Th-17 responses, enabling targeted immunomodulatory strategies to improve TB control and develop successful TB vaccines.

5.2 The role of $CD8^+$ T cells in host defense against *Mtb*

$CD8^+$ T cells are T cells that express the CD8 receptor. These cells recognize antigens presented on the surface of infected host cells by MHC class I molecules, leading to host cell killing and making them also known as cytotoxic T cells. $CD8^+$ T cells activated by antigen-presenting cells (APCs) through MHC class I molecules play an essential role in eliminating *Mtb* during the early stages of infection. Cross-presentation of *Mtb* antigens with MHC class I molecules leads to $CD8^+$ T-cell activation. Shortly after infection, these $CD8^+$ T cells migrate to infected tissues, where they produce IFN-γ and induce apoptosis in infected cells by releasing perforin, granzymes, and granulysin, as well as through Fas–FasL interactions [50].

Although protection against *Mtb* has traditionally been attributed primarily to Th-1-type CD4⁺ T lymphocytes, there is growing evidence that CD8⁺ T cells perform critical, non-redundant functions in controlling infection at both the early and late stages of the disease [50].

During infection, CD8⁺ T cells recognize mycobacterial antigens presented by infected cells in the context of major histocompatibility complex class I (MHC-I) molecules, including macrophages, dendritic cells, and pulmonary epithelial cells [51, 52]. This recognition triggers cytotoxic mechanisms that eliminate cells harboring viable bacilli, thereby limiting the intracellular niche of *Mtb* and contributing to the control of bacterial load [50].

One of the main effector mechanisms of CD8⁺ T cells in TB is granule-mediated cytotoxicity, dependent on perforin and granzymes. Perforin facilitates the formation of pores in the target cell membrane, allowing the entry of granzymes that induce apoptosis [53]. This process not only eliminates the infected cell but can also promote the exposure of the bacillus to extracellular microbicidal mechanisms and secondary phagocytosis [54]. Additionally, while mice do not express granulysin, human CD8⁺ T cells do. This molecule has direct antimicrobial activity, which can damage the mycobacterial cell wall. This is a particularly relevant mechanism for containing intracellular pathogens, such as Mtb [55, 56].

In addition to their cytotoxic function, CD8⁺ T cells contribute significantly to the immune response by producing pro-inflammatory cytokines. Among these, IFN-γ is essential for the classical activation of macrophages, promoting the production of reactive oxygen and nitrogen species, as well as phagolysosome maturation [57, 58]. TNF-α, as mentioned before, participates in the organization and maintenance of the granuloma [59]. Thus, CD8⁺ T cells not only act as cytotoxic effector cells but also as promoters of the innate and adaptive immune response.

In the context of tuberculous granuloma, CD8⁺ T cells play a relevant role in the balance between bacterial containment and tissue damage. During latent infection, these cells contribute to the control of persistent bacilli and help prevent disease reactivation [60, 61]. Studies in animal models and humans have shown that a functional or numerical decrease in CD8⁺ T cells is associated with an increased risk of progression to active TB, underscoring their importance in long-term immunosurveillance [62].

However, CD8⁺ T cell activity must be finely regulated. Excessive or uncontrolled activation can contribute to the characteristic immunopathology of pulmonary TB, promoting tissue necrosis, cavitation, and impaired lung function [26, 63]. This phenomenon is particularly evident in advanced stages of active disease, where the intense cytotoxic response can indirectly benefit the bacillus by facilitating its dissemination and transmission [64].

Finally, CD8⁺ T cells generate immunological memory populations that enable a faster, more efficient response to reinfection [65]. Although the BCG vaccine predominantly induces CD4⁺ T cell-mediated responses, robust CD8⁺ T cell responses are considered a key objective in the development of new TB vaccines [65, 66]. In this regard, a deeper understanding of the role of CD8⁺ T cells in TB is essential for the design of more effective immunotherapeutic and vaccination strategies.

Overall, current evidence indicates that $CD8^+$ T cells are fundamental components of the immune response against *Mtb*, participating in both the direct elimination of infected cells and the regulation of the inflammatory microenvironment (**Figure 3**). Their integrated, protective, yet potentially pathogenic function reinforces the idea that the outcome of TB depends on the delicate balance between defense mechanisms and tissue damage [20, 67].

5.3 γ/δ T cells at the interface of early immunity and granuloma formation during pulmonary TB

Gamma/delta T lymphocytes (γ/δ T cells) exhibit less variability than α/β T cells and are, therefore, classified as non-conventional cells, possessing γ and δ chains rather than α and β chains [68]. This population is considered an intermediary between innate and adaptive immunity [68–70], and several mycobacterial peptidic and nonpeptidic antigens can be recognized by γ/δ T cells [71, 72].

γ/δ T cells were first identified in granulomas over 30 years ago and appear to contribute to granuloma formation and development (**Figure 3**) [73]. Moreover, the disruption of γ/δ T cells in mice does not affect host resistance but does influence the response in early granulomas [74].

The precise role of γ/δ T cells in mycobacterial infections is still uncertain. It has been reported that γ/δ T cells have a protective function during early TB in mice lacking both α/β and γ/δ T cells, while highlighting the necessity of α/β T cells for protection [75]. In contrast, depleting γ/δ T cells in BCG-infected mice did not alter the development of the CD4 T cell response in the lung but decreased the cytotoxic activity and IFN-γ production by CD8 T cells [70]. These multiple findings suggest context-dependent roles for γ/δ T cells in immune responses to mycobacteria. The hypothesis that environmental or experimental conditions can influence the activity of these cells suggests that future research may identify essential variables that affect their function.

It has been shown that gamma/delta T cells support the development of epithelioid granulomas in a mouse model of bovine paratuberculosis. However, they do not restrict mycobacterial growth [76]. Moreover, the removal of γ/δ T cells in *Mtb*-infected young mice does not affect host resistance or surface marker expression. Differences were observed compared with other knockout animal models, but it does influence the integrity of the early granulomatous response [77].

In the context of diabetes and latent TB, γ/δ T cells show decreased frequencies of cells expressing Th-1/Th-17 cytokines, such as IFN-γ and IL-17, as well as cytotoxic and immune markers [78]. This evidence needs further investigation, as it may represent a novel biological marker in latent TB. In IFN-γ release assay (IGRA)-negative patients with higher lesion severity scores, fewer Vγ2Vδ2 T cells are observed, suggesting that increased Fas/FasL expression triggers Vγ2Vδ2 T-cell apoptosis [79].

Recent reports have shown that Vd1/3 T cells are induced by BCG vaccination in humans and non-human primates [80, 81]. In macaques, Vd1/3 T cells are activated and induce pro-inflammatory cytokines and cytotoxic responses in the airway. This activation suggests that the BCG vaccine enhances granuloma maturation by facilitating a robust airway immune response, which, in turn, may reinforce the granuloma structure, highlighting the interconnected roles of T cells in immune defense.

5.4 The role of T cells in granuloma development during *Mtb* infection

T lymphocytes constitute a significant population in granulomas, accounting for approximately 15–50% of the total leukocyte population. While α/β T cells are the most frequently studied, a distinct subset accounts for about 2% of the T lymphocyte population [82]. Building on this foundation, the roles and recruitment of different T cell subsets during granuloma maturation are discussed below.

Granuloma maturation involves a sequential recruitment of diverse immune cells, with T cell subsets serving an essential role. These subsets include $CD4^+$ effector cells, $CD4^+$ regulatory cells, $CD8^+$ cytotoxic cells, and other phenotypes [64]. Evidence shows that T cells are important to granuloma function. Mogues T et al. (2001) reported that bacterial growth persisted for more than 20 days in class II –/– mice lacking CD4 immunity [83]. In contrast, the absence of $CD8^+$ T cells did not affect bacterial control or extend survival, demonstrating the key role of $CD4^+$ T cells. This finding may be attributed to the critical role of $CD4^+$ T cells in activating macrophages via cytokine signaling, which is key to effective bacterial clearance.

This population also undergoes dynamic cellular processes. Egen et al. (2008) showed that this dynamism is mediated by cytokines such as TNF-α. Their results show that T cells linger within granulomas but remain restricted, forming a barrier at the surface. T cells may briefly patrol the surrounding sinusoidal space. Upon entry, T cells adhere to the granuloma core, which is composed mostly of macrophages via specific interactions [84].

6. Immunoregulation and pathological responses during pulmonary TB

In TB, the protective immune response must be maintained under strict immunoregulatory balance to prevent excessive tissue damage. Although T-cell and macrophage activation is essential for controlling the infection, a dysregulated inflammatory response can lead to severe pulmonary immunopathology. In this context, various immunoregulatory pathways modulate the intensity of the response, including the production of anti-inflammatory cytokines such as IL-10 and TGF-β and the activity of regulatory T cells (Tregs), which limit excessive inflammation. Th2 cells also play a modulatory role by producing cytokines such as IL-4, IL-5, and IL-13, which promote immune responses more closely associated with humoral immunity and alternative macrophage activation. Although these responses can contribute to the regulation of inflammation, a predominance of Th2 polarization can antagonize the protective Th1 response, reduce the microbicidal capacity of macrophages, and promote the persistence of the bacillus. Furthermore, during chronic infection, inhibitory pathways such as PD-1/PD-L1, CTLA-4, and other immune checkpoint molecules are activated, decreasing T-cell activation. Taken together, these mechanisms reflect a delicate balance between immune control and pathology: while limiting tissue damage, they can also facilitate the survival and persistence of the pathogen in the host.

6.1 The influence of Th2 cytokines on the outcome of *Mtb* infection

Th-2 cells are characterized by the expression of the transcription factor GATA3 (GATA-binding protein 3) and by the production of cytokines IL-4, IL-5, IL-9, and

IL-13. The Th-2 response is associated with allergic reactions and protective immunity against helminths [85]. This response is essential for humoral immunity, as it promotes B-cell growth and differentiation, IgE class switching, and macrophage polarization toward an M2 phenotype [86]. Among these cytokines, IL-4 is critical for Th-2 cell development because its binding to its receptor activates the signaling pathway needed for the expression of a group of genes, including GATA3, which regulates Th-2 cytokine production and suppresses proteins like IL-12Rβ2 and T-bet that are necessary for Th-1 differentiation [87].

There is an ongoing debate about the role of Th-2 cells in controlling *Mtb* infection. Some studies have linked the Th-2 response to a harmful effect on protection against *Mtb* [88]. In contrast, other studies have found no such link and suggest that insufficient IFN-γ production, rather than increased IL-4 levels, is the main factor impairing infection control [89, 90]. However, this discrepancy might be due to the challenge of measuring IL-4 levels, since it is a labile cytokine that requires only a small number of mRNA copies to be biologically active; thus, it is produced in small amounts and can be hard to detect [91]. Furthermore, results may vary depending on the detection method employed. The study of IL-4 is further complicated by the existence of the alternatively spliced variant IL-4δ2, which acts as an IL-4 antagonist, and by the presence of soluble IL-4 receptors that modulate its bioavailability [92]. It is also important to consider the substantial heterogeneity among studies, including differences in the clinical form of the disease evaluated and the type of biological sample analyzed (plasma, serum, or bronchoalveolar lavage fluid). Environmental factors must also be considered, such as exposure to other pathogens, such as helminths, that may influence preexisting immune responses prior to infection with *Mtb*, as well as the genetic background of the populations. Additionally, mycobacterial factors, including virulence and drug resistance, may contribute to variability in IL-4 levels [91]. Despite the heterogeneity across studies and the multiple factors that may influence IL-4 concentrations, a meta-analysis including 51 studies conducted between 1995 and 2022 that evaluated IL-4 levels in patients with tuberculosis (TB) compared with healthy controls concluded that IL-4 levels were significantly higher in both serum and bronchoalveolar lavage fluid from patients with pulmonary TB relative to healthy controls.

During *Mtb* infection, a Th-2 immune response may regulate inflammation. Still, it may also contribute to infection persistence, as Th-2 cytokines antagonize and inhibit IFN-γ activity and production by Th-1 cells [93], as well as other antimycobacterial mechanisms described below.

It is well established that Th-1 cytokine production predominates during the early stages of infection, whereas Th-2 cytokine production is associated with later stages and the active phase of the disease. The predominance of a Th-2 response and the decrease in the Th-1 response have been shown by comparing samples from healthy individuals and those with active TB, in which higher IL-4 levels were found in the latter [94], along with increased levels of other Th-2 cytokines such as IL-13 and IL-5 [95]. An increase in IL-4, together with the C–C motif chemokine ligand 4 (CCL4) (which encourages the Th-2 immune response), has also been observed in samples from patients with moderate-to-severe TB [94]. Similarly, increased IL-4 expression has been reported in individuals with TB-related lung cavitations [96].

In addition to these observations, the role of IL-4δ2, an IL-4 variant produced by alternative splicing and known to have antagonistic effects on IL-4, has been examined. Therefore, the IL-4 delta 2 splice variant (IL-4δ2) may inhibit the Th-2 response [91]. It has been observed that healthy individuals infected with, or previously infected by, *Mtb* show higher IL-4δ2 expression than those with active TB, implying that IL-4δ2 might help control *Mtb* infection [89].

In murine studies, an association has been identified between the Th-2 immune response and the evasion of antimycobacterial mechanisms. The virulence factor early secreted antigenic target 6 kDa (ESAT-6) from the virulent *Mtb* strain H37Rv has been shown to induce IL-1β production in dendritic cells, which, in turn, promotes T-cell differentiation toward a Th-2 phenotype, in contrast to the vaccine strain *Mycobacterium bovis* Bacillus Calmette–Guérin (BCG) [97]. Similarly, in mice lacking a functional IL-4 gene, the pathological manifestations of infection with the H37Rv strain are attenuated [98]. Moreover, the absence of IL-4 activity also led to less fibrosis, a significant tissue-damaging problem in chronic active TB. Indeed, IL-13 and IL-4 stimulate the production of TGF, a strong pro-fibrogenic and anti-inflammatory cytokine [98].

Moreover, the virulence of *Mtb* strains has been linked to their ability to induce polarization toward a Th-2 immune response. For example, some highly virulent *Mtb* strains, such as those from the W-Beijing lineage, promote Th-2 polarization, and multidrug-resistant (MDR) strains of the Haarlem lineage have been shown to increase the number of IL-4–producing T cells [99]. The highly virulent clinical isolate A96, which is resistant to the antibiotic rifampicin (RIF), causes early polarization of the immune response toward Th-2, and this virulence decreases when infecting mice lacking one of the IL-4 receptor chains [100]. Therefore, inducing Th-2 immune polarization has been suggested as an immune-evasion strategy used by *Mtb* to evade host effector mechanisms [4].

In vitro studies using THP-1 macrophages have shown that *Mtb* secretes the ESX-1 secretion-associated protein regulator (EspR), which promotes IL-4 expression, thereby inducing macrophage polarization toward the M2 phenotype and increasing mycobacterial survival, as M2 macrophages are inefficient at eliminating *Mtb* [101]. Additionally, IL-4 and IL-13 have been shown to inhibit autophagy in murine and human macrophages, a protective mechanism against *Mtb*; their inhibition reduces processes such as antigen presentation and T-cell clonal expansion [102].

Finally, an association has been demonstrated between helminth infection, which induces a Th-2 immune response, and increased susceptibility to *Mtb* infection, as observed in populations from regions with a high prevalence of helminth and *Mtb* coinfection [103]. In mice infected with the *helminth Nippostrongylus brasiliensis* and subsequently coinfected with *Mtb*, the mycobacterial burden and alternative macrophage activation increase relative to controls infected only with *Mtb* [104].

In conclusion, the failure of the Th-1 immune response may be partially attributable to an inappropriate Th-2 response, characterized by increased expression and production of cytokines such as IL-4, in combination with other factors that downregulate essential Th-1 mechanisms required to combat intracellular pathogens such as *Mtb* (**Figure 3**).

6.2 Regulatory T cells in tuberculosis: Balancing inflammation and immune suppression

During *Mtb* infection, not only pro-inflammatory responses, such as those mediated by Th-1 and Th-17 cells, are involved, but also modulatory Th-2 and regulatory T cells (Tregs) are activated. Tregs are $CD4^+$ T lymphocytes that constitutively express the alpha chain of the IL-2 receptor (CD25) and the specific transcription factor forkhead box P3 (FoxP3). Together with T cell receptor (TCR) stimulation, FoxP3 is associated with the acquisition of the regulatory phenotype and function characteristic of $CD4^{+}CD25^{+}$ cells, which exhibit high expression levels of CTLA-4, glucocorticoid-induced tumor necrosis factor receptor–related protein (GITR), and CD25 [105].

Tregs can arise through two distinct pathways: those generated directly in the thymus, known as natural regulatory T cells (nTregs), and cells that differentiate in the periphery from naïve T cells, referred to as inducible regulatory T cells (iTregs) [106]. The mechanisms by which Tregs modulate immune responses include the production of anti-inflammatory cytokines such as IL-10, TGF-β, and IL-35; cytolysis mediated by the release of granzymes A and B and perforin; metabolic disruption through IL-2 consumption, the production of adenosine and cAMP; and suppression mediated via dendritic cells (DCs) through the cytotoxic T-lymphocyte–associated protein 4 (CTLA-4) interaction with CD80/CD86 [106–108].

During TB infection, a highly pro-inflammatory microenvironment is generated that favors the activation of regulatory responses, which are essential for limiting tissue damage. This environment gives rise to distinct profiles of balance between regulatory and effector immune responses [109, 110]. However, an imbalance characterized by the predominance of Tregs and Th-2 responses over Th-1 and Th-17 responses has been associated with increased disease severity [111–116]. Importantly, Treg activation does not depend solely on the inflammatory milieu, as the mycobacteria can actively modulate immunoregulatory responses to their own advantage. During *Mtb* infection, antigen-specific Tregs are activated and drive dendritic cells toward a tolerogenic state through interactions, such as CTLA-4–CD80/CD86 and PD-1–PD-L1, thereby impairing antigen presentation to effector $CD4^{+}$ and $CD8^{+}$ T cells. These tolerogenic dendritic cells are also an important source of indoleamine 2,3-dioxygenase (IDO), which, in turn, promotes the polarization of naïve T cells toward a regulatory phenotype. Collectively, the suppressive effects of Tregs, the limitation of antigen presentation, and the immunosuppressive activity of IDO delay effector T-cell activation and migration to the lung. In addition, the accumulation of Tregs in the lung disrupts the Th-17/Treg axis, limiting early neutrophil recruitment [109, 117–121]. While mycobacterial antigens such as ESAT-6 or culture filtrate protein 10 (CFP-10) induce robust protective Th-1 and Th-17 responses, other antigens, such as antigen 85B (Ag85B), act as potent activators of $FoxP3^{+}$ T cells. Tregs bearing TCRs specific for this antigen are particularly efficient at limiting effector T-cell activation and delaying their migration from the lymph nodes to the lung. Moreover, these Tregs can induce a tolerogenic state in dendritic cells, thereby restricting antigen presentation to effector cells and contributing to an immunosuppressive environment; in the lung, they also reduce macrophages' ability to eliminate *Mtb* [117, 122, 123]. Another example of this phenomenon is Rv1272c, an ATP-binding cassette transporter required for mycobacterial survival under hypoxic conditions. This protein increases linoleic acid production, which promotes CTLA-4 trafficking in Tregs and, consequently, inhibits ROS production in macrophages, thereby favoring intracellular mycobacterial survival [124]. Finally, within the granuloma, an immunoregulatory microenvironment enriched in Tregs and characterized by high IDO production can disrupt the granuloma, permitting mycobacterial growth and ultimately promoting disease reactivation [112, 125–127].

Tregs play a dual, but predominantly detrimental, role in active TB. Although they help to limit excessive inflammation, their expansion, spatial organization, and enhanced functional activity promote immune suppression, bacterial persistence, and disease progression (**Figure 3**). Understanding Treg-mediated immune regulation in TB is, therefore, essential for developing host-directed therapies and vaccination strategies that avoid reinforcing regulatory pathways associated with poor disease control.

7. Mechanisms of T-cell immune evasion by *Mtb*

Evasion of the T-cell-mediated immune response is one of the cornerstones of *Mtb* remarkable persistence in the human host. Unlike many intracellular pathogens that evade immunity primarily through antigenic variation, *Mtb* has evolved a complex and redundant set of strategies that modulate T-cell activation, recognition, and effector function without completely abolishing the adaptive response. These strategies include delayed T-cell priming, interference with antigen presentation, functional diversion of cytotoxic responses, manipulation of the immunoregulatory microenvironment, and exploitation of inhibitory pathways of the immune system (**Figure 4**). Collectively, these mechanisms allow the bacillus to maintain a delicate balance between immune control and bacterial persistence, favoring latency, disease progression, and transmission. Understanding these evasion pathways in an integrated way is fundamental for the rational design of new vaccines and host-directed therapies that can restore an effective T-cell response without exacerbating pulmonary immunopathology.

7.1 Deliberate delay in the onset of adaptive immunity (late T-cell priming)

A key feature of TB is that, even though *Mtb* expresses highly immunogenic antigens early on, the adaptive response appears to be delayed: in aerosol infection models, T-cell priming occurs in draining mediastinal lymph nodes and depends on transport by migrating DCs. However, this migration of infected DCs to the lymph node is not detected until approximately 11–12 days, leaving an initial "window" during which the bacillus establishes itself in a protected niche before facing effective T-cell pressure. This delay suggests an evasion strategy that does not completely prevent the immune response but instead postpones it long enough to allow infection and persistence to consolidate; in fact, it has been proposed that part of this delay is due to specific inhibitory effects on pulmonary APCs, aligning with Mtb's adaptation to its natural infection route. Furthermore, bacterial factors, such as NuoG, contribute to this delay by inhibiting the apoptosis of infected neutrophils, thereby affecting antigen capture and the initiation of an effective T-cell response, supporting the idea of a time-dependent rather than an absolute evasion [128, 129].

7.2 Inhibition of antigen presentation by MHC-II via TLR2-CIITA

Mtb follows a homeostatic regulatory principle: prolonged TLR stimulation in macrophages can decrease protein presentation, thereby limiting tissue damage, and the bacillus sequesters the proteins to reduce recognition by $CD4^+$ cells. Cell wall components, such as the 19 kDa lipoprotein (LpqH), which acts as a TLR2 agonist,

DOI: http://dx.doi.org/10.5772/intechopen.1015455

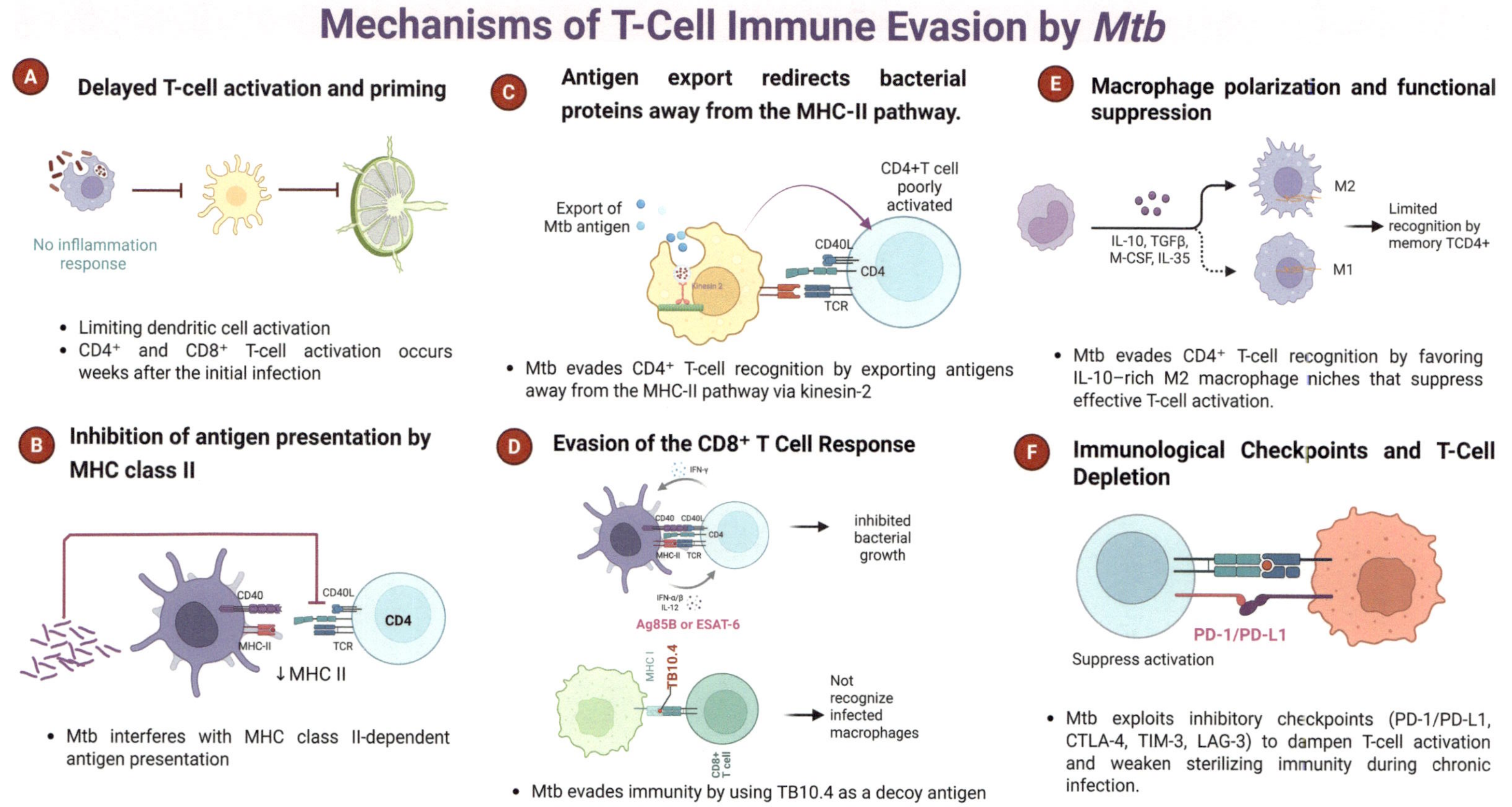

Figure 4.
Mechanisms of T-cell immune evasion by Mtb. *(a)* Mtb *delays dendritic cell activation and t-cell priming. (b) It impairs MHC-II antigen presentation, limiting CD4⁺ recognition. (c) Kinesin-2–dependent antigen export diverts proteins from the MHC-II pathway. (d) TB10.4 acts as a decoy, expanding CD8⁺ T cells that poorly recognize infected macrophages. (e) Survival in IL-10–rich M2-like macrophages weakens memory CD4⁺ responses. (f) During chronic infection, inhibitory checkpoints (PD-1/PD-L1, CTLA-4, TIM-3, LAG-3) suppress T-cell activation. Together, these mechanisms promote persistence while sustaining transmission. Created in BioRender. Barrios, J. (2026) https://biorender.Com/52zinoo.*

are associated with a decrease in MHC-II expression on infected macrophages. Mechanistically, this is linked to reduced CIITA transactivator activity and interference with IFN-γ-induced responses, thus lowering the macrophage's ability to recognize effector $CD4^+$ molecules in the tissue. This inhibition involves prolonged TLR2 signaling, activation of MAPK pathways, and induction of repressive factors that block CIITA promoters, resulting in less MHC-II and, therefore, fewer peptide-MHC-II complexes on the surface. The expected functional outcome is that, even in the presence of competent Th-1 lymphocytes, the bacillus reduces the likelihood of recognition at the site of infection by hijacking macrophages and using them as a niche to persist, promote chronic infection, and decrease inflammation [128, 130, 131].

7.3 Kinesin-2-dependent antigen export diverts bacterial proteins away from the MHC-II pathway

In addition to blocking presentation, *Mtb* can redirect antigens away from the MHC-II loading pathway. In infected DCs and macrophages, bacterial antigens are exported via microtubule-associated vesicular transport that depends on kinesin-2, thereby reducing the amount of antigen entering the MHC-II presentation pathway. Although these exported antigens can be taken up and presented by neighboring uninfected cells, the overall effect favors the pathogen because export reduces CD4 activation by the infected cell, an interaction essential for effective control in vivo. In fact, when export is blocked through kinesin-2 depletion, activation of specific CD4 cells by Mtb antigen, such as Ag85B, increases, leading to better control of intracellular infection. Therefore, the bacillus uses export as an active evasion tactic to diminish direct recognition by infected cells [132].

7.4 Evasion of the $CD8^+$ T cell response and decoy antigens

An important mechanism of *Mtb* evasion is the presentation of antigens to T lymphocytes. It has been observed that $TCD4^+$ cells specific for Ag85B or ESAT-6 recognize infected macrophages and inhibit bacterial growth, but TB10.4-specific $TCD8^+$ cells do not recognize infected macrophages or restrict Mtb. Paradoxically, $TCD8^+$ cells can recognize TB10.4 if the antigen reaches the cytosol. Therefore, *Mtb* interferes with the effective presentation and recognition of this antigen during infection. TB10.4 induces a massive and persistent expansion of TCD8 +, but with a low capacity to detect the infected cell itself, disrupting the response to subdominant antigens that could be presented on infected macrophages [133].

7.5 Macrophage polarization and functional suppression

Mtb can select or prefer the cellular niche where it is least detectable. In humans with latent infection, autologous memory $CD4^+$ cells strongly recognize Mtb-infected M1-like macrophages but poorly recognize Mtb-infected M2-like macrophages, even though both types can activate $CD4^+$ cells when loaded with exogenous or inactivated antigen. Infected M2 cells express IL-10 and increased PD-L1. Neutralizing IL-10 enhances memory $CD4^+$ activation against infected M2 macrophages, suggesting that IL-10 acts as a dominant brake that reduces effective recognition and activation. High levels of IL-10 and TGFβ in granulomas can inhibit T cell effector functions, which is related to granuloma microarchitecture [129, 134].

7.6 Immunological checkpoints and T-cell depletion

During chronic infection, the immune system activates inhibitory pathways to limit immunopathology, but these pathways can also decrease effector potency against *Mtb*. TCR-MHC recognition and CD28-CD80/86 costimulation trigger activation, while PD-1/PD-L1 and other molecules, such as CTLA-4, TIM-3, and LAG-3, suppress this activation, either as a host strategy to prevent excessive responses or as part of pathological states where immunity is suppressed. Mtb maintains an environment of chronic inflammation and regulation that benefits from checkpoints that lower the efficiency of sterilizing control [135].

7.7 Antigenic conservation and evolutionary benefit of the T-cell response

Mtb exhibits a remarkable pattern of T-cell epitope conservation. Human T-cell epitopes in *Mtb* are highly conserved, display minimal sequence variability, and show strong signatures of purifying selection, indicating that the bacillus is not under substantial evolutionary pressure to diversify these regions to evade immune recognition. Rather, accumulating evidence suggests that *Mtb* may derive a selective advantage from maintaining recognition by specific T-cell repertoires. $CD4^+$ T-cell responses are essential for the establishment and maintenance of latency, a state that enables long-term bacterial persistence, while certain forms of T-cell–driven immunopathology, such as pulmonary cavitation, facilitate transmission by enhancing aerosol spread. In this context, partial immune control may represent an evolutionarily favorable equilibrium, sufficient immune activation to sustain transmission, yet insufficient for sterilizing bacterial clearance. Importantly, *Mtb* can further attenuate effective T-cell pressure by limiting direct recognition of infected cells through mechanisms including antigen export and impaired antigen presentation. Because T cells frequently recognize antigens released from infected cells rather than peptides presented directly on infected macrophages, the intensity of cognate immune pressure acting on the bacillus is reduced. As a result, the evolutionary incentive for mutations within dominant T-cell epitopes is weakened, thereby indirectly reinforcing their long-term conservation in the *Mtb* genome [132, 136].

8. Immunoregulatory pathways, immune evasion, and therapeutic opportunities in tuberculosis

During advanced stages of active TB, even in the absence of overt immunosuppressive conditions, a profound and sustained suppression of *Mtb*-specific protective immune responses is observed. Multiple immunoregulatory pathways attenuate host defense, thereby facilitating bacillary persistence and disease progression. Many of these mediators are potent anti-inflammatory molecules that are overproduced as a compensatory attempt to limit tissue injury; however, this regulatory environment weakens protective immunity and enhances bacterial replication. Understanding the balance between protective and nonprotective immune responses provides a rational basis for therapeutic intervention, either by restoring deficient protective mediators or by inhibiting suppressive pathways that impair antimycobacterial immunity [137]. This strategy underlies the concept of host-directed therapy (HDT) [138]. From a translational perspective, these insights highlight the potential to develop targeted immunomodulatory interventions that complement antimicrobial therapy, improve immune-mediated bacterial control, and ultimately enhance clinical outcomes in TB.

Importantly, *Mtb's* capacity to evade effective T-cell recognition also has implications for vaccination. Evasion of the T-cell response partially explains the limited efficacy of the Bacillus Calmette–Guérin (BCG) vaccine and many vaccine candidates targeting highly immunodominant antigens. Many of these antigens elicit strong T-cell responses but fail to promote efficient recognition of infected macrophages, allowing bacilli to persist despite robust immunogenicity. Consequently, future vaccine strategies should prioritize antigens and formulations that promote effective T-cell recognition of infected cells while avoiding dysfunctional or evasive T-cell responses [128, 139]. Recent studies have proposed a conceptual shift in TB vaccine development, emphasizing rational antigen selection based on protective efficacy rather than on immunogenicity alone. Using systematic approaches to evaluate *Mtb* antigens recognized by human $CD4^+$ T lymphocytes, investigators identified substantial heterogeneity in the protective capacity of different antigens and demonstrated that several of the most protective targets had not been previously considered in clinical vaccine trials. Based on these findings, a trivalent vaccine comprising mRNA encoding selected protective antigens, encapsulated in lipid nanoparticles, was developed. This formulation induced robust, multifunctional, and durable cellular immune responses and provided superior protection compared with BCG in both high-dose and ultra-low-dose murine infection models, while also enhancing BCG-induced immunity. These findings highlight that the future of TB vaccination will likely depend on integrated strategies that combine rational antigen selection with innovative vaccine platforms capable of generating protective immune responses that more closely mimic those required for effective control of infection [140, 141].

During TB, the progression from controlled infection to active disease is heavily influenced by immunosuppressive pathways that weaken protective cellular immunity. Although many of these regulatory mechanisms initially develop to limit excessive inflammation and tissue damage, their ongoing activation can weaken antimycobacterial defenses, allowing bacilli to persist. Several cytokines and inhibitory signaling pathways, including Th2-related cytokines, anti-inflammatory mediators, and immune checkpoint molecules, play key roles in regulating T-cell responses, macrophage activation, and granuloma stability. Increasing experimental and clinical evidence shows that targeting these immunosuppressive networks could restore effective Th1-driven immunity and enhance the host's ability to control infection. The following studies demonstrate how specific regulatory pathways contribute to disease progression and highlight their potential as targets for host-directed therapeutic strategies.

Several immunosuppressive pathways contribute to disease progression during *Mtb* infection by dampening protective cellular immunity and promoting bacterial persistence. IL-4 drives polarization toward a nonprotective Th2 phenotype, antagonizing Th1-mediated antimycobacterial responses and facilitating disease progression; accordingly, IL-4 blockade preserves a Th1-dominant immune profile and significantly reduces pulmonary bacterial burden, either alone or in combination with antimycobacterial IgA monoclonal antibodies targeting α-crystalline antigens [142]. Similarly, IL-10 promotes TB progression by inhibiting macrophage activation and suppressing Th1 responses; in CBA/J–M mice overexpressing IL-10, blockade of the IL-10 receptor during chronic infection enhanced pulmonary T cell recruitment and IFN-γ production, reduced bacillary load, and improved survival [143]. The Th17 cytokine IL-17A also exhibits a dual role: although it synergizes with IFN-γ to support granuloma formation, excessive IL-17A activity drives massive neutrophil recruitment and tissue damage [86]; accordingly, neutralization of IL-17A in murine TB reduced inflammatory pathology without significantly affecting bacillary burden, highlighting the need for a balanced Th1–Th17 axis [144]. In addition, inhibitory checkpoint pathways contribute to immune dysfunction, as PD-1 is upregulated in patients with active TB, together with its ligand PD-L1 [145], reflecting T cell exhaustion; blockade of PD-1 enhances the survival of IFN-γ–producing T cells and improves protective immunity against *Mtb* [146].

Another major regulatory pathway involves TGF-β, which suppresses cell-mediated immunity while acting as both an anti-inflammatory and profibrotic mediator. Elevated TGF-β levels have been detected in blood mononuclear cells from TB patients and in tuberculous lung lesions, and increased TGF-β expression during disease progression in BALB/c mice impairs protective immunity. Blockade using soluble recombinant receptor type III to TGF-β or β-glycan enhanced IFN-γ and IL-2 expression, reduced IL-4 levels, and significantly decreased pulmonary bacterial load, although increased lung consolidation highlighted the important anti-inflammatory role of TGF-β [147]. Notably, during chronic infection, niflumic acid, a selective cyclooxygenase-2 inhibitor, administered with β-glycan produced synergistic effects, enhancing Th-1 responses, suppressing Th-2 cytokines, increasing iNOS expression, and reducing pulmonary inflammation, fibrosis, and bacillary load. This approach achieved disease control comparable to that of antimicrobial therapy alone and, when combined with antimicrobials, accelerated bacillary clearance [147].

Beyond inhibiting suppressive pathways, HDT strategies may also aim to restore deficient protective mediators that are essential for effective antimycobacterial immunity. IFN-γ is a central cytokine in TB control, promoting macrophage activation, enhancing MHC class II expression, and stimulating TNF-α and iNOS production, thereby strengthening antimycobacterial mechanisms [21]. In advanced experimental TB (60 days post-infection), when extensive pneumonia and high bacillary burden are established, a single dose of recombinant adenovirus encoding IFN-γ (AdIFN-γ) significantly reduced bacterial load and pulmonary inflammation in mice infected with either the drug-sensitive H37Rv strain or the multidrug-resistant CIBIN99 strain. When combined with standard antimicrobial therapy (isoniazid [INH], PIR, RIF), AdIFN-γ further reduced bacillary burden and lung pathology compared with antibiotics alone, suggesting that gene therapy may shorten treatment duration [148]. Similarly, inhaled plasmids expressing murine IFN-γ, administered weekly for 4 weeks in aerosol-infected Swiss mice, significantly reduced pulmonary bacterial burden and improved lung histopathology and gross morphology [149]. IL-12, produced by macrophages, NK cells, and dendritic cells in response to infection [150], drives Th-1 differentiation and suppresses anti-inflammatory cytokine production. Given its central role in Th-1 polarization, IL-12 has been evaluated for therapeutic use. Prophylactic administration of adenovirus encoding IL-12 (AdIL-12) one day before infection with H37Rv significantly reduced bacillary load, diminished pneumonia, and enhanced IFN-γ, TNF-α, and iNOS expression compared to controls [151]. In a transmission model, a single intratracheal dose of an adenovirus encoding IL-12 (AdIL-12) administered to healthy mice co-housed with animals infected with a highly virulent Beijing strain (9,001,000) completely prevented infection. Therapeutically, four intranasal doses of AdIL-12 administered during late-stage progressive TB (60 days post-infection) significantly reduced pulmonary bacillary burden [151].

Collectively, these findings indicate that the immune landscape of TB is governed by a delicate balance between protective immunity and immunopathology. Effective HDT strategies must carefully modulate this equilibrium. The evidence suggests a therapeutic window where immune responses can be selectively enhanced to restore Th1-mediated antimicrobial mechanisms while simultaneously limiting excessive inflammation that causes lung damage. In this framework, HDT strategies are unlikely to rely on a single intervention; instead, combination approaches that inhibit immunosuppressive pathways, such as IL-4, IL-10, TGF-β, and PD-1 signaling, while restoring key protective mediators, such as IFN-γ and IL-12, are likely to be most effective. When combined with conventional antimicrobial therapy, these immunomodulatory interventions could improve bacterial clearance, stabilize granuloma function, reduce tissue damage, and shorten treatment time. These immunological principles also have important implications for vaccine development. The limited effectiveness of BCG and many candidate vaccines highlights the need to design immunization strategies that overcome immune evasion and promote effective recognition of infected macrophages. Therefore, next-generation TB vaccines will likely require rational antigen selection based on protective efficacy rather than immunogenicity alone, along with advanced platforms capable of eliciting long-lasting, functionally effective T-cell responses. In this context, integrating vaccination strategies with therapeutic immunomodulation may serve as a complementary approach to both prevent infection and improve disease management, ultimately offering a more comprehensive framework for TB prevention and treatment.

9. Conclusion

TB results from a dynamic interaction between the bacillus and the host's immune system. Throughout this chapter, it has been shown that T lymphocytes constitute the central axis of this interaction, performing both protective and potentially pathogenic functions. Experimental and clinical evidence demonstrates that the Th-1 response, primarily mediated through the IL-12/IFN-γ axis, is essential for macrophage activation, granuloma formation and maintenance, and the control of bacillary replication. However, this response does not act in isolation but is integrated with other cell populations, such as Th-17, $CD8^+$, Treg, and γ/δ T cells, whose combined contributions determine the balance between bacterial containment and immunopathology.

The clinical outcome of the infection depends on the quality, intensity, location, and regulation of these cellular responses. While a balanced Th-1/Th-17 response favors antimicrobial control, a shift toward Th-2 or regulatory profiles, or excessive activation of inhibitory mechanisms such as PD-1, IL-10, or TGF-β, can facilitate bacterial persistence and disease progression. Similarly, dysregulated cytotoxic responses can contribute to tissue necrosis and pulmonary cavitation, promoting transmission.

Furthermore, it has been highlighted that *Mtb* does not completely evade the immune response but rather modulates it strategically, delaying T-cell activation, interfering with antigen presentation, and promoting regulatory microenvironments that allow its survival. This understanding has driven the development of host-directed therapies aimed at both enhancing protective mechanisms (such as IFN-γ or IL-12) and attenuating immunosuppressive pathways. Integrating these strategies with conventional antimicrobial chemotherapy represents a promising approach to improve bacterial control, reduce lung damage, and potentially shorten treatment duration.

In general, TB should be understood not only as an infectious disease but also as a complex immunoregulatory disease, in which the balance between activation and control determines the clinical outcome. A deeper understanding of the immunological networks that govern the T-cell response will enable the design of more effective vaccines and more precise immunomodulatory therapies capable of eliminating bacterial persistence without exacerbating immunopathology.

Acronyms and abbreviations

AdIFN-γ	adenovirus encoding interferon gamma
AdIL-12	adenovirus encoding interleukin 12
Ag85B	antigen 85B
APCs	antigen-presenting cells
BCG	Bacillus Calmette–Guérin
CCL4	C-C motif chemokine ligand 4
CCL20	C-C motif chemokine ligand 20
CCR6	C-C chemokine receptor type 6
$CD4^+$	cluster of differentiation 4
$CD8^+$	cluster of differentiation 8
CFP-10	culture filtrate protein 10
CIITA	class II transactivator
CTLA-4	cytotoxic T-lymphocyte–associated protein 4
CXCL1	C-X-C motif chemokine ligand 1
CXCL8	C-X-C motif chemokine ligand 8
CXCR5	C-X-C chemokine receptor type 5
DCs	dendritic cells
ESAT-6	early secreted antigenic target 6 kDa
EspR	ESX-1 secretion-associated protein regulator
FoxP3	forkhead box P3
GATA3	GATA-binding protein 3
GITR	glucocorticoid-induced tumor necrosis factor receptor–related protein
GM-CSF	granulocyte-macrophage colony-stimulating factor
HDT	host-directed therapy
IDO	indoleamine 2,3-dioxygenase
IFN-γ	interferon gamma
IGRA	interferon gamma release assay

IL	interleukin
IL-1β	interleukin 1 beta
IL-2	interleukin 2
IL-4δ2	interleukin 4 delta 2 splice variant
IL-6	interleukin 6
IL-10	interleukin 10
IL-12	interleukin 12
IL-13	interleukin 13
IL-17A	interleukin 17A
IL-21	interleukin 21
IL-23	interleukin 23
IL-35	interleukin 35
ILCs	innate lymphoid cells
INH	isoniazid
iNOS	inducible nitric oxide synthase
iTregs	inducible regulatory T cells
LAM	lipoarabinomannan
M1	classically activated macrophage phenotype
M2	alternatively activated macrophage phenotype
MDR	multidrug-resistant
MHC-I	major histocompatibility complex class I
MHC-II	major histocompatibility complex class II
Mtb	*Mycobacterium tuberculosis*
MTBC	Mycobacterium tuberculosis Complex
NK cells	natural killer cells
nTregs	natural regulatory T cells
PD-1	programmed cell death protein 1
PD-L1	programmed death-ligand 1
PE	proline-glutamic acid protein family
PIR	pyrazinamide
PPE	proline-proline-glutamic acid protein family
RIF	rifampicin
RORγt	retinoic acid receptor-related orphan receptor gamma t
ROS	reactive oxygen species
STAT3	signal transducer and activator of transcription 3
STAT4	signal transducer and activator of transcription 4
TB	Tuberculosis
TB10.4	tuberculosis antigen 10.4
TCR	T cell receptor
TDM	trehalose dimycolate
TGF-β	transforming growth factor beta
Th-1	T helper type 1
Th-2	T helper type 2
Th-17	T helper type 17
Th-22	T helper type 22
TLR2	toll-like receptor 2
TNF-α	tumor necrosis factor alpha
VEGF	vascular endothelial growth factor
γ/δ T cells	gamma/delta T lymphocytes

Acknowledgments

The authors used Grammarly to assist with English grammar correction and improve the clarity and readability of the manuscript. Additionally, ChatGPT (OpenAI) was used solely to generate the list of abbreviations included in this document. All scientific content, interpretations, and conclusions were developed and reviewed by the authors, who take full responsibility for the accuracy and integrity of the work.

Conflict of Interest

The authors declare no conflict of interest.

Author details

Jacqueline V. Lara-Espinosa[1], Mayra Silva Miranda[1,2,3,4], María Fernanda Arce-Aceves[2,5], Vasti Lozano-Ordaz[2,6], Yadira Rodríguez- Miguez[7] and Rogelio Hernández-Pando[1,4*]

1 Experimental Pathology Section, Department of Pathology, National Institute of Medical Sciences and Nutrition "Salvador Zubirán", Tlalpan, Mexico

2 Secretariat of Science, Humanities, Technology and Innovation (SECIHTI), Colonia Crédito Constructor, Mexico City, Mexico

3 National Institute of Respiratory Diseases "Ismael Cosío Villegas" (INER), Tlalpan, Mexico

4 Mexican Network for Research on Tuberculosis and Other Mycobacterioses A.C. (REMexTB), Tuxtla Gutiérrez, Mexico

5 Department of Immunology, Institute of Biomedical Research, National Autonomous University of Mexico, Mexico City, Mexico

6 Research and Assistance Center in Technology and Design of the State of Jalisco (CIATEJ), Jalisco, Mexico

7 Autonomous University of the State of Hidalgo (UAEH), Institute of Agricultural Sciences, Tulancingo, Mexico

*Address all correspondence to: rogelio.hernandezp@incmnsz.mx

References

[1] Juhás M, Bouz G, Pang L, Weeks SD, Jandourek O, Konečná K, Paterová P, Bárta P, Halířová M, Kučerová-Chlupáčová M, Doležal M, Zitko J, et al. Targeting Mycobacterium tuberculosis: The Role of Alkyl Substitution in Pyrazinamide Derivatives. ACS Omega. 2026;**11**(3):3937–3948. DOI: 10.1021/acsomega.5c07249

[2] Global tuberculosis report 2025. Geneva: World Health Organization; 2025. Licence: CC BY-NC-SA 3.0 IGO

[3] Sabt A, Korycka-Machala M, Kassem AF, The Son N, Ha NX, Brzostek A, et al. Investigation of Potent Anti-Mycobacterium tuberculosis Agents Derived from Pyridine Derivatives Targeting the Enoyl Acyl Carrier Protein Reductase (InhA): Design, Synthesis, and Computational Analysis. Drug Design Devel Ther. 2026;**20**:1–17

[4] Zhuang L, Yang L, Li L, Ye Z, Gong W. Mycobacterium Tuberculosis: Immune Response, Biomarkers, and Therapeutic Intervention. MedComm. 2024;**5**(1):e419. DOI: 10.1002/mco2.419

[5] Bhat KH, Ahmed A, Kumar S, Sharma P, Mukhopadhyay S. Role of PPE18 Protein in Intracellular Survival and Pathogenicity of Mycobacterium tuberculosis in Mice. PLoS One. 2012;7 (12). DOI: 10.1371/journal.pone.0052601

[6] Warner DF, Barczak AK, Gutierrez MG, Mizrahi V. Mycobacterium tuberculosis biology, pathogenicity and interaction with the host. Nature Reviews Microbiology. Nature Research. 2025;788–804. DOI: 10.1038/s41579-025-01201-x

[7] Koch A, Mizrahi V. Mycobacterium tuberculosis. Trends in microbiology. 2018;**26**(6):555–556. DOI: 10.1016/j.tim.2018.02.012

[8] Jacobo-Delgado YM, Rodríguez-Carlos A, Serrano CJ, Rivas-Santiago B. Mycobacterium tuberculosis cell-wall and antimicrobial peptides: A mission impossible?. Frontiers in Immunology. 2023;**14**(5):1–18. DOI: 10.3389/fimmu.2023.1194923

[9] Juhás M, Bouz G, Pang L, Weeks SD, Jandourek O, Konečná K, et al. Targeting Mycobacterium tuberculosis: The Role of Alkyl Substitution in Pyrazinamide Derivatives. ACS Omega. 2026. DOI: 10.1021/acsomega.5c07249

[10] Warner DF, Barczak AK, Gutierrez MG, Mizrahi V. Mycobacterium tuberculosis biology, pathogenicity and interaction with the host. Nature Reviews, Microbiology. 2025;**23**(12):788–804. DOI: 10.1038/s41579-025-01201-x

[11] Maison DP. Tuberculosis pathophysiology and anti-VEGF intervention. J. Clin. Tuberc. Other Mycobact. Dis. 2022;**27**:100300. DOI: 10.1016/j.jctube.2022.100300

[12] Carabalí-Isajar ML, Rodríguez-Bejarano OH, Amado T, Patarroyo MA, Izquierdo MA, Lutz JR, et al. Clinical manifestations and immune response to tuberculosis. World Journal of Microbiology & Biotechnology. 2023;**39** (8):1–26. DOI: 10.1007/s11274-023-03636-x

[13] van Meijgaarden KE, Grace PS, Freund NT, Achkar JM, Lindenstrøm T, Tan J, et al. Antibodies in tuberculosis:

functional capacity as key determinant. Infection and immunity; 2026;**94**(2): e0039425. DOI: 10.1128/iai.00394-25

[14] Thakur A, Mikkelsen H, Jungersen G. Intracellular pathogens: Host immunity and microbial persistence strategies. Journal of Immunology Research. Hindawi Limited. 2019. DOI: 1 0.1155/2019/1356540

[15] Sankar P, Mishra BB. Early innate cell interactions with Mycobacterium tuberculosis in protection and pathology of tuberculosis. Frontiers in Immunology. 2023;**14**(10):1–21. DOI: 10.3389/fimmu.2023.1260859

[16] Krug S, Parveen S, Bishai WR. Host-Directed Therapies: Modulating Inflammation to Treat Tuberculosis. Frontiers in Immunology. 2021;**12** (April):1–10. DOI: 10.3389/fimmu.2021.660916

[17] Swain SL, McKinstry KK, Strutt TM. Expanding roles for CD4$^+$ T cells in immunity to viruses. Nat Rev Immuno. 2012;**12**(2):136–148. DOI: 10.1038/nri3152

[18] Barber-Mayer KD, Barber DL. Innate and adaptive cellular immune responses to Mycobacterium tuberculosis infection. Cold Spring Harb. Perspect. Med. 2015;**5**(12):1–19. DOI: 10.1101/cshperspect.a018424

[19] Kolloli A, Subbian S. Host-directed therapeutic strategies for tuberculosis. Frontiers in Medicine. Frontiers Media S.A. 2017. DOI: 10.3389/fmed.2017.00171

[20] O'Garra A, Redford PS, McNab FW, Bloom CI, Wilkinson RJ, Berry MPR. The Immune Response in Tuberculosis. Annual Review of Immunology. 2013;475–527. DOI: 10.11 46/annurev-immunol-032712-095939

[21] Flynn JAL, Chan J, Triebold KJ, Dalton DK, Stewart TA, Bloom BR. An essential role for interferon γ in resistance to mycobacterium tuberculosis infection. Journal of Experimental Medicine. 1993;**178** (6):2249–2254. DOI: 10.1084/jem.178.6.2249

[22] Szabo SJ, Kim ST, Costa GL, Zhang X, Fathman CG, Glimcher LH. A novel transcription factor, T-bet, directs Th1 lineage commitment. Cell. 2000;**100**(6):655–669. DOI: 10.1016/S0 092-8674(00)80702-3

[23] Imran M, Alshrari AS, Khan A, Alzahrani AR. IFN-γ-Driven macrophage responses in the immunity to Mycobacterium tuberculosis and Mycobacterium leprae. Frontiers in Cellular Infection and Microbiology. 2025;**15**(November). DOI: 10.3389/fcimb.2025.1679691

[24] Dalton D. IFN-γ and IFN-γ Receptor Knockout Mice. Cytokine Knockouts. 2003;347–360. DOI: 10.1385/1-59259-405-0

[25] da Silva Da A, V. DSM, Oliveira Barros CC, Dias Alexandre PB, Timóteo RP, Catarino JS, et al. TNF-α blockade impairs in vitro tuberculous granuloma formation and down modulate Th1, Th17 and Treg cytokines. PLoS One. 2018;**13**(3):1–13. DOI: 10.1371/journal.pone.0194430

[26] Dheda K, Schwander SK, Zhu B, Van Zyl-Smit RN, Zhang Y. The immunology of tuberculosis: From bench to bedside. Respirology. 2010;**15** (3):433–450. DOI: 10.1111/j.1440-1843.2010.01739.x

[27] Wang H, Ruan G, Li Y, Liu X. The Role and Potential Application of IL-12 in the Immune Regulation of Tuberculosis. International Journal of

Molecular Sciences. 2025;**26**(7):1–26. DOI: 10.3390/ijms26073106

[28] Salgame P. Host innate and Th1 responses and the bacterial factors that control Mycobacterium tuberculosis infection. Curr. Opin. Immunol. 2005;**17**(4):374–380. DOI: 10.1016/j.coi.2005.06.006

[29] Olive AJ. strategies and protective immunity during Mycobacterium tuberculosis infection [Internet]. 2025;10.1128/msphere.00517-24

[30] Li HM, Wang LJ, Huang Q, Pan HF, Zhang TP. Exploring the association between Th17 pathway gene polymorphisms and pulmonary tuberculosis. Frontiers in Immunology. 2022;**13**(November):1–12. DOI: 10.3389/fimmu.2022.994247

[31] Wang J, Zhao X, Wan YY. Intricacies of TGF-β signaling in Treg and Th17 cell biology. Cell. Mol. Immunol. 2023;**20**(9):1002–1022. DOI: 10.1038/s41423-023-01036-7

[32] Zhang W, Liu X, Zhu Y, Liu X, Gu Y, Dai X, et al. Transcriptional and posttranslational regulation of Th17/Treg balance in health and disease. Eur. J. Immunol. 2021;**51**(9):2137–2150. DOI: 10.1002/eji.202048794

[33] Schnell A, Littman DR, Kuchroo VK. TH17 cell heterogeneity and its role in tissue inflammation. Nat. Immunol. 2023;**24**(1):19–29. DOI: 10.1038/s41590-022-01387-9

[34] Wang C, Kang SG, Lee J, Sun Z, Kim CH. The roles of CCR6 in migration of Th17 cells and regulation of effector T-cell balance in the gut. Mucosal Immunol. 2009;**2**(2):173–183. DOI: 10.1038/mi.2008.84

[35] Shanmugasundaram U, Bucsan AN, Ganatra SR, Ibegbu C, Quezada M, V. BR, et al. Pulmonary Mycobacterium tuberculosis control associates with CXCR3- And CCR6-expressing antigen-specific Th1 and Th17 cell recruitment. JCI Insight. 2020;**5**(14):1–18. DOI: 10.1172/JCI.INSIGHT.137858

[36] Torrado E, Cooper AM. IL-17 and Th17 cells in tuberculosis. Cytokine & Growth Factor Reviews. 2010;**21**(6):455–462. DOI: 10.1016/j.cytogfr.2010.10.004

[37] Ogongo P, Tran A, Marzan F, Gingrich D, Krone M, Aweeka F, et al. High-parameter phenotypic characterization reveals a subset of human Th17 cells that preferentially produce IL-17 against M. tuberculosis antigen. Frontiers in Immunology. 2024;**15**(April):1–11. DOI: 10.3389/fimmu.2024.1378040

[38] Rodríguez-Míguez Y, Lozano-Ordaz V, Ortiz-Cabrera AE, Barrios-Payan J, Mata-Espinosa D, Huerta-Yepez S, et al. Effect of IL-17A on the immune response to pulmonary tuberculosis induced by high- and low-virulence strains of Mycobacterium bovis. PLoS One. 2024;**19**(7):1–22. DOI: 10.1371/journal.pone.0307307

[39] Ritter K, Behrends J, Rückerl D, Hölscher A, Volz J, Prinz I, et al. High-Dose Mycobacterium tuberculosis H37rv Infection in IL-17A- and IL-17A/F-Deficient Mice. Cells. 2022;**11**(18):1–17. DOI: 10.3390/cells11182875

[40] Li Y, Wei C, Xu H, Jia J, Wei Z, Guo R, et al. The immunoregulation of Th17 in host against intracellular bacterial infection. Mediators Inflamm. 2018;**2018**. DOI: 10.1155/2018/6587296

[41] Fan X, Shu P, Wang Y, Ji N, Zhang D. Interactions between neutrophils and T-helper 17 cells. Frontiers in Immunology. 2023;**14**(10):1–11. DOI: 10.3389/fimmu.2023.1279837

[42] Monin L, Griffiths KL, Slight S, Lin Y, Rangel-Moreno J, Khader SA. Immune requirements for protective Th17 recall responses to Mycobacterium tuberculosis challenge. Mucosal Immunol. 2015;**8**(5):1099–1109. DOI: 10.1038/mi.2014.136

[43] Paroli M, Caccavale R, Fiorillo MT, Spadea L, Gumina S, Candela V, et al. The Double Game Played by Th17 Cells in Infection: Host Defense and Immunopathology. Pathogens. 2022;**11**(12). DOI: 10.3390/pathogens11121547

[44] Pollara G, Turner CT, Rosenheim J, Chandran A, Bell LCK, Khan A, et al. Exaggerated IL-17A activity in human in vivo recall responses discriminates active tuberculosis from latent infection and cured disease. Sci. Transl. Med. 2021;**13**(592). DOI: 10.1126/scitranslmed.abg7673

[45] Zhang Q, Zhang Y, Guo Z, Wang Z, Hu H, Song S, et al. CCR4$^+$ memory Tregs and PD-1$^+$ T cells as novel immunodiagnostic biomarkers for active tuberculosis. BMC Infect. Dis. 2025;**25**(1). DOI: 10.1186/s12879-025-11623-w

[46] Starshinova A, Kudryavtsev I, Rubinstein A, Malkova A, Dovgaluk I, Kudlay D. Tuberculosis and COVID-19 Dually Affect Human Th17 Cell Immune Response. Biomedicines. 2023;**11**(8):2123. DOI: 10.3390/biomedicines11082123

[47] Wang J, Fan XY, Hu Z. Immune correlates of protection as a game changer in tuberculosis vaccine development. npj Vaccines. Nature Research. 2024. DOI: 10.1038/s41541-024-01004-w

[48] Choi HG, Kwon KW, Choi S, Back YW, Park HS, Kang SM, et al. Antigen-specific IFN-γ/IL-17-co-producing CD4$^+$ T-cells are the determinants for protective efficacy of tuberculosis subunit vaccine. Vaccines (Basel). 2020;**8**(2):1–22. DOI: 10.3390/vaccines8020300

[49] Woodworth JS, Clemmensen HS, Battey H, Dijkman K, Lindenstrøm T, Laureano RS, et al. A Mycobacterium tuberculosis-specific subunit vaccine that provides synergistic immunity upon co-administration with Bacillus Calmette-Guérin. Nature Communications. 2021;**12**(1). DOI: 10.1038/s41467-021-26934-0

[50] Lin PL, Flynn JAL. CD8 T cells and Mycobacterium tuberculosis infection. Seminars in Immunopathology. 2015;**37**:239–249. DOI: 10.1007/s00281-015-0490-8

[51] Caccamo N, Pietra G, Sullivan LC, Brooks AG, Prezzemolo T, La Manna MP, et al. Human CD8 T lymphocytes recognize Mycobacterium tuberculosis antigens presented by HLA-E during active tuberculosis and express type 2 cytokines. Eur. J. Immunol. 2015;**45**(4):1069–1081. DOI: 10.1002/eji.201445193

[52] Woodworth JS, Behar SM. Mycobacterium tuberculosis-specific CD8$^+$ T cells and their role in immunity. Critical Reviews™ in Immunology. 2006;**26**(4). DOI: 10.1615/critrevimmunol.v26.i4.30

[53] Lieberman J. The ABCs of granule-mediated cytotoxicity: New

weapons in the arsenal. Nature Reviews Immunology. 2003;361–370. DOI: 10.1038/nri1083

[54] Alenzi FQ, Alotaibi AQ, Almotiri GM, Alanazi AM, Alanazi FM, Alenazi MS, et al. Role of Apoptosis in Microbial Infection. Open J Apoptosis. 2014;**03**(02):32–38. DOI: 10.4236/ojapo.2014.32004

[55] Qin Y, Xu J, Wang Q, Shi J. Cytotoxic granules and effector molecules from immune cells in tuberculosis: Mechanisms of host defense and therapeutic potential. Virulence. 2025;**16**(1):2542466. DOI: 10.1080/21505594.2025.2542466

[56] Stenger S, Hanson DA, Teitelbaum R, Dewan P, Niazi KR, Froelich CJ, et al. An antimicrobial activity of cytolytic T cells mediated by granulysin. Science (1979). 1998;**282**(5386):121–125. DOI: 10.1126/science.282.5386.121

[57] Cavalcanti YVN, Brelaz MCA, Jkdal N, Ferraz JC, Pereira VRA. Role of TNF-alpha, IFN-gamma, and IL-10 in the development of pulmonary tuberculosis. Pulmonary Medicine. 2012. DOI: 10.1155/2012/745483

[58] Nathan C, Shiloh MU. Reactive oxygen and nitrogen intermediates in the relationship between mammalian hosts and microbial pathogens. The National Academy of Sciences. 2000;**97**(16):8841–8848. DOI: 10.1073/pnas.97.16.8841

[59] Mohan VP, Scanga CA, Yu K, Scott HM, Tanaka KE, Tsang E, et al. Effects of tumor necrosis factor alpha on host immune response in chronic persistent tuberculosis: Possible role for limiting pathology. Infect and Immun. 2001;**69**(3):1847–1855. DOI: 10.1128/IAI.69.3.1847-1855.2001

[60] Barry CE, Boshoff HI, Dartois V, Dick T, Ehrt S, Flynn JA, et al. The spectrum of latent tuberculosis: Rethinking the biology and intervention strategies. Nature Reviews, Microbiology. 2009;7(12):845–855. DOI: 10.1038/nrmicro2236

[61] Gideon HP, Flynn JL. Latent tuberculosis: What the host "sees"?. Immunologic Resaerch. 2011;**50**(2–3):202–212. DOI: 10.1007/s12026-011-8229-7

[62] Van Pinxteren LAH, Cassidy JP, Smedegaard BHC, Agger EM, Andersen P. Control of latent Mycobacterium tuberculosis infection is dependent on CD8 T cells. Eur. J. Immunol. 2000;**30**(12):3689–3698. DOI: 10.1002/1521-4141(200012)30:12

[63] Tobin DM. Host-directed therapies for tuberculosis. Cold Spring Harb. Perspect. Med. 2015;**5**(10). DOI: 10.1101/cshperspect.a021196

[64] Pagán AJ, Ramakrishnan L. The Formation and Function of Granulomas. Annual review of immunology. 2018;**36**:639–665. DOI: 10.1146/annurev-immunol

[65] Butler NS, Nolz JC, Harty JT. Immunologic considerations for generating memory CD8 T cells through vaccination. Cellular Microbiology. 2011;925–933. DOI: 10.1111/j.1462-5822.2011.01594.x

[66] Tait DR, Hatherill M, Van Der Meeren O, Ginsberg AM, Van Brakel E, Salaun B, et al. Final Analysis of a Trial

of M72/AS01 E Vaccine to Prevent Tuberculosis . New England Journal of Medicine. 2019;**381**(25):2429–2439. DOI: 10.1056/nejmoa1909953

[67] V. SN, Flynn JL. CD8⁺ T cells participate in the memory immune response to Mycobacterium tuberculosis. Infect and Immun. 2001;**69**(7):4320–4328. DOI: 10.1128/IAI.69.7.4320-4328.2001

[68] Chien YH, Jores R, Crowley MP. Recognition by γ/δ T cells. Ann Rev Immunol. 1996;**14**:511–532. DOI: 10.1146/annurev.immunol.14.1.511

[69] Shen Y, Zhou D, Qiu L, Lai X, Simon M, Shen L, et al. Adaptive immune response of Vγ2Vδ2⁺ T cells during mycobacterial infections. Science. 2010;**295**(5563):2255–2258. DOI: 10.1126/science.1068819.Adaptive

[70] Dieli F, Ivanyi J, Marsh P, Williams A, Naylor I, Sireci G, et al. Characterization of Lung γδ T Cells Following Intranasal Infection with Mycobacterium bovis Bacillus Calmette-Guérin . The Journal of Immunology. 2003;**170**(1):463–469. DOI: 10.4049/jimmunol.170.1.463

[71] Tanaka Y, Morita CT, Tanaka Y, Nieves E, Brenner MB, Bloom BR. Natural and synthetic non-peptide antigens recognized by human γδ T cells. Nature. 1995;**375**(6527):155–8. DOI: 10.1038/375155a0

[72] Li Y, Wang X, Teng D, Chen H, Wang M, Wang J, et al. Identification of the Ligands of TCRγδ by Screening the Immune Repertoire of γδT Cells From Patients With Tuberculosis. Frontiers in Immunology. 2019;**10**. DOI: 10.3389/fimmu.2019.02282

[73] Silva Miranda M, Breiman A, Allain S, Deknuydt F, Altare F. The tuberculous granuloma: an unsuccessful host defence mechanism providing a safety shelter for the bacteria? Journal of Immunology Research. 2012;**2012**(1):139127. DOI: 10.1155/2012/139127

[74] Turner J, Frank AA, V BJ, Marietta PM, Vesosky B, Orme IM. Tuberculosis in aged gd T cell gene disrupted mice [Internet]. Report. Available from: www.elsevier.nl/locate/expgero

[75] Ladel CH, Blum C, Dreher A, Reifenberg K, Kaufmann SH. Protective role of γ/δ T cells and α/β T cells in tuberculosis. European journal of immunology. 1995;**25**(10):2877–81. DOI: 10.1002/eji.1830251025

[76] Tanaka S, Itohara S, Sato M, Taniguchi T, Yokomizo Y. Reduced formation of granulomata in γδ T cell knockout BALB/c mice inoculated with Mycobacterium avium subsp. paratuberculosis. Vet Pathol. 2000;**37**(5):415–421. DOI: 10.1354/vp.37-5-415

[77] Turner J, Frank AA, V. Brooks JV, Marietta PM, Vesosky B, Orme IM. Tuberculosis in aged γδ T cell gene disrupted mice. Exp Gerontol. 2001;**36**(2):245–254. DOI: 10.1016/S0531-5565(00)00199-6

[78] Kathamuthu GR, Kumar NP, Moideen K, Menon PA, Babu S. Decreased Frequencies of Gamma/Delta T Cells Expressing Th1/Th17 Cytokine, Cytotoxic, and Immune Markers in Latent Tuberculosis-Diabetes/Pre-Diabetes Comorbidity. Frontiers in Cellular Infection and Microbiology. 2021;**11**. DOI: 10.3389/fcimb.2021.756854

[79] Yan L, Shen H, Xiao H. Characteristics of peripheral Vγ2Vδ2 T cells in interferon-γ release assay negative pulmonary tuberculosis patients. BMC Infect. Dis. 2018;**18**(1). DOI: 10.1186/s12879-018-3328-x

[80] Sadeghi M, Khan, N, Chen Y, Jurado LF, Sinha A, Couto K, et al. Neonatal BCG Vaccination Engages the Vasculature to Elicit γδ T Cell–Mediated Protection against Tuberculosis. bioRxiv. 2025. DOI: 10.64898/2025.12.08.693020

[81] Maerz MD, Makatsa MS, Bucsan AN, Sutton MS, Bishop E, Tian Z, et al. BCG vaccination induces antibacterial effector functions among Vδ1/3 T cells that are associated with protection against tuberculosis. Cell Reports Medicine. 2026;**7**(1):102536. DOI: 10.1016/j.xcrm.2025.102536

[82] Ordway D, Henao-Tamayo M, Orme IM, Gonzalez-Juarrero M. Foamy Macrophages within Lung Granulomas of Mice Infected with Mycobacterium tuberculosis Express Molecules Characteristic of Dendritic Cells and Antiapoptotic Markers of the TNF Receptor-Associated Factor Family . The Journal of Immunology. 2005;**175**(6):3873–3881. DOI: 10.4049/jimmunol.175.6.3873

[83] Mogues T, Goodrich ME, Ryan L, LaCourse R, North RJ. The relative importance of T cell subsets in immunity and immunopathology of airborne Mycobacterium tuberculosis infection in mice. Journal of Experimental Medicine. 2001;**193**(3):271–280. DOI: 10.1084/jem.193.3.271

[84] Egen JG, Rothfuchs AG, Feng CG, Winter N, Sher A, Germain RN. Macrophage and T Cell Dynamics During the Development and Disintegration of Mycobacterial Granulomas. Report

[85] Kokubo K, Onodera A, Kiuchi M, Tsuji K, Hirahara K, Nakayama T. Conventional and pathogenic Th2 cells in inflammation, tissue repair, and fibrosis. Frontiers in Immunology. 2022;**13**(August):1–17. DOI: 10.3389/fimmu.2022.945063

[86] Walker JA, McKenzie ANJ. TH2 cell development and function. Nat Rev Immuno. 2018;**18**(2):121–133. DOI: 10.1038/nri.2017.118

[87] Nakayama T, Hirahara K, Onodera A, Endo Y, Hosokawa H, Shinoda K, et al. Th2 cells in health and disease. Ann Rev Immunol. 2017;**35**:53–84

[88] V. DSM, Massaro Junior VJ, Machado JR, Silva DAA, Castellano LR, Alexandre PBD, et al. Expression pattern of transcription factors and intracellular cytokines reveals that clinically cured tuberculosis is accompanied by an increase in mycobacterium-specific Th1, Th2, and Th17 cells. BioMed Research International, Hindawi. 2015;**2015**:5–10

[89] Demissie A, Abebe M, Aseffa A, Rook G, Fletcher H, Zumla A, et al. Healthy Individuals That Control a Latent Infection with Mycobacterium tuberculosis Express High Levels of Th1 Cytokines and the IL-4 Antagonist IL-4δ2 . The Journal of Immunology. 2004;**172**(11):6938–6943. DOI: 10.4049/jimmunol.172.11.6938

[90] Saini M, Nagarajan K, Bhardwaj S, Ghai R, Mishra A. Immune biomarkers as key targets in managing tuberculosis: A systematic review. Curr Proteomics.

2025;**22**(5). DOI: 10.1016/j.curpro.2025.100050

[91] Rook GAW, Hernandez-Pando R, Dheda K, Teng Seah G. IL-4 in tuberculosis: Implications for vaccine design. Trends Immuol. 2004;**25**(9):483–488. DOI: 10.1016/j.it.2004.06.005

[92] Pooran A, Davids M, Nel A, Shoko A, Blackburn J, Dheda K. IL-4 subverts mycobacterial containment in Mycobacterium tuberculosis-infected human macrophages. European Respiratory Journal. 2019;**54**(2). DOI: 10.1183/13993003.02242-2018

[93] Liu Q, Que S, Qiu Y, Tang M, Liu S, Yang G, et al. Host Immune Response to Mycobacterium tuberculosis Infection: Implications for Vaccine Development. Journal of Inflammation Research . 2025;**18**:8429–8445

[94] Ashenafi S, Aderaye G, Bekele A, Zewdie M, Aseffa G, Hoang ATN, et al. Progression of clinical tuberculosis is associated with a Th2 immune response signature in combination with elevated levels of SOCS3. Clinical Immunology. 2014;**151**(2):84–99. DOI: 10.1016/j.clim.2014.01.010

[95] Hao L, Imran QM, Ullah N. CD39 dynamics in tuberculosis: A potential biomarker of immune dysregulation and T cell exhaustion. Frontiers in Immunology. 2025;**16**(August):1–23. DOI: 10.3389/fimmu.2025.1601637

[96] He J, Song L, Zheng P. Interleukin-4 expression is increased in patients with tuberculosis: A systematic review and meta-analysis. Medicine (United States). 2023;**102**(24):E34041. DOI: 10.1097/MD.0000000000034041

[97] Dwivedi VP, Bhattacharya D, Chatterjee S, Prasad DVR, Chattopadhyay D, Van Kaer L, et al. Mycobacterium tuberculosis directs T helper 2 cell differentiation by inducing interleukin-1β production in dendritic cells. Journal of Biological Chemistry. 2012;**287**(40):33656–33663. DOI: 10.1074/jbc.M112.375154

[98] Immunol EJ - 2003 - Hernandez-Pando-Pulmonary tuberculosis in BALB c mice with non-functional IL-4 genes changes in.pdf

[99] Brighenti S, Ordway DJ. Regulation of immunity to tuberculosis. Tuberculosis and the Tubercle Bacillus. Second Edition. 2017;73–93. DOI: 10.1128/9781555819569.ch3

[100] Arce-Aceves MF, Espinosa-Neira R, Mata-Espinosa DA, Barrios-Payan JA, Castelán-Sánchez HG, Alcaraz-Estrada SL, et al. Fitness costs of Mycobacterium tuberculosis resistant to rifampicin is compensated by rapid Th2 polarization mediated by early and high IL-4 production during mice infection. Scientific Reports. 2025;**15**(1):1–15. DOI: 10.1038/s41598-024-81446-3

[101] Yandrapally S, Agarwal A, Chatterjee A, Sarkar S, Mohareer K, Banerjee S. Mycobacterium tuberculosis EspR modulates Th1-Th2 shift by transcriptionally regulating IL-4, steering increased mycobacterial persistence and HIV propagation during co-infection. Frontiers in Immunology. 2023;**14**(October):1–13. DOI: 10.3389/fimmu.2023.1276817

[102] Harris J, De Haro SA, Master SS, Keane J, Roberts EA, Delgado M, et al. T Helper 2 Cytokines Inhibit

Autophagic Control of Intracellular Mycobacterium tuberculosis. Immunity. 2007;**27**(3):505–517. DOI: 10.1016/j.immuni.2007.07.022

[103] Bhengu KN, Naidoo P, Singh R, Mpaka-Mbatha MN, Nembe N, Duma Z, et al. Immunological Interactions between Intestinal Helminth Infections and Tuberculosis. Diagnostics. 2022;**12**(11). DOI: 10.3390/diagnostics12112676

[104] Potian JA, Rafi W, Bhatt K, McBride A, Gause WC, Salgame P. Preexisting helminth infection induces inhibition of innate pulmonary anti-tuberculosis defense by engaging the IL-4 receptor pathway. Journal of Experimental Medicine. 2011;**208**(9):1863–1874. DOI: 10.1084/jem.20091473

[105] Kitagawa Y, Ohkura N, Sakaguchi S. Molecular determinants of regulatory T cell development: The essential roles of epigenetic changes. Frontiers in Immunology. 2013;**4**(MAY):1–10. DOI: 10.3389/fimmu.2013.00106

[106] Arce-Sillas A, Álvarez-Luquín DD, Tamaya-Domínguez B, Gomez-Fuentes S, Trejo-Garciá A, Melo-Salas M, et al. Regulatory T Cells: Molecular Actions on Effector Cells in Immune Regulation. J Immunol Res. 2016;**2016**. DOI: 10.1155/2016/1720827

[107] Vignali DAA, Collison LW, Workman CJ. How regulatory T cells work. Nat Rev Immuno. 2008;**8**(7):523–532. DOI: 10.1038/nri2343

[108] Wing JB, Sakaguchi S. Multiple Treg suppressive modules and their adaptability. Frontiers in Immunology. 2012;**3**(JUN):1–6. DOI: 10.3389/fimmu.2012.00178

[109] Lozano-Ordaz V, Rodriguez-Miguez Y, Ortiz-Cabrera AE, Hernandez-Bazan S, Mata-Espinosa D, Barrios-Payan J, et al. Beneficial or detrimental activity of regulatory T cells, indoleamine 2,3-dioxygenase, and heme oxygenase-1 in the lungs is influenced by the level of virulence of Mycobacterium tuberculosis strain infection. Frontiers in Cellular Infection and Microbiology. 2023;**13**(May):1–14. DOI: 10.3389/fcimb.2023.1105872

[110] D'Alessio FR, Tsushima K, Aggarwal NR, West EE, Willett MH, Britos MF, et al. $CD4^+CD25^+Foxp3^+$ Tregs resolve experimental lung injury in mice and are present in humans with acute lung injury. Journal of Clinical Investigation. 2009;**119**(10):2898–2913. DOI: 10.1172/JCI36498

[111] Wang X, Tang G, Huang Y, Song H, Zhou S, Mao L, et al. Using immune clusters for classifying Mycobacterium tuberculosis infection. Int. Immunopharmacol. 2024;**128**(October 2023):111572. DOI: 10.1016/j.intimp.2024.111572

[112] Gideon HP, Hughes TK, Tzouanas CN, Wadsworth MH, Tu AA, Gierahn TM, et al. Multimodal profiling of lung granulomas in macaques reveals cellular correlates of tuberculosis control. Immunity. 2022;**55**(5):827–846.e10. DOI: 10.1016/j.immuni.2022.04.004

[113] Gao W, Yang N, Ji S, Zeng Y. Frequency of $CD4^+$ regulatory T cells and modulation of $CD4^+$ T lymphocyte activation in pleural tuberculoma. Tuberculosis. 2022;**134**:102210. DOI: 10.1016/j.tube.2022.102210

[114] Wang L, Jiang W, Wang X, Tong L, Song Y. Regulatory T cells in

inflammation and resolution of acute lung injury. Clinical Respiratory Journal. 2022;**16**(9):587–595. DOI: 10.1111/crj.13527

[115] Lim HJ, Park JS, Cho YJ, Il YH, Park KU, Lee CT, et al. $CD4^+FoxP3^+$ T regulatory cells in drug-susceptible and multidrug-resistant tuberculosis. Tuberculosis. 2013;**93**(5):523–528. DOI: 10.1016/j.tube.2013.06.001

[116] Ferrian S, Ross M, Conradie F, Omar JV, Ismail N, Little F, et al. Frequency of circulating $CD4^+KI67^+HLA\text{-}DR\text{-}T$ regulatory cells prior to treatment for multidrug resistant tuberculosis can differentiate the severity of disease and predict time to culture conversion. Frontiers in Immunology. 2018;**9**(OCT):1–12. DOI: 10.3389/fimmu.2018.02438

[117] Shafiani S, Tucker-Heard G, Kariyone A, Takatsu K, Urdahl KB. Pathogen-specific regulatory T cells delay the arrival of effector T cells in the lung during early tuberculosis. Journal of Experimental Medicine. 2010;**207**(7):1409–1420. DOI: 10.1084/jem.20091885

[118] Scott-Browne JP, Shafiani S, Tucker-Heard G, Ishida-Tsubota K, Fontenot JD, Rudensky AY, et al. Expansion and function of Foxp3-expressing T regulatory cells during tuberculosis. Journal of Experimental Medicine. 2007;**204**(9):2159–2169. DOI: 10.1084/jem.20062105

[119] Li N, Xie WP, Kong H, Min R, Hu CM, Zhou XB, et al. Enrichment of regulatory T-cells in blood of patients with multidrug-resistant tuberculosis. International Journal of Tuberculosis and Lung Disease. 2015;**19**(10):1230–1238. DOI: 10.5588/ijtld.15.0148

[120] Quinn KM, Rich FJ, Goldsack LM, de Lisle GW, Buddle BM, Delahunt B, et al. Accelerating the secondary immune response by inactivating $CD4^+CD25^+$ T regulatory cells prior to BCG vaccination does not enhance protection against tuberculosis. Eur. J. Immunol. 2008;**38**(3):695–705. DOI: 10.1002/eji.200737888

[121] Quinn KM, McHugh RS, Rich FJ, Goldsack LM, De Lisle GW, Buddle BM, et al. Inactivation of $CD4^+CD25^+$ regulatory T cells during early mycobacterial infection increases cytokine production but does not affect pathogen load. Immunol Cell Biol. 2006;**84**(5):467–474. DOI: 10.1111/j.1440-1711.2006.01460.x

[122] Piccaro G, Aquino G, Gigantino V, Tirelli V, Sanchez M, Iorio E, et al. Mycobacterium tuberculosis antigen 85B modifies BCG-induced antituberculosis immunity and favors pathogen survival. J Leukoc Biol. 2024;**115**(6):1053–1069. DOI: 10.1093/jleuko/qiae014

[123] Sun M, Phan JM, Kieswetter NS, Huang H, Kkq Y, Smith MT, et al. Specific $CD4^+$ T cell phenotypes associate with bacterial control in people who ‘resist’ infection with Mycobacterium tuberculosis. Nat. Immunol. 2024;**25**(8):1411–1421. DOI: 10.1038/s41590-024-01897-8

[124] Cheng H, Li S, Liu H, Yan M, Wang J, Huang J, et al. Mycobacterium tuberculosis-derived linoleic acid increases regulatory T cell function to promote bacterial survival within macrophages. Nature Microbiology. 2025:2949–2965. DOI: 10.1038/s41564-025-02140-2

[125] Peyron P, Vaubourgeix J, Poquet Y, Levillain F, Botanch C,

Bardou F, et al. Foamy macrophages from tuberculous patients' granulomas constitute a nutrient-rich reservoir for M. tuberculosis persistence. PLoS Pathog. 2008;**4**(11):1–14. DOI: 10.1371/journal.ppat.1000204

[126] Garcia-Jimenez WL, Villarreal-Ramos B, Grainger D, Hewisnon RG, Vordermeier HM, Salguero FJ. The expression of Indoleamine 2, 3-dioxygenase (IDO) is reduced in granulomas from BCG vaccinated cattle compared to granulomas from unvaccinated controls after experimental challenge with Mycobacterium bovis. Vet Immunol Immunopathol. 2018;**203**(July):52–56. DOI: 10.1016/j.vetimm.2018.08.002

[127] McCaffrey EF, Donato M, Keren L, Chen Z, Delmastro A, Fitzpatrick MB, et al. The immunoregulatory landscape of human tuberculosis granulomas. Nat. Immunol. 2022;**23**(2):318–329. DOI: 10.1038/s41590-021-01121-x

[128] Goldberg MF, Saini NK, Porcelli SA. Evasion of innate and adaptive immunity by Mycobacterium tuberculosis. Molecular Genetics of Mycobacteria. 2015;747–772. DOI: 10.1128/9781555818845.ch36

[129] Chandra P, Grigsby SJ, Philips JA. Immune evasion and provocation by Mycobacterium tuberculosis. Nature Reviews, Microbiology. 2022;**20**(12):750–766. DOI: 10.1038/s41579-022-00763-4

[130] V. HC, Boom WH. Regulation of antigen presentation by Mycobacterium tuberculosis: A role for Toll-like receptors. Nature Reviews, Microbiology. 2010;**8**(4):296–307. DOI: 10.1038/nrmicro2321

[131] AA RT, Potter NS, Ramachandra L, Pai RK, Convery M, Henry Boom W, et al. Alternate Class I MHC Antigen Processing Is Inhibited by Toll-Like Receptor Signaling Pathogen-Associated Molecular Patterns: Mycobacterium tuberculosis 19-kDa Lipoprotein, CpG DNA, and Lipopolysaccharide. The Journal of Immunology. 2003;**1**(171):1413–22. DOI: 10.4049/jimmunol.171.3.1413

[132] Srivastava S, Grace PS, Ernst JD. Antigen Export Reduces Antigen Presentation and Limits T Cell Control of M. tuberculosis. Cell Host & Microbe. 2016;**19**(1):44–54. DOI: 10.1016/j.chom.2015.12.003

[133] Yang JD, Mott D, Sutiwisesak R, Lu YJ, Raso F, Stowell B, et al. Mycobacterium tuberculosis-specific $CD4^{+}$and $CD8^{+}$ T cells differ in their capacity to recognize infected macrophages. PLoS Pathog. 2018;**14**(5). DOI: 10.1371/journal.ppat.1007060

[134] Gail DP, Suzart VG, Du W, Kaur Sandhu A, Jarvela J, Nantongo M, et al. Mycobacterium tuberculosis impairs human memory $CD4^{+}$ T cell recognition of M2 but not M1-like macrophages. iScience. 2023;**26**(9). DOI: 10.1016/j.isci.2023.107706

[135] Ahmed M, Tezera LB, Elkington PT, Leslie AJ. The paradox of immune checkpoint inhibition re-activating tuberculosis. European Respiratory Journal. 2022;**60**(5). DOI: 10.1183/13993003.02512-2021

[136] Comas Ĩ, Chakravartti J, Small PM, Galagan J, Niemann S, Kremer K, et al. Human T cell epitopes of Mycobacterium tuberculosis are evolutionarily hyperconserved. Nature

Genetics [Internet]. 2010;**42**(6): 498–503. DOI: 10.1038/ng.590

[137] Doherty TM. Immunotherapy for TB. Immunotherapy. 2012;**4** (6):629–647. DOI: 10.2217/imt.12.52

[138] Xu J, Wang B, Hu M, Huo F, Guo S, Jing W, et al. Primary Clofazimine and Bedaquiline Resistance among Isolates from Patients with Multidrug-Resistant Tuberculosis. Antimicrobial agents and chemotherapy. 2017;**61**(6): e00239–17. DOI: 10.1128/AAC

[139] Ernst JD. Mechanisms of M. tuberculosis Immune Evasion as Challenges to TB Vaccine Design. Cell Host & Microbe. 2018;**24**(1):34–42. DOI: 10.1016/j.chom.2018.06.004

[140] Seshadri C. A systematic approach to tuberculosis vaccine development. Cell. 2025;**188**(24):6698–6699. DOI: 10.1016/j.cell.2025.10.024

[141] Vidal SJ, Lasrado N, Tostanoski LH, Chaudhari J, Mbiwan ER, Neka GD, et al. Mining the CD4 antigen repertoire for next-generation tuberculosis vaccines. Cell. 2025;**188**(24):6791–6803.e13. DOI: 10.1016/j.cell.2025.08.027

[142] Buccheri S, Reljic R, Caccamo N, Ivanyi J, Singh M, Salerno A, et al. IL-4 depletion enhances host resistance and passive IgA protection against tuberculosis infection in BALB/c mice. Eur. J. Immunol. 2007;**37**(3):729–737. DOI: 10.1002/eji.200636764

[143] Beamer GL, Flaherty DK, Assogba BD, Stromberg P, Gonzalez-Juarrero M, De Waal R, et al. Interleukin-10 Promotes Mycobacterium tuberculosis Disease Progression in CBA/J Mice 1. Report

[144] Segueni N, Tritto E, Bourigault ML, Rose S, Erard F, Le Bert M, et al. Controlled Mycobacterium tuberculosis infection in mice under treatment with anti-IL-17A or IL-17F antibodies, in contrast to TNFα neutralization. Scientific Reports. 2016;**6**. DOI: 10.1038/srep36923

[145] Shen L, Shi H, Gao Y, Ou Q, Liu Q, Liu Y, et al. The characteristic profiles of PD-1 and PD-L1 expressions and dynamic changes during treatment in active tuberculosis. Tuberculosis. 2016;**101**:146–150

[146] Singh A, Mohan A, Dey AB, Mitra DK. Inhibiting the programmed death 1 pathway rescues Mycobacterium tuberculosis-specific interferon γ-producing T cells from apoptosis in patients with pulmonary tuberculosis. Journal of Infectious Diseases. 2013;**208**(4):603–615. DOI: 10.1093/infdis/jit206

[147] Hernández-Pando R, Orozco-Esteves H, Maldonado HA, Aguilar-León D, Vilchis-Landeros MM, Mata-Espinosa DA, et al. A combination of a transforming growth factor-β antagonist and an inhibitor of cyclooxygenase is an effective treatment for murine pulmonary tuberculosis. Clinical and Experimental Allergy. 2006;**144**(2):264–272. DOI: 10.1111/j.1365-2249.2006.03049.x

[148] Mata-Espinosa DA, Mendoza-Rodríguez V, Aguilar-León D, Rosales R, López-Casillas F, Hernández-Pando R. Therapeutic effect of recombinant adenovirus encoding interferon-γ in a murine model of

progressive pulmonary tuberculosis. Molecular Therapy. 2008;**16**(6):1065–1072. DOI: 10.1038/mt.2008.69

[149] Bharti R, Srivastava A, Roy T, Verma K, Reddy DVS, Shafi H, et al. Transient Transfection of the Respiratory Epithelium with Gamma Interferon for Host-Directed Therapy in Pulmonary Tuberculosis. Mol Ther-Nucleic Acids. 2020;**22**:1121–1128

[150] Cheng EM, Tsarovsky NW, Sondel PM, Rakhmilevich AL. Interleukin-12 as an in situ cancer vaccine component: a review. Cancer immunology, immunotherapy: CII. 2022;**71**(9):2057–2065. DOI: 10.1007/s00262-022-03144-1

[151] Mata-Espinosa DA, Francisco-Cruz A, Marquina-Castillo B, Barrios-Payan J, Ramos-Espinosa O, Bini EI, et al. Immunotherapeutic effects of recombinant adenovirus encoding interleukin 12 in experimental pulmonary tuberculosis. Scand. J. Immunol. 2019;**89**(3). DOI: 10.1111/sji.12743

Section 2

T Cell Dysfunction in Tumor and Chronic Inflammatory Disorders

Chapter 4

RNA Methylation and T Cells in Tumor Immunity: Functions, Therapeutic Strategies, and Prospections

Shuang Shang and Lifang Ma

Abstract

RNA methylation is an important post-transcriptional regulatory mechanism that influences gene expression in cancer and immune cells. Dysregulation of RNA methylation has been linked to tumor progression, immune evasion, and therapeutic resistance. In tumor immunity, immune cells function under conditions of persistent antigen stimulation and immunosuppressive signaling, requiring dynamic regulation of RNA metabolism. This chapter summarizes major RNA methylation mechanisms and outlines their regulatory enzymes and immune-related functions. Particular emphasis is placed on the roles of RNA methylation in T cells across different functional stages, including development, activation, expansion, and exhaustion, and how these processes affect antitumor immune responses. These findings highlight RNA methylation as a regulatory layer influencing immunotherapy response and suggest that targeting RNA methylation may provide new strategies to overcome immunotherapy resistance.

Keywords: RNA methylation, T cells, tumor microenvironment, cancer immunotherapy, immunotherapy resistance, therapeutic strategies

1. Introduction

T cells are central components of adaptive immunity and play a critical role in antitumor immune responses [1]. Effective tumor control relies on proper T-cell development, activation, and sustained effector function within the tumor microenvironment [2]. However, in many cancers, T-cell responses are compromised due to persistent antigen stimulation and immunosuppressive signals, resulting in functional impairment and limited therapeutic efficacy [3].

T-cell function is regulated at multiple levels, including transcriptional and epigenetic levels [4, 5]. Nevertheless, effective immune responses also require rapid and flexible regulation of gene expression at the post-transcriptional level. This layer of regulation enables immune cells to adjust protein output without initiating new transcription, which is particularly important during rapid activation and under chronic stimulation conditions commonly observed in tumors.

RNA methylation represents a major post-transcriptional regulatory mechanism that influences RNA stability, translation efficiency, and RNA turnover [6, 7]. Increasing evidence indicates that RNA methylation contributes to immune regulation in cancer by shaping immune-related gene expression programs. Therefore, studying RNA methylation in immune cells provides important insights into the regulation of tumor immunity and may reveal new opportunities for therapeutic intervention.

2. RNA methylation in tumor immunity

RNA methylation comprises a group of post-transcriptional RNA modifications that regulate RNA metabolism and gene expression [8]. By modulating RNA stability, translation, and turnover, these modifications add a dynamic regulatory layer beyond transcriptional control. Dysregulation of RNA methylation has been widely reported in cancer and is associated with tumor progression, immune evasion, and therapeutic resistance [9–11].

Tumor immunity occurs within a complex microenvironment characterized by persistent antigen exposure, metabolic stress, and immunosuppressive signaling [12–14]. Immune cells operating in this context require adaptable regulatory mechanisms to maintain functionality. RNA methylation contributes to this adaptability by regulating immune-related transcripts involved in cytokine signaling, immune activation, and cell survival. Multiple RNA methylation types have been implicated in tumor immunity, among which N6-methyladenosine (m^6A), 5-methylcytosine (m^5C), and N1-methyladenosine (m^1A) are the most extensively studied.

2.1 N6-methyladenosine

N6-methyladenosine is the most abundant internal modification in eukaryotic messenger RNA [15]. It is deposited by a methyltransferase complex centered on METTL3 and METTL14 [16] and can be removed by demethylases such as FTO and ALKBH5 [17, 18]. Reader proteins recognize m^6A-modified transcripts and regulate their stability and translation [19, 20].

In tumor immunity, m^6A has been linked to the regulation of immune-related gene expression across multiple immune cell types [21]. Altered m^6A landscapes are associated with changes in cytokine signaling, antigen presentation, and immune cell activation within the tumor microenvironment [22–24]. Dysregulation of m^6A regulators in tumors can reshape immune responses, contributing to either immune suppression or enhanced antitumor immunity, depending on the context.

Importantly, m^6A has also been associated with responses to immune checkpoint blockade (ICB). Several studies have reported that modulation of m^6A-related enzymes influences sensitivity to PD-1 or PD–L1 blockade by affecting tumor-immune interactions. For example, YTHDF1 exerts a detrimental effect on antitumor immunity through the m^6A–p65-CXCL1/CXCR2 axis, thereby facilitating the progression of colorectal cancer (CRC) [21]. Another study showed that the circCCAR1/miR-127-5p/WTAP feedback loop promotes hepatocellular carcinoma

(HCC) growth and metastasis, causing immunosuppression by impairing $CD8^+$ T cell function and inducing anti-PD1 resistance [25]. These findings suggest that m^6A acts as a key epi-transcriptomic regulator linking RNA metabolism to antitumor immune responses and immunotherapeutic outcomes.

Overall, m^6A exerts broad regulatory effects on immune-related transcripts and has the most direct evidence linking it to immunotherapy response. Its reversible nature and well-characterized regulatory enzymes make it a central node in epi-transcriptomic control of tumor immunity.

2.2 5-Methylcytosine

5-Methylcytosine is an RNA modification found in messenger RNA, as well as in transfer and ribosomal RNAs [26]. 5-Methylcytosine is primarily catalyzed by enzymes of the NSUN family and DNMT2 and it has been implicated in RNA stability and translational regulation [27, 28]. Compared with m^6A, the immune-related functions of m^5C remain less well-characterized.

Emerging evidence suggests that m^5C participates in tumor immunity by modulating immune-related gene expression and cellular stress responses [29, 30]. Aberrant expression of m^5C-associated enzymes has been linked to altered immune signaling pathways and immune cell infiltration in multiple cancer types. The NSUN2/ALYREF axis promotes immune evasion and tumor progression in NSCLC by stabilizing PD–L1 mRNA through m^5C methylation, representing a promising novel target for lung cancer immunotherapy [31]. NSUN2 is recruited to Il17a/Il17f chromatin in mouse $CD4^+$ T cells, promoting Th17 differentiation via m^5C-mediated mRNA stabilization [32]. These changes may influence how immune cells adapt to metabolic and inflammatory stress within the tumor microenvironment.

In addition, m^5C-related gene signatures have been correlated with immune activation states and clinical outcomes in cancer patients. Although mechanistic insights remain limited, current findings support a contributory role for m^5C in shaping immune phenotypes in tumors.

2.3 N1-methyladenosine

N1-methyladenosine is a relatively low-abundance RNA modification detected in both coding and non-coding RNAs. N1-methyladenosine is catalyzed by methyltransferases of the TRMT family and can be reversed by ALKBH family demethylases [33, 34]. This modification is often associated with structured RNA regions and translational control.

The role of m^1A in tumor immunity is still emerging. Dysregulation of m^1A-associated regulators has been reported in several cancers and is associated with changes in metabolic and stress-response pathways, which are critical for immune cell function in tumors [35]. In gastric cancer (GC), m^1A level of SFRP2 regulates the NFAT/TOX-mediated immune evasion axis, and targeting SFRP2 represents a promising strategy to overcome ICB resistance [36]. These alterations may indirectly influence immune activity within the tumor microenvironment. Although direct evidence connecting m^1A to immunotherapy response is currently limited, existing observations suggest that m^1A may contribute to immune regulation in cancer and merits further investigation.

While m^6A, m^5C, and m^1A differ in abundance, regulatory enzymes, and molecular targets, they share a common functional feature in tumor immunity: the modulation of immune-related transcript stability and translation. Among them, m^6A is currently the most extensively characterized in immune regulation, with clearer links to T-cell function and immunotherapy response. In contrast, m^5C and m^1A remain less defined but appear to contribute to immune adaptation and tumor-immune interactions. Together, these modifications form an integrated epi-transcriptomic network that influences antitumor immune responses at multiple levels.

3. RNA methylation in different periods of T cells

T cells undergo dynamic functional transitions during antitumor immune responses, including development, activation, expansion, and exhaustion under chronic antigen stimulation [37–39]. These transitions require precise regulation of gene expression programs to support proliferation, effector function, and long-term persistence. In tumor settings, sustained antigen exposure and immunosuppressive signals further challenge T-cell functionality [40, 41].

RNA methylation has emerged as an important post-transcriptional regulatory mechanism contributing to T-cell fate decisions across these functional periods by modulating RNA stability and translation [42]. RNA methylation influences how T cells respond to activation cues and adapt to the tumor microenvironment.

3.1 T cell development

T-cell development is a tightly regulated process that ensures the generation of a functional and self-tolerant T-cell repertoire. This process depends on coordinated transcriptional and post-transcriptional control of gene expression [43, 44].

Previous studies have shown that m^6A modification mediated by METTL3 influences the stability of transcripts involved in lymphocyte differentiation and survival. Loss of METTL3 in developing T cells impairs maturation and alters homeostasis, highlighting the importance of RNA methylation in establishing a competent T-cell pool [42]. N6-methyladenosine modification on the 3′-UTR (untranslated region) of Tcf7 mRNA, catalyzed by METTL3, also enhances the stability of Tcf7 mRNA and thereby ensures TCF-1 expression, which is essential for sustaining T follicular helper (Tfh) cell differentiation [45]. METTL14-dependent m^6A modification facilitates the splicing process and production of miR-149-3p, which in turn regulates Th17 cell differentiation [46].

Although these effects are not tumor-specific, defects in T-cell development may ultimately limit effective antitumor immune responses.

3.2 T cell activation and expansion

Following antigen recognition, naïve T cells undergo rapid activation and clonal expansion, accompanied by extensive transcriptional and metabolic reprogramming. Efficient post-transcriptional regulation is required to sustain high biosynthetic demands during this phase.

RNA methylation has been reported to regulate the stability and translation of transcripts involved in T-cell receptor signaling, cytokine responses, and cell cycle progression. For example, METTL3-dependent m^6A modification promotes T-cell proliferation by facilitating the timely turnover of negative regulators of activation pathways [47]. Deficiency of METTL3 and m^6A modification in Treg cells elevated SOCS mRNA expression, which in turn caused deactivation of the IL-2/STAT5 signaling pathway, an essential pathway for preserving the functions and stability of Treg cells [48]. Dysregulation of m^6A erasers, such as ALKBH5 has been associated with altered activation dynamics. ALKBH5 reduces m^6A modification of *CXCL2* and *IFNG* mRNA, boosting their stability and translation to drive $CD4^+$ T cell responses [49]. Tumor-intrinsic FTO constrained the activation and effector phenotypes of $CD8^+$ T cells; silencing FTO attenuated the glycolytic capacity of tumor cells, which in turn restored the functional activity of $CD8^+$ T cells [50]. In colon cancer, m^1A levels were inversely associated with the proliferation of $CD8^+$ T effector cells [51]. In HCC, NSUN2 inhibits the activity and cytotoxicity of $CD8^+$ T cells, contributing to immune evasion [52].

However, in tumor immunity, aberrant RNA methylation during T-cell activation may impair expansion or skew differentiation, thereby limiting effective antitumor responses.

3.3 T cell exhaustion

In the tumor microenvironment, persistent antigen exposure and chronic inflammatory signaling drive T cells into a dysfunctional state known as T cell exhaustion [53]. Exhausted T cells are characterized by sustained expression of inhibitory receptors, reduced cytokine production, impaired proliferative capacity, and distinct transcriptional and epigenetic programs. This dysfunctional differentiation state represents a major barrier to durable responses to ICB and contributes to immunotherapy resistance. Epigenetic and post-transcriptional mechanisms are increasingly recognized as important regulators of exhaustion-associated gene expression programs.

Emerging evidence indicates that RNA methylation contributes to the regulation of exhaustion-associated gene expression programs. Dysregulated m^6A modification has been linked to altered stability of transcripts involved in effector function and inhibitory signaling. N6-methyladenosine mediates the process of T cell exhaustion and can be recognized as a biomarker and therapeutic target for advancing cancer immunotherapy [54]. Loss of METTL14 function results in abnormal differentiation of $CD8^+$ T cells, which, in turn, induces $CD8^+$ T cell dysfunction and impairs the activation of $CD8^+$ T effector cells [50]. While NSUN1 binds HIV-1 TAR RNA (5′-LTR [long terminal repeat]) to induce m^5C methylation, it competes with Tat–TAR interaction and impairs HIV-1 transcriptional elongation, thereby promoting viral latency in $CD4^+$ T cells [55].

These findings suggest that RNA methylation influences both the establishment and potential reversibility of T-cell exhaustion, thereby affecting responses to ICB. Moreover, RNA methylation has been implicated in modulating responses to ICB, suggesting a potential role in determining the reversibility of T-cell exhaustion.

4. Therapeutic strategies and future prospections

The involvement of RNA methylation in regulating T-cell function and tumor immunity highlights its potential as a therapeutic target. Modulation of RNA methylation enzymes, including METTL3, ALKBH5, and FTO, has been shown in preclinical models to influence antitumor immune responses and sensitivity to ICB.

Combining RNA methylation–targeted strategies with existing immunotherapies, such as PD-1/PD–L1 inhibitors, cancer vaccines, or adoptive cell therapies, may enhance therapeutic efficacy by improving immune cell functionality within tumors [56]. For example, a low level of METTL3 can lead to resistance to anti-PD1 antibodies in thyroid cancer [57]. The development of selective modulators and a deeper understanding of cell-type-specific effects will be essential for clinical translation. Several RNA methylation-targeting agents are currently under preclinical or early clinical evaluation. For example, small-molecule FTO inhibitors have demonstrated enhanced sensitivity to ICB in melanoma and HCC [24, 58]. In addition, NSUN2 inhibitors have been developed, providing potential pharmacological tools for targeting m^5C-dependent pathways. Research has shown that NSUN2 knockdown potentiated the cytotoxicity of $CD8^+$ T cells *in vitro* and promoted TNF-α^+ T-cell infiltration [59]. Although most agents remain in early development stages, these advances support the translational feasibility of targeting RNA methylation in cancer immunotherapy.

Future studies integrating RNA methylation profiling with genomic and immunological analyses may enable patient stratification and precision immunotherapy. Continued investigation into RNA methylation-mediated immune regulation is expected to expand the therapeutic landscape and improve outcomes for cancer patients.

Acknowledgements

This study was supported by the Excellent Talents Nurture Project of Shanghai Chest Hospital (2021YNZYY02).

The authors acknowledge the use of DeepSeek for the review framework and language polishing of the manuscript.

Author details

Shuang Shang and Lifang Ma*
Department of Clinical Laboratory, Shanghai Chest Hospital, Shanghai Jiao Tong University School of Medicine, Shanghai, China

*Address all correspondence to: mlf2281@sjtu.edu.cn

References

[1] Zajac AJ, Blattman JN, Murali-Krishna K, Sourdive DJ, Suresh M, Altman JD, Ahmed R. Viral immune evasion due to persistence of activated T cells without effector function. Journal of Experimental Medicine. 1998;**188**(12):2205–2213

[2] Woo SR, Fuertes MB, Corrales L, Spranger S, Furdyna MJ, Leung MY, Duggan R, Wang Y, Barber GN, Fitzgerald KA, Alegre ML, Gajewski TF. STING-dependent cytosolic DNA sensing mediates innate immune recognition of immunogenic tumors. Immunity. 2014;**41**(5):830–842

[3] Wang K, Coutifaris P, Brocks D, Wang G, Azar T, Solis S, Nandi A, Anderson S, Han N, Manne S, Kiner E, Sachar C, Lucas M, George S, Yan PK, Kier MW, Laughlin AI, Kothari S, Giles J, Mathew D, Ghinnagow R, Alanio C, Flowers A, Xu W, Tenney DJ, Xu X, Amaravadi RK, Karakousis GC, Schuchter LM, Buggert M, Oldridge D, Minn AJ, Blank C, Weber JS, Mitchell TC, Farwell MD, Herati RS, Huang AC. Combination anti-PD-1 and anti-CTLA-4 therapy generates waves of clonal responses that include progenitor-exhausted CD8(+) T cells. Cancer Cell. 2024;**42**(9):1582–1597.e10

[4] Sumida TS, Lincoln MR, He L, Park Y, Ota M, Oguchi A, Son R, Yi A, Stillwell HA, Leissa GA, Fujio K, Murakawa Y, Kulminski AM, Epstein CB, Bernstein BE, Kellis M, Hafler DA. An autoimmune transcriptional circuit drives FOXP3(+) regulatory T cell dysfunction. Science Translational Medicine. 2024;**16**(762):eadp1720

[5] Chaudhry MZ, Chen E, Man HO, Jones A, Denman R, Yu H, Huang Q, Ilich A, Schreuder J, Navarro S, Tuong ZK, Belz GT. GFI1-driven transcriptional and epigenetic programs maintain CD8(+) T cell stemness and persistence. Nature Immunology. 2025;**26**(6):894–907

[6] Wang H, Hu X, Huang M, Liu J, Gu Y, Ma L, Zhou Q, Cao X. Mettl3-mediated mRNA m(6)A methylation promotes dendritic cell activation. Nature Communications. 2019; **10**(1):1898

[7] Zheng H, Aihaiti Y, Cai Y, Yuan Q, Yang M, Li Z, Xu K, Xu P. The m6A/m1A/m5C-related methylation modification patterns and immune landscapes in rheumatoid arthritis and osteoarthritis revealed by microarray and single-cell transcriptome. Journal of Inflammation Research. 2023;**16**: 5001–5025

[8] De Kesel J, Fijalkowski I, Pieters T, Borin C, Christensen KT, Wittouck M, Van Laere J, Guerrero L, Reunes L, Caruso M, Thakkar B, Sleeckx W, Xu LK, Van Nieuwerburgh F, Deforce D, De Keersmaecker K, Lammens T, Goossens S, Taghon T, Han C, Veltri G, Serafin V, Palhais B, Sharma ND, Huang H, Liu H, Matlawska-Wasowska K, Milovanovic A, Novoa EM, Wang E, Ntziachristos P. HNRNPC and m6A RNA methylation control oncogenic transcription and metabolism in T-cell leukemia. Blood. 2025;**146** (3):275–290

[9] Yan W, Liu X, Qiu X, Zhang X, Chen J, Xiao K, Wu P, Peng C, Hu X, Wang Z, Qin J, Sun L, Chen L, Wu D, Huang S, Yin L, Li Z. PRMT5-mediated FUBP1 methylation accelerates prostate cancer progression. Journal of Clinical Investigation. 2024;**134**(18):e175023

[10] Xiao S, Ma S, Sun B, Pu W, Duan S, Han J, Hong Y, Zhang J, Peng Y, He C, Yi P, Caligiuri MA, Yu J. The tumor-intrinsic role of the m(6)A reader YTHDF2 in regulating immune evasion. Science Immunology. 2024;**9**(95):eadl2171

[11] Lu Y, Zhu J, Zhang Y, Li W, Xiong Y, Fan Y, Wu Y, Zhao J, Shang C, Liang H, Zhang W. Lactylation-driven IGF2BP3-mediated serine metabolism reprogramming and RNA m6A-modification promotes lenvatinib resistance in HCC. Advanced Science (Weinheim). 2024;**11**(46):e2401399

[12] Carnevale J, Shifrut E, Kale N, Nyberg WA, Blaeschke F, Chen YY, Li Z, Bapat SP, Diolaiti ME, O'Leary P, Vedova S, Belk J, Daniel B, Roth TL, Bachl S, Anido AA, Prinzing B, Ibañez-Vega J, Lange S, Haydar D, Luetke-Eversloh M, Born-Bony M, Hegde B, Kogan S, Feuchtinger T, Okada H, Satpathy AT, Shannon K, Gottschalk S, Eyquem J, Krenciute G, Ashworth A, Marson A. RASA2 ablation in T cells boosts antigen sensitivity and long-term function. Nature. 2022;**609**(7925):174–182

[13] Liu Y, Lin J, Yu Z, Li X, Lv X, Liu P, Sun X, Zhang Z, Gao X, Sun K, Li D, Li J, Liu Y, Jiang Y, Zou S, Lin J, Sun B, Fu D, Shen B. Tumor-associated Schwann cell remodeling under metabolic stress via lactate sensing orchestrates pancreatic ductal adenocarcinoma development. Cell Metabolism. 2025;**37**(9):1907–1925.e14

[14] Lai P, Liu L, Bancaro N, Troiani M, Calì B, Li Y, Chen J, Singh PK, Arzola RA, Attanasio G, Pernigoni N, Pasquini E, Mosole S, Rinaldi A, Sgrignani J, Qiu S, Song P, Li Y, Desbats MA, Ángel AR, Mestre RP, Cavalli A, Barile L, de Bono J, Alimonti A. Mitochondrial DNA released by senescent tumor cells enhances PMN-MDSC-driven immunosuppression through the cGAS-STING pathway. Immunity. 2025;**58**(4):811–825.e7

[15] Wang X, Lu Z, Gomez A, Hon GC, Yue Y, Han D, Fu Y, Parisien M, Dai Q, Jia G, Ren B, Pan T, He C. N6-methyladenosine-dependent regulation of messenger RNA stability. Nature. 2014;**505**(7481):117–120

[16] Lin Z, Hsu PJ, Xing X, Fang J, Lu Z, Zou Q, Zhang KJ, Zhang X, Zhou Y, Zhang T, Zhang Y, Song W, Jia G, Yang X, He C, Tong MH. Mettl3-/Mettl14-mediated mRNA N(6)-methyladenosine modulates murine spermatogenesis. Cell Research. 2017;**27**(10):1216–1230

[17] Zhou H, Xie Z, Qian Y, Ni W, Cui L, Fang X, Wan S, Zhao X, Qin A, Fan S, Wu Y. FTO-mediated SMAD2 m6A modification protects cartilage against Osteoarthritis. Exp Mol Med. 2024;**56**(10):2283–2295

[18] Hu Y, Gong C, Li Z, Liu J, Chen Y, Huang Y, Luo Q, Wang S, Hou Y, Yang S, Xiao Y. Demethylase ALKBH5 suppresses invasion of gastric cancer via PKMYT1 m6A modification. Molecular Cancer. 2022;**21**(1):34

[19] Liu T, Wei Q, Jin J, Luo Q, Liu Y, Yang Y, Cheng C, Li L, Pi J, Si Y, Xiao H, Li L, Rao S, Wang F, Yu J, Yu J, Zou D, Yi P. The m6A reader YTHDF1 promotes ovarian cancer progression via augmenting EIF3C translation. Nucleic Acids Research. 2020;**48**(7):3816–3831

[20] Zhou Y, Ćorović M, Hoch-Kraft P, Meiser N, Mesitov M, Körtel N, Back H, Naarmann-de Vries IS, Katti K, Obrdlík A, Busch A, Dieterich C,

Vaňáčová Š, Hengesbach M, Zarnack K, König J. m6A sites in the coding region trigger translation-dependent mRNA decay. Molecular Cell. 2024;**84**(23):4576–4593.e12

[21] Bao Y, Zhai J, Chen H, Wong CC, Liang C, Ding Y, Huang D, Gou H, Chen D, Pan Y, Kang W, To KF, Yu J. Targeting m(6)A reader YTHDF1 augments antitumour immunity and boosts anti-PD-1 efficacy in colorectal cancer. Gut. 2023;**72**(8):1497–1509

[22] Luo S, Liao C, Zhang L, Ling C, Zhang X, Xie P, Su G, Chen Z, Zhang L, Lai T, Tang J. METTL3-mediated m6A mRNA methylation regulates neutrophil activation through targeting TLR4 signaling. Cell Reports. 2023;**42**(3):112259

[23] Han D, Liu J, Chen C, Dong L, Liu Y, Chang R, Huang X, Liu Y, Wang J, Dougherty U, Bissonnette MB, Shen B, Weichselbaum RR, Xu MM, He C. Anti-tumour immunity controlled through mRNA m(6)A methylation and YTHDF1 in dendritic cells. Nature. 2019;**566**(7743):270–274

[24] Chen A, Zhang VX, Zhang Q, Sze KM, Tian L, Huang H, Wang X, Lee E, Lu J, Lyu X, Lee MJ, Wong CM, Ho DW, Ng IO. Targeting the oncogenic m6A demethylase FTO suppresses tumourigenesis and potentiates immune response in hepatocellular carcinoma. Gut. 2024;**74**(1):90–102

[25] Hu Z, Chen G, Zhao Y, Gao H, Li L, Yin Y, Jiang J, Wang L, Mang Y, Gao Y, Zhang S, Ran J, Li L. Exosome-derived circCCAR1 promotes CD8+ T-cell dysfunction and anti-PD1 resistance in hepatocellular carcinoma. Molecular Cancer. 2023;**22**(1):55

[26] Gonskikh Y, Tirrito C, Bommisetti P, Mendoza-Figueroa MS, Stoute J, Kim J, Wang Q, Song Y, Liu KF. Spatial regulation of NSUN2-mediated tRNA m5C installation in cognitive function. Nucleic Acids Research. 2025;**53**(2):gkae1169

[27] Yang S, Li J, Mao S, Zhao X, Liu D, Chen J, Fu J, Bu Y, Wu X, Liu S, Yu Q, Dong Q, Tang Z, Fang Y, Shi Y. DNMT2-m5C-ACLY axis promotes lenvatinib resistance in hepatocellular carcinoma through histone acetylation-mediated notch pathway. Advanced Science (Weinheim). 2026;**3**(13):e15931

[28] Tao Y, Felber JG, Zou Z, Njomen E, Remsberg JR, Ogasawara D, Ye C, Melillo B, Schreiber SL, He C, Remillard D, Cravatt BF. Chemical proteomic discovery of isotype-selective covalent inhibitors of the RNA methyltransferase NSUN2. Angewandte Chemie International Edition in English. 2023;**62**(51):e202311924

[29] Chen Z, Zeng C, Yang L, Che Y, Chen M, Sau L, Wang B, Zhou K, Chen Y, Qing Y, Shen C, Zhang T, Wunderlich M, Wu D, Li W, Wang K, Leung K, Sun M, Tang T, He X, Zhang L, Swaminathan S, Mulloy JC, Müschen M, Huang H, Weng H, Xiao G, Deng X, Chen J. YTHDF2 promotes ATP synthesis and immune evasion in B cell malignancies. Cell. 2025;**188**(2):331–351.e30

[30] Chen B, Hong Y, Zhai X, Deng Y, Hu H, Tian S, Zhang Y, Ren X, Zhao J, Jiang C. m6A and m5C modification of GPX4 facilitates anticancer immunity via STING activation. Cell Death Dis. 2023;**14**(12):809

[31] Yang Y, Cao L, Xu X, Li D, Deng Y, Li L, Zeng B, Jiang H, Shan L, Huang Y, Xu Y, Ma L. NSUN2/ALYREF axis-driven m(5)C methylation enhances

PD-L1 expression and facilitates immune evasion in non-small-cell lung cancer. Cancer Immunol Immunother. 2025;**74**(4):132

[32] Yang WL, Qiu W, Zhang T, Xu K, Gu ZJ, Zhou Y, Xu HJ, Yang ZZ, Shen B, Zhao YL, Zhou Q, Yang Y, Li W, Yang PY, Yang YG. Nsun2 coupling with RoR γ t shapes the fate of Th17 cells and promotes colitis. Nature Communications. 2023;**14**(1):863

[33] Hu CK, Huang WZ, He L, Chang C, Ren YL, Dai RX, Wu Q, Su Q. De-succinylation-induced accumulation of TRMT10C in the nucleus plays a detrimental role in coronary microembolization via its m1A modification function. International Journal of Biological Sciences. 2025; **21**(7):2891–2920

[34] Gu X, Zhuang A, Yu J, Yang L, Ge S, Ruan J, Jia R, Fan X, Chai P. Histone lactylation-boosted ALKBH3 potentiates tumor progression and diminished promyelocytic leukemia protein nuclear condensates by m1A demethylation of SP100A. Nucleic Acids Research. 2024;**52**(5):2273–2289

[35] Miao S, Li H, Song X, Liu Y, Wang G, Kan C, Ye Y, Liu RJ, Li HB. tRNA m1A modification regulates cholesterol biosynthesis to promote antitumor immunity of CD8+ T cells. Journal of Experimental Medicine. 2025;**222**(3):e20240559

[36] Liu Y, Liu G, Wang X, Zhang X, Wu J, Li Y, Lu Y, Shi C, Ye F, Sun R. The m(1)A-SFRP2-NFAT/TOX axis governs T cell exhaustion in gastric cancer. Cellular Oncology (Dordrecht). 2025;**48**(5):1553–1569

[37] Jneid B, Bochnakian A, Hoffmann C, Delisle F, Djacoto E, Sirven P, Denizeau J, Sedlik C, Gerber-Ferder Y, Fiore F, Akyol R, Brousse C, Kramer R, Walters I, Carlioz S, Salmon H, Malissen B, Dalod M, Piaggio E, Manel N. Selective STING stimulation in dendritic cells primes antitumor T cell responses. Science Immunology. 2023;**8**(79):eabn6612

[38] Elia I, Rowe JH, Johnson S, Joshi S, Notarangelo G, Kurmi K, Weiss S, Freeman GJ, Sharpe AH, Haigis MC. Tumor cells dictate anti-tumor immune responses by altering pyruvate utilization and succinate signaling in CD8(+) T cells. Cell Metabolism. 2022;**34**(8):1137–1150.e6

[39] Tay C, Tanaka A, Sakaguchi S. Tumor-infiltrating regulatory T cells as targets of cancer immunotherapy. Cancer Cell. 2023;**41**(3):450–465

[40] Globig AM, Zhao S, Roginsky J, Maltez VI, Guiza J, Avina-Ochoa N, Heeg M, Araujo Hoffmann F, Chaudhary O, Wang J, Senturk G, Chen D, O'Connor C, Pfaff S, Germain RN, Schalper KA, Emu B, Kaech SM. The β(1)-adrenergic receptor links sympathetic nerves to T cell exhaustion. Nature. 2023; **622**(7982):383–392

[41] Waibl Polania J, Hoyt-Miggelbrink A, Tomaszewski WH, Wachsmuth LP, Lorrey SJ, Wilkinson DS, Lerner E, Woroniecka K, Finlay JB, Ayasoufi K, Fecci PE. Antigen presentation by tumor-associated macrophages drives T cells from a progenitor exhaustion state to terminal exhaustion. Immunity. 2025;**58**(1):232–246.e6

[42] Li HB, Tong J, Zhu S, Batista PJ, Duffy EE, Zhao J, Bailis W, Cao G, Kroehling L, Chen Y, Wang G, Broughton JP, Chen YG, Kluger Y, Simon MD, Chang HY, Yin Z,

Flavell RA. m(6)A mRNA methylation controls T cell homeostasis by targeting the IL-7/STAT5/SOCS pathways. Nature. 2017;**548**(7667):338–342

[43] Li N, Kang Y, Wang L, Huff S, Tang R, Hui H, Agrawal K, Gonzalez GM, Wang Y, Patel SP, Rana TM. ALKBH5 regulates anti-PD-1 therapy response by modulating lactate and suppressive immune cell accumulation in tumor microenvironment. Proceedings of the National Academy of Sciences of the USA (PNAS). 2020;**117**(33):20159–20170

[44] Li H, Zhang MJ, Zhang B, Lin WP, Li SJ, Xiong D, Wang Q, Wang WD, Yang QC, Huang CF, Deng WW, Sun ZJ. Mature tertiary lymphoid structures evoke intra-tumoral T and B cell responses via progenitor exhausted CD4(+) T cells in head and neck cancer. Nature Communications. 2025;**16**(1):4228

[45] Yao Y, Yang Y, Guo W, Xu L, You M, Zhang YC, Sun Z, Cui X, Yu G, Qi Z, Liu J, Wang F, Liu J, Zhao T, Ye L, Yang YG, Yu S. METTL3-dependent m (6)A modification programs T follicular helper cell differentiation. Nature Communications. 2021;**12**(1):1333

[46] Cao Y, Wang Z, Yan Y, Ji L, He J, Xuan B, Shen C, Ma Y, Jiang S, Ma D, Tong T, Zhang X, Gao Z, Zhu X, Fang JY, Chen H, Hong J. Enterotoxigenic bacteroidesfragilis promotes intestinal inflammation and malignancy by inhibiting exosome-packaged miR-149-3p. Gastroenterology. 2021;**161**(5): 1552–1566.e12

[47] Fang M, Li Y, Wang P, Wang Y, Wang X, Wa X, Zhang Y, He Z, Li J, Li L, Su Y, Zhou H, He J, Liu Y. METTL3 inhibition restores PD-L1 expression and CD8+ T-cell cytotoxic function in immunotherapy-treated gastric cancer. Cancer Immunology Research. 2025;**13** (7):1037–1052

[48] Tong J, Cao G, Zhang T, Sefik E, Amezcua Vesely MC, Broughton JP, Zhu S, Li H, Li B, Chen L, Chang HY, Su B, Flavell RA, Li HB. m(6)A mRNA methylation sustains Treg suppressive functions. Cell Research. 2018;**28** (2):253–256

[49] Zhou J, Zhang X, Hu J, Qu R, Yu Z, Xu H, Chen H, Yan L, Ding C, Zou Q, Ye Y, Wang Z, Flavell RA, Li HB. m(6)A demethylase ALKBH5 controls CD4(+) T cell pathogenicity and promotes autoimmunity. Science Advances. 2021;**7**(25):eabg0470

[50] Liu Y, Liang G, Xu H, Dong W, Dong Z, Qiu Z, Zhang Z, Li F, Huang Y, Li Y, Wu J, Yin S, Zhang Y, Guo P, Liu J, Xi JJ, Jiang P, Han D, Yang CG, Xu MM. Tumors exploit FTO-mediated regulation of glycolytic metabolism to evade immune surveillance. Cell Metabolism. 2021; **33**(6):1221–1233.e11

[51] Gao Y, Wang H, Li H, Ye X, Xia Y, Yuan S, Lu J, Xie X, Wang L, Zhang J. Integrated analyses of m(1)A regulator-mediated modification patterns in tumor microenvironment-infiltrating immune cells in colon cancer. Oncoimmunology. 2021;**10**(1):1936758

[52] Jiang J, Liu F, Cui D, Xu C, Chi J, Yan T, Guo F. Novel molecular mechanisms of immune evasion in hepatocellular carcinoma: NSUN2-mediated increase of SOAT2 RNA methylation. Cancer Commun (Lond). 2025;**45**(7):846–879

[53] Chow A, Perica K, Klebanoff CA, Wolchok JD. Clinical implications of T cell exhaustion for cancer

immunotherapy. Nature Reviews Clinical Oncology. 2022;**19**(12):775–790

[54] Ji W, Fang Y, Chen L, Zheng Y, Pei Y, Mei C, Zhou M. Pan-cancer characterization of m6A-mediated regulation of T cell exhaustion dynamics and clinical relevancies in human cancers. Molecular Therapy – Nucleic Acids. 2025;**36**(1):102465

[55] Kong W, Biswas A, Zhou D, Fiches G, Fujinaga K, Santoso N, Zhu J. Nucleolar protein NOP2/NSUN1 suppresses HIV-1 transcription and promotes viral latency by competing with Tat for TAR binding and methylation. PLoS Pathog. 2020;**16**(3): e1008430

[56] Yin H, Zhang X, Yang P, Zhang X, Peng Y, Li D, Yu Y, Wu Y, Wang Y, Zhang J, Ding X, Wang X, Yang A, Zhang R. RNA m6A methylation orchestrates cancer growth and metastasis via macrophage reprogramming. Nature Communications. 2021;**12**(1):1394

[57] Liu Z, Wang T, She Y, Wu K, Gu S, Li L, Dong C, Chen C, Zhou Y. N(6)-methyladenosine-modified circIGF2BP3 inhibits CD8(+) T-cell responses to facilitate tumor immune evasion by promoting the deubiquitination of PD-L1 in non-small cell lung cancer. Molecular Cancer. 2021;**20**(1):105

[58] Xiao Z, Li T, Zheng X, Lin L, Wang X, Li B, Huang J, Wang Y, Shuai X, Zhu K. Nanodrug enhances post-ablation immunotherapy of hepatocellular carcinoma via promoting dendritic cell maturation and antigen presentation. Bioactive Materials. 2023;**21**:57–68

[59] Wang K, Kong F, Han X, Zhi Y, Wang H, Ren C, Wang H. Integrative multi-omics reveal NSUN2 facilitates glycolysis and histone lactylation-driven immune evasion in renal carcinoma. Genes and Immunity. 2025;**26**(4):312–323

Chapter 5

T Cell Exhaustion in Chronic Infectious Diseases: Mechanisms, Tissue-Specific Programming and Therapeutic Opportunities

Vanessa Carregaro

Abstract

T cell exhaustion has emerged as a distinct differentiation program that arises in settings of sustained antigenic stimulation, chronic tissue remodeling, and complex regulatory tissue microenvironments. In chronic infectious diseases, including persistent viral infections, tuberculosis, visceral leishmaniasis, and Chagas disease, this functional state does not merely represent a loss of immunological competence but an evolutionary adaptation aimed at limiting tissue damage in the face of long-lasting inflammation. Advances in transcriptomics and epigenomics have revealed that exhaustion comprises hierarchical cellular trajectories in which $TCF\text{-}1^{+}$ progenitor cells retain plasticity and rescue potential, whereas terminally exhausted populations exhibit epigenetic rigidity and irreversible dysfunction. These states are shaped by the integration of multiple axes, including altered antigen presentation, persistent innate signaling (such as TLR–type I interferon (IFN-I) pathways), tissue-imposed metabolic pressures, and regulatory circuits mediated by adenosine, IL-10, PD-1/PD-L1, and other immune checkpoints. Understanding these circuits has direct implications for therapeutic interventions. Although checkpoint blockade shows partial efficacy in some viral infections, its application in parasitic and bacterial diseases can exacerbate immunopathology, highlighting that exhaustion fulfills an essential tissue-protective role in certain contexts. Emerging strategies include the selective modulation of progenitor niches, metabolic interventions, and the fine-tuning of innate pathways that sustain profound states of dysfunction. Thus, integrating cellular mechanisms, tissue microenvironments, and systemic pathophysiology is crucial for developing safe and precise approaches to the management of chronic infections.

Keywords: T cell exhaustion, chronic infectious diseases, inhibitory receptors, transcriptional programming, host–pathogen interactions

1. Introduction

Modern understanding of T cell exhaustion has profoundly reshaped how immune responses in chronic infectious diseases are interpreted. Exhaustion is no longer viewed simply as a progressive loss of function but as an adaptive cellular program induced by persistent antigenic stimulation and continuous regulatory cues present in long-standing inflammatory environments [1]. In prolonged infections such as chronic viral hepatitis, HIV, tuberculosis, and various parasitic diseases, this program involves sustained expression of inhibitory receptors, engagement of transcriptional circuits dominated by factors such as TOX, and the reconfiguration of metabolic pathways. The result is T cells that retain residual effector activity yet remain insufficient to achieve full pathogen control [2].

The tissue microenvironments in which these infections unfold exert a decisive influence on the depth and quality of exhaustion. Tuberculous granulomas, inflamed hepatosplenic regions, hypoxic niches, or tissue microenvironments rich in IL-10, TGF-β, and persistent type I interferons stabilize exhausted phenotypes by reinforcing epigenetic profiles that are difficult to reverse [3]. These factors determine not only the effectiveness of local immune responses but also the clinical course of infection, pathogen burden, extent of tissue damage, and responsiveness to antimicrobial therapies.

A particularly relevant aspect that has emerged in recent years stems from advances in immunobiologics and the study of immune checkpoint pathways. Work in other areas of immunology has refined our understanding of the regulatory functions exerted by molecules such as PD-1, CTLA-4, TIM-3, LAG-3, and TIGIT. These advances have shown that the mechanisms sustaining exhaustion are not restricted to a single disease context but rather reflect general principles of immune regulation. Thus, although chronic infectious diseases exhibit their own specific features, many of the inflammatory processes that support exhaustion, such as persistent activation, low-grade inflammation, metabolic remodeling, and loss of coordination between effector and regulatory pathways, are comparable to those observed in other immune-mediated conditions. This has opened space to consider that strategies originally developed to modulate T cell responses in other settings may offer promising avenues in the context of chronic infections as well [4].

This translational perspective has fueled growing interest in approaches aimed at modulating or reversing exhaustion in infectious diseases. In experimental models, the blockade of inhibitory pathways can partially restore the production of key cytokines, recover cytotoxicity, expand less dysfunctional progenitor populations, and improve pathogen control in specific situations [5]. Clinical evidence in chronic viral hepatitis, tuberculosis, and parasitic infections also suggests that the degree of exhaustion influences treatment responses and relapse risk, indicating that immunomodulatory interventions may play a complementary role alongside conventional antimicrobial therapy [6].

However, this therapeutic potential demands caution. Reactivating T cells within chronically inflamed tissues may have paradoxical effects, including exacerbation of immunopathology, disruption of protective structures such as granulomas, or increased tissue damage driven by uncontrolled inflammation. Recent literature reinforces that exhaustion is a complex regulatory program, strongly shaped by the tissue, the pathogen, and the stage of infection [1]. Consequently, the use of checkpoint inhibitors in chronic infections should not be seen as a simple extension of established approaches but as a field that requires a finely tuned understanding of local biology and the nuances of host–pathogen interactions.

Comprehending T cell exhaustion in chronic infectious diseases, therefore, requires integrating molecular mechanisms, microenvironmental features, clinical implications, and therapeutic limitations. This introduction lays the conceptual foundation for the chapter, which examines how these elements converge to shape immune responses in persistent infections and how accumulated knowledge can guide therapeutic strategies that are safe, effective, and truly capable of advancing the treatment of these diseases (**Figure 1**).

2. Molecular architecture of T cell exhaustion

T cell exhaustion is a sustained functional state supported by a complex, integrated, and relatively stable molecular architecture resulting from the combination of persistent signals derived from the TCR, regulatory cytokines, and adverse metabolic conditions present in chronic infections. Rather than representing a linear loss of effector activity, exhaustion reflects the establishment of a new transcriptional and epigenetic equilibrium that redefines T cell identity. The expression of inhibitory receptors, often used as an operational marker of exhaustion, represents only the most accessible dimension of this phenomenon, since profound changes in intracellular signaling pathways maintain dysfunction even when antigenic stimulation is partially reduced [7].

At the core of this program lies a transcriptional network profoundly reshaped by chronic stimulation. Continuous antigen exposure favors sustained activation of NFAT, uncoupled from AP-1 – a condition that induces genes associated with the exhausted phenotype, such as PDCD1, HAVCR2, and LAG3, while impairing the transcription of effector genes that depend on NFAT–AP-1 cooperation. In parallel, the transcription factor TOX plays a central role in reconfiguring chromatin accessibility and stabilizing exhausted identity. Additional regulators, including the NR4A family, BATF, and EOMES, contribute to the establishment and maintenance of this state by modulating differentiation, survival, and functional suppression [2, 8].

These alterations give rise to a continuum of dysfunctional states composed of progenitor-like and terminally exhausted compartments. Progenitor-like exhausted cells, characterized by TCF-1 expression and a less deeply committed epigenetic profile, retain proliferative capacity and respond more effectively to immunomodulatory interventions. In contrast, terminally exhausted cells exhibit strong epigenetic repression, high co-expression of multiple inhibitory receptors, and severely restricted function. In chronic infections, the balance between these compartments determines whether the host sustains partially effective control or progresses to deeper states of dysfunction [9].

Epigenetic remodeling is another defining element of the exhaustion architecture. Chromatin accessibility studies demonstrate that exhausted T cells present a highly specific epigenetic landscape distinct from that of effector or memory cells. This reconfiguration includes the opening of enhancers associated with the exhaustion program, the closure of regulatory elements linked to memory differentiation, and the consolidation of a remarkably rigid transcriptional identity. Such rigidity helps

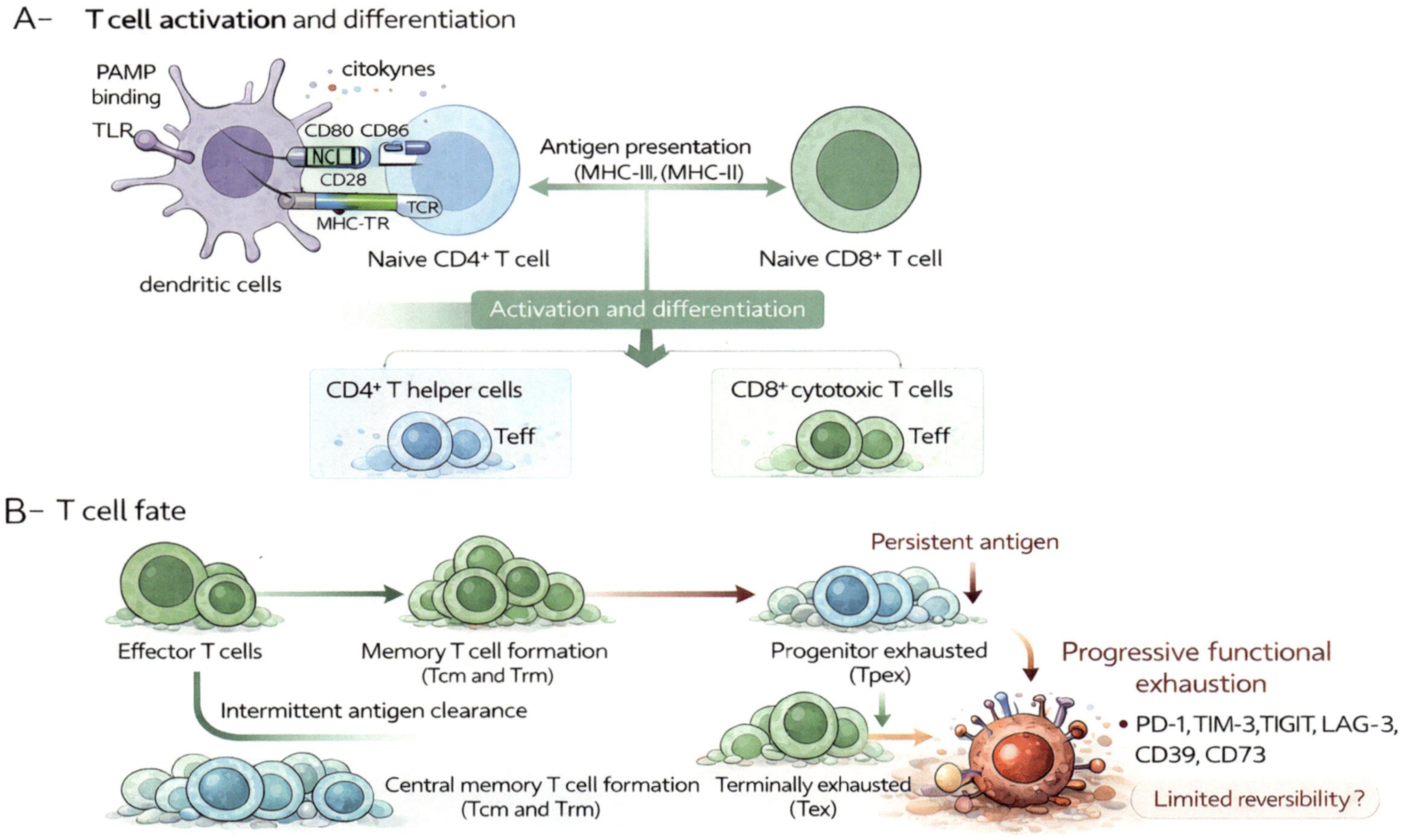

Figure 1.
Activation, differentiation, and fate decisions of T cells under transient versus persistent antigen exposure. (a) Antigen-presenting cells, particularly dendritic cells, sense pathogen-associated molecular patterns (PAMPs) through toll-like receptors (TLRs), inducing cytokine production and upregulation of costimulatory molecules (CD80, CD86). Antigen presentation via MHC-II to CD4+ T cells and MHC-I to CD8⁺ T cells, together with CD28-mediated costimulation and inflammatory cues, initiates naïve T-cell activation and differentiation into helper or cytotoxic effector subsets. (b) T-cell fate is determined by the duration and intensity of antigenic stimulation. Under intermittent antigen exposure, activated CD4⁺ and CD8⁺ T cells undergo clonal expansion, acquire effector functions (IL-2, IFN-γ, TNF), and, after contraction, generate central memory (TCM) and tissue-resident memory (TRM) populations that sustain long-term immunity. In contrast, persistent antigen stimulation induces progressive expression of inhibitory receptors (e.g., PD-1, CTLA-4, TIM-3, TIGIT, LAG-3, CD39, CD73), reduced proliferative capacity, and functional decline in both CD4⁺ and CD8⁺ compartments, culminating in T-cell exhaustion (TEX).

explain the difficulty of fully reversing dysfunction, even after antigen reduction or checkpoint blockade [9].

In summary, the molecular architecture of exhaustion integrates sustained microenvironmental cues with transcriptional and epigenetic circuits that progressively reshape T-cell identity. Understanding these structural components is essential for interpreting the depth of dysfunction observed in chronic infectious diseases and for guiding therapeutic strategies aimed at safely modulating this state.

3. Induction mechanisms and intracellular signaling pathways

T cell exhaustion in chronic infections arises from the sustained convergence of antigenic, cytokine-mediated, and microenvironmental signals that progressively reprogram T cell identity. Continuous antigenic stimulation is the primary initiating event. Unlike acute activation, where TCR signaling is transient and accompanied by strong costimulation, chronic exposure maintains NFAT activity for extended periods under conditions in which AP-1 is insufficiently induced. This imbalance drives a transcriptional profile dominated by NFAT-dependent induction of dysfunction-associated genes such as PDCD1, HAVCR2, and LAG3, while limiting the coordinated expression of effector genes that require NFAT–AP-1 cooperation [10].

A second upstream driver is the decline in CD28-mediated costimulatory signaling, which is critical for sustaining survival and cytotoxic programs. During chronic infections, CD28 pathways become progressively impaired due to reduced receptor expression and microenvironmental suppression of PI3K–AKT signaling. Parallel engagement of inhibitory receptors, such as PD-1, intensifies this suppression through recruitment of phosphatases, including SHP-2, which antagonize key phosphorylation events downstream of the TCR. The resulting reduction in ZAP-70 activation and CD3ζ phosphorylation contributes to the attenuated intracellular signaling cascade characteristic of exhaustion [7].

Regulatory cytokines further consolidate the induction of dysfunctional states. IL-10 signaling limits inflammatory cytokine production and fosters transcriptional profiles associated with reduced effector capacity, whereas TGF-β restricts proliferation and differentiation into robust effector phenotypes. Persistent type I interferons, common in antigen-rich tissues, act synergistically with these cytokines by heightening regulatory tone, diminishing TCR sensitivity, and contributing to proliferative decline [11].

Metabolic and second messenger dynamics also support the induction of exhaustion. Sustained calcium flux leads to prolonged calcineurin activation and persistent NFAT recruitment, reinforcing the exhaustion-associated transcriptional program. Energy restriction, hypoxia, and inflammatory stress favor activation of AMPK and HIF-1α pathways, promoting a shift toward catabolic metabolism and reduced biosynthetic capacity. These pressures facilitate the induction of transcriptional regulators such as NR4A and TOX, which contribute to the establishment of the epigenetic rigidity characteristic of the exhausted state [12].

Together, these signals demonstrate that exhaustion is not a passive consequence of antigen persistence but the result of a coordinated network of upstream pressures that drive and stabilize dysfunctional differentiation. Understanding these induction mechanisms is essential for identifying therapeutic points of intervention and for anticipating contexts in which modulation may exacerbate inflammation or disrupt tissue homeostasis.

4. Immunometabolism and mitochondrial dysfunction in T cell exhaustion

Cellular metabolism is a central determinant of T cell function, and its reconfiguration in chronic infections is a key driver of exhaustion. After acute activation, effector T cells rely heavily on aerobic glycolysis to sustain rapid proliferation, cytokine production, and cytotoxicity. In contrast, memory T cells favor oxidative phosphorylation and lipid metabolism, supporting longevity and robust recall responses. Exhausted T cells, however, do not mirror either of these physiological states. They exhibit fragmented mitochondria, impaired ATP generation, increased reactive oxygen species, and limited replenishment of biosynthetic precursors – features that reflect profound mitochondrial dysfunction induced by the chronically inflamed environment [13].

The tissue microenvironments of persistent infections exert strong pressure on T-cell metabolism. In tuberculous granulomas, for example, the combination of hypoxia, lactate accumulation, intense glucose competition, and high energetic demands of microbicidal phagocytes directly affects T-cell bioenergetics. Chronic activation also leads to reduced expression of glucose transporters and an inability to maintain sustained glycolytic flux, compromising essential effector functions. Diminished mTOR activity, together with increased AMPK signaling, shifts metabolism toward a predominantly catabolic state incompatible with robust effector responses. This imbalance is further exacerbated when inhibitory receptors, such as PD-1, directly modulate metabolic signaling by suppressing PI3K–AKT activation and attenuating anabolic stimuli required for clonal expansion and effector function [14].

Mitochondrial dysfunction in exhausted T cells is not merely a consequence of energy deprivation but a structuring element of cellular identity. Reduced mitochondrial membrane potential, disrupted cristae architecture, and limited capacity to utilize fatty acids collectively impair the efficiency of oxidative phosphorylation. In parallel, the accumulation of oxidative stress impacts ROS-sensitive pathways, including NFAT and calcineurin, thereby perpetuating transcriptional circuits associated with dysfunction. Failure to remodel mitochondrial metabolism prevents T cells from regaining functional plasticity, even in the presence of external stimuli such as antimicrobial therapy or checkpoint blockade [9].

In addition, specific metabolic pathways associated with chronic inflammation profoundly influence the degree and stability of exhaustion. Sustained HIF-1α activation in hypoxic microenvironments enforces a glycolytic bias even when cells are unable to maintain it, aggravating the mismatch between metabolic demand and capacity. Reduced availability of essential amino acids, notably tryptophan and arginine, due to the activity of enzymes such as IDO and arginase, common in regulatory inflammatory settings, limits proliferation and promotes functional decline. Persistent interference with biosynthetic pathways favors the expression of transcriptional regulators such as TOX, NR4A, and BATF, which consolidate the epigenetic rigidity characteristic of exhaustion [15, 16].

Thus, immunometabolism emerges as a fundamental component in the understanding of T-cell exhaustion during chronic infectious diseases. Mitochondrial dysfunction, disruption of anabolic–catabolic balance, nutrient scarcity, and inhibitory receptor signaling converge to shape a deeply constrained functional state. Integrating these elements not only offers a mechanistic explanation for the loss of T-cell efficacy in persistent infections but also reveals potential metabolic points of intervention to partially restore host immunity (**Figure 2**).

5. Tissue microenvironments in chronic infections

T cell exhaustion in chronic infectious diseases cannot be fully understood without considering the tissue microenvironments in which these cells operate. The persistence of infection is associated with inflamed niches where immunological, metabolic, and structural factors converge to shape the depth of dysfunction. In tuberculous granulomas, for instance, the layered architecture, composed of

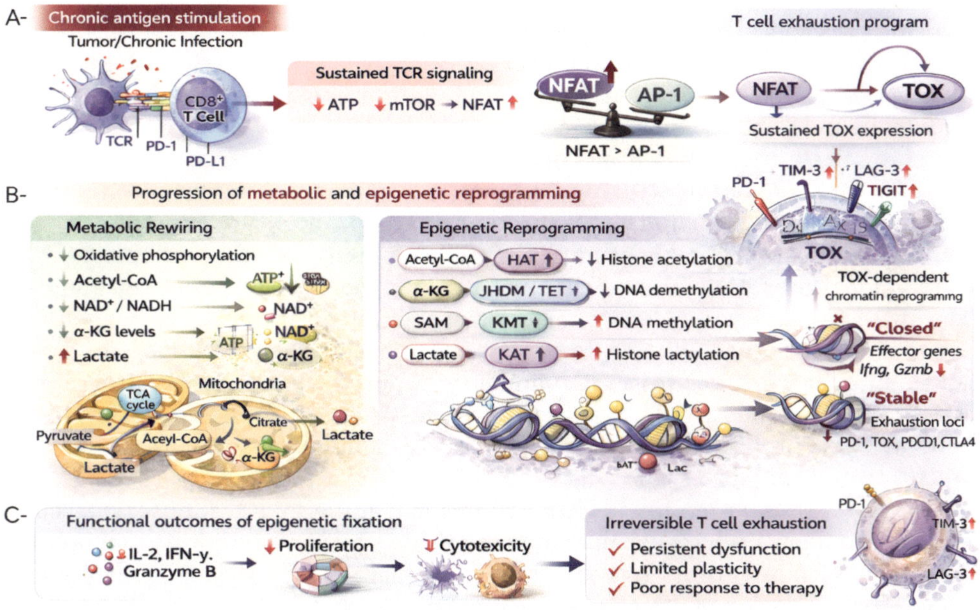

Figure 2.
Signaling–metabolic–epigenetic integration in T cell exhaustion. (a) Chronic antigen stimulation in cancer and persistent infection sustains TCR signaling in the context of reduced mTOR activity and PD-1 engagement. Sustained NFAT activation in the absence of balanced AP-1 cooperation (NFAT > AP-1) promotes TOX induction, establishing the transcriptional circuitry of exhaustion and progressive inhibitory receptor expression. (b) Metabolic rewiring is depicted by colored gradients, which represent the shift from an oxidative, acetyl-CoA–rich state to a hypoxic, lactate-accumulating, α-ketoglutarate (α-KG)–limited environment as exhaustion deepens. These metabolites directly regulate epigenetic enzymes: • Acetyl-CoA sustains histone acetyltransferase activity, • α-KG supports TET and JMJ demethylases, • Lactate promotes histone lactylation and limits α-KG-dependent demethylation, restricting plasticity.these changes remodel enhancers via TOX and increase accessibility at exhaustion-associated loci (e.g., TOX, PDCD1, CTLA4) while constraining effector gene enhancers (e.g., IFNG, GZMB). (c) This epigenetic consolidation enforces reduced cytokine production, impaired proliferation and diminished cytotoxicity, stabilizing a TEX state with limited responsiveness to therapeutic reinvigoration.

differentiated macrophages, fibroblasts, residual neutrophils, and T cells positioned in peripheral zones, creates a singular milieu. High metabolic demands and oxygen consumption by microbicidal phagocytes generate regions of hypoxia, lactate accumulation, and glucose limitation. These metabolic constraints, together with the sustained production of regulatory cytokines such as IL-10, TGF-β, and type I interferons, foster deeply exhausted phenotypes marked by limited proliferation, co-expression of multiple inhibitory receptors, and reduced cytotoxicity. The spatial positioning of T cells within granulomas further shapes this phenomenon: cells located in inner regions tend to display more severe functional impairment than those in peripheral zones, where oxygen and nutrient availability are relatively higher [17, 18].

The liver offers another emblematic example of a microenvironment prone to promoting exhaustion in persistent infections. Even under homeostatic conditions, the liver is highly tolerogenic due to constant exposure to antigens from the portal circulation and the presence of regulatory cells, such as Kupffer cells and stromal cells that produce IL-10 and TGF-β. In chronic infections with hepatotropic viruses or visceral parasites, these characteristics are amplified, creating a scenario in which inhibitory signaling predominates. Continuous type I interferon activity, low-grade inflammatory remodeling, and altered antigen presentation by hepatic dendritic cells collectively drive progressive loss of function in resident T cells. In this setting, $CD8^+$ T cells within the liver parenchyma typically express high levels of PD-1 and exhibit pronounced dysfunction, with minimal residual IFN-γ production and severely compromised cytotoxicity [19].

In the spleen, exhaustion arises in an environment shaped by ongoing systemic inflammation and chronic structural remodeling. In many persistent infections, disruption of germinal centers, expansion of red pulp zones, and alterations in dendritic cell subsets capable of providing full costimulation all contribute to dysfunctional activation. These phenomena reduce the quality of initial priming and perpetuate regulatory signals that favor exhausted phenotypes. The prolonged presence of circulating antigens, together with imbalanced activation of interferon-dependent pathways, creates a predominantly suppressive environment that limits clonal expansion and favors progenitor-like exhausted populations that, despite retaining some proliferative potential, are poorly equipped to generate robust effector responses [20–22].

Mucosal tissues, especially in chronic intestinal and viral infections, represent microenvironments where exhaustion is intensified by persistent inflammation and loss of epithelial integrity. Imbalance among regulatory cells, dysbiotic microbiota, and continuous influx of microbial antigens leads to sustained production of IL-10, IL-27, TGF-β, and tolerogenic mediators such as IDO. These factors, combined with high metabolic demands and competition for essential nutrients imposed by microbiota and local inflammatory cells, create an environment that favors the rapid installation of exhausted states. T cells in these regions often display transcriptional signatures compatible with profound dysfunction, including high expression of TOX, NR4A, and multiple inhibitory receptors, along with progressive loss of IL-2 production and effective cytotoxicity [15].

Therefore, tissue microenvironments in chronic infections modulate not only T-cell functionality but also the degree and qualitative nature of exhaustion. The convergence of metabolic signals, regulatory cytokines, persistent interferons, and structural particularities of each tissue generates conditions in which dysfunction becomes not only probable but biologically advantageous to limit excessive inflammation. Understanding this diversity of niches is crucial for interpreting the heterogeneity of exhaustion across infections and for guiding therapeutic approaches that account for the specificities of each infected tissue.

6. Exhaustion across different classes of chronic infections

T cell exhaustion is a conserved adaptive program across chronic infections, but its dominant drivers and phenotypic consequences vary according to pathogen biology and the tissue microenvironment. Despite these differences, viruses, bacteria, and parasites converge on shared molecular features, including sustained NFAT signaling, induction of TOX and NR4A family members, and progressive loss of proliferative and cytotoxic potential, coupled with regulatory cytokine circuits and metabolic stress.

6.1 Viral infections

In persistent viral infections such as HIV and chronic hepatitis, continuous TCR stimulation and sustained type I interferon production shape T-cell populations marked by PD-1, TOX, and NR4A expression, with progressive loss of clonal expansion and cytotoxicity [23, 24]. These environments are typically rich in IFN-I and regulatory cytokines, which consolidate the transcriptional and epigenetic programs characteristic of exhaustion.

6.2 Bacterial infections: The granuloma as a metabolic–spatial organizer

In tuberculosis, granuloma formation creates highly structured microenvironments characterized by hypoxia, glucose scarcity, and lactate accumulation. These metabolic pressures, combined with persistent antigen load, favor exhaustion, with functional impairment strongly influenced by the spatial localization of T cells within granulomas [1, 3, 25]. Unlike viral infections, where exhaustion emerges primarily from systemic antigenemia and cytokine exposure, granulomas impose tissue-imposed constraints that limit T-cell access to nutrients and oxygen.

6.3 Parasitic infections: Chronicity, regulation, and mixed inflammatory tone

Chronic parasitic diseases introduce additional layers of complexity due to extreme pathogen persistence and intense microenvironmental modulation.

In leishmaniasis, the early response to *Leishmania infantum*, dominated by IFN-γ, IL-1α/β, and IL-18, rapidly evolves into an immunoregulatory milieu enriched with IL-10, TGF-β, IL-27, and type I interferons. This coexistence of protective and suppressive forces fosters exhausted $CD4^+$ and $CD8^+$ T-cell phenotypes characterized by PD-1, CTLA-4, TIGIT, CD39/CD73, and BLIMP-1 expression [25, 26].

Innate immunity plays a structuring role in shaping exhaustion trajectories during *L. infantum* infection. TLR2 is essential for initiating the early inflammatory response, driving myeloid recruitment that subsequently influences T-cell priming and polarization [27]. TLR9 expressed by dendritic cells, further modulates this process by regulating neutrophil recruitment and refining the quality of antigen presentation, thereby impacting T-cell activation and differentiation [28]. In parallel, TLR4 activation engages a TRIF–IRF-1–IFN-β signaling axis that suppresses IL-12 production and limits Th1 responses, an adaptive mechanism that protects tissues but simultaneously allows parasite persistence and deepens T-cell exhaustion [29].

Metabolic constraints further influence T-cell trajectories. The adenosine A2A receptor, highly expressed on exhausted $CD4^{+}CD39^{+}$ T cells, senses adenosine-rich inflamed tissues and diminishes Th1 responses, facilitating parasite escape and contributing to long-lasting dysfunction [30, 31].

6.4 Chronic Chagas disease: Exhaustion as a double-edged sword

In chronic *Trypanosoma cruzi* infection, the persistence of the parasite in the myocardium leads to prolonged inflammation and sustained PD-1 expression on $CD4^{+}$ and $CD8^{+}$ T cells, along with PD-L1/PD-L2 expression on myeloid cells. Experimental blockade of this pathway reduces parasitemia but exacerbates cardiac immunopathology and shortens survival, illustrating the dual character of exhaustion: tissue-protective yet permissive to chronic infection [32, 33].

6.5 Convergent mechanisms across pathogen classes

Endosomal sensors, such as TLR3, TLR7, and TLR9, which are potent inducers of type I interferons, provide a mechanistic bridge linking innate recognition to the stabilization of exhausted T-cell states. These pathways reduce IL-12, increase PD-L1/PD-L2, favor the expansion of Tregs and MDSCs, and may consolidate dysfunctional profiles in prolonged infections caused by *L. infantum* and *L. braziliensis* [34, 35].

Thus, although viruses, bacteria, and parasites engage exhaustion through partially distinct routes – viral antigenemia, spatial metabolic restriction in granulomas, and parasite-driven immunoregulation – they converge on the formation of regulatory tissue microenvironments that balance pathogen control with tissue preservation (**Table 1**).

7. Exhaustion trajectories and reversal potential

T cell exhaustion is no longer regarded as a uniform terminal state of dysfunction but as a continuous program composed of distinct cellular trajectories that emerge as antigenic stimulation persists and microenvironmental conditions evolve. Recent high-resolution transcriptomic and epigenomic studies have demonstrated that exhausted populations include progenitor-like cells with preserved proliferative capacity and terminally differentiated cells that are rigidly fixed in deeply dysfunctional states [5, 36]. This hierarchical organization helps explain why some interventions selectively rescue specific cellular compartments, whereas others fail or amplify undesirable inflammatory responses [37].

Progenitor-like exhausted cells represent the most plastic segment of this continuum. Characterized by TCF-1 expression and intermediate PD-1 levels, they retain epigenetic features associated with memory and proliferation, allowing

Category	Viral infections	Bacterial infections (TB)	Parasitic infections
Dominant drivers	Persistent antigenemia; type I IFN; prolonged NFT.	Granuloma-imposed antigen persistence, hypoxia, metabolic stress	Extreme pathogen persistence; IL-10, TGF-β, IL-27; type I IFN
Transcriptional modules	TOX, NR4A, BATF, Eomes	TOX, NR4A, HIF-1α	BLIMP-1, TOX, NR4A: inhibitory receptor programs
Metabolic constraints	Mitochondrial dysfunction; reduced OXPHOS	Hypoxia; glucose scarcity; lactate; AMPK activation	Adenosine-rich microenvironment (A2a); nutrient depletion
Microenvironment	Systemic IFN-I inflammation	Spatial metabolic and oxygen gradients within granulomas	Liver/spleen remodeling; immunoregulatory cytokines; TLR-driven pressures
Innate sensing pathways	TLR7/9 → IFN-I; plasmacytoid DCs	Macrophage/DC PRRs shaping granuloma metabolism	TLR2, TLR9; TLR4–TRIF–IRF-1 → PD-L1
Exhaustion phenotype	High PD-1, TOX, NR4A; reduced cytotoxicity.	Heterogeneous; location-dependent	Deep dysfunction: PD-1, CTLA-4, TIGIT, CD39/CD73; BLIMP-1 high
Reversibility	Moderate–high	Limited	Very low; high risk upon rescue
Functional consequences	Impaired viral control; partial restoration with PD-1 therapy.	Preserves tissue integrity but restricts bacterial clearance.	Exhaustion balances parasite control and tissue protection; blockade is risky

Table 1.
Comparative features of T-cell exhaustion across chronic viral, bacterial, and parasitic infections.

them to respond more robustly to rescue stimuli such as antimicrobial therapy or checkpoint blockade. Localization of these cells within specialized niches, often near dendritic cells that provide limited costimulation, protects them from excessive antigenic exposure and favors the maintenance of their functional potential [38].

Terminally exhausted cells, by contrast, express high levels of PD-1, TIM-3, TIGIT, and ectoenzymes such as CD39/CD73, together with strong activity of transcription factors such as TOX and NR4A which consolidate stable epigenetic states of dysfunction [38, 39]. These lymphocytes accumulate in highly inflamed regions exposed to hypoxia, oxidative stress, nutrient deprivation, and elevated IL-10, TGF-β, and type I interferons – conditions that reinforce a predominantly regulatory functional profile [19, 26]. The robustness of this program likely underlies their refractoriness to checkpoint blockade and the risk of precipitating immunopathology if such cells are broadly reactivated.

The dynamics of these trajectories reflect interactions among antigenic load, metabolism, and tissue inflammation. In the liver and spleen during *L. infantum* infection, for instance, the combination of sustained type I interferons, adenosine, IL-10, and reduced costimulation imposes pressures that drive progression toward deeply exhausted states. In chronic Chagas disease, the heterogeneity observed among T cells infiltrating the myocardium mirrors local parasite distribution and the intensity of inflammation, demonstrating that exhaustion functions as a self-protective mechanism to limit cardiac damage, even at the cost of suboptimal parasite control [40].

Therapeutic responses may depend, at least in part, on this architecture. The functional restoration observed after PD-1/PD-L1 blockade in some experimental models primarily derives from the expansion of TCF-1⁺ progenitor cells, whereas terminally exhausted cells contribute little to recovery. In chronic parasitic infections, this discrepancy is even more pronounced: although PD-1 blockade can reduce parasite burden, it frequently triggers exuberant inflammation, as seen in models of Chagas cardiomyopathy, where such interventions exacerbate tissue damage and decrease survival [40, 41].

Bioenergetic aspects also decisively influence these trajectories. Progenitor-like cells maintain metabolic flexibility and mitochondrial integrity, whereas terminally exhausted cells exhibit marked dysfunction, accumulation of reactive oxygen species, and limited substrate utilization [42, 43]. Pathways such as A2AR, type I interferons, and innate receptors directly modulate this metabolism and determine how quickly progenitor compartments progress toward epigenetically irreversible states [44].

Thus, the potential reversibility of exhaustion depends less on the removal of a single inhibitory brake and more on the ability to selectively modulate the environment in which T cells differentiate. Promising strategies include the preservation of progenitor niches, fine-tuning antigen presentation, and metabolic interventions that alleviate adverse tissue pressures. In chronic diseases such as visceral leishmaniasis and Chagas disease, any approach must respect the delicate balance between restoring function and avoiding immunopathology – a principle that encapsulates the adaptive role of exhaustion in chronic infections (**Figure 3**).

8. Therapeutic implications and future perspectives

Contemporary understanding of T cell exhaustion has profoundly reshaped the landscape of immunological interventions in chronic infectious diseases. What was once viewed as an irreversible failure of adaptive immunity is now recognized as a regulated differentiation program that balances pathogen control with the preservation of host tissues. This conceptual shift explains why therapeutic strategies borrowed from oncology, particularly checkpoint blockade, often yield heterogeneous and sometimes deleterious outcomes in persistent infections.

The potential reversibility of exhaustion depends fundamentally on the presence of TCF-1⁺ progenitor cells, which retain epigenetic plasticity and relative metabolic integrity [5]. In chronic viral infections, this compartment is frequently preserved, enabling treatments such as anti-PD-1 therapy to promote clonal expansion and partial recovery of effector function. In parasitic and bacterial infections, however, where microenvironments are characterized by sustained inflammation, high type I interferon signaling, elevated adenosine levels, and extensive tissue remodeling, T-cell trajectories tend to shift toward terminal exhaustion. In such settings, therapeutic rescue becomes limited and may even be hazardous [31, 39].

Visceral leishmaniasis exemplifies this dilemma. Excessive IL-10, TGF-β, type I interferons, and PD-L1 expression in the liver and spleen generate rigidly dysfunctional T-cell states, and broad attempts to "reinvigorate" these cells risk disrupting compensatory mechanisms that prevent immunopathology [26]. Chronic

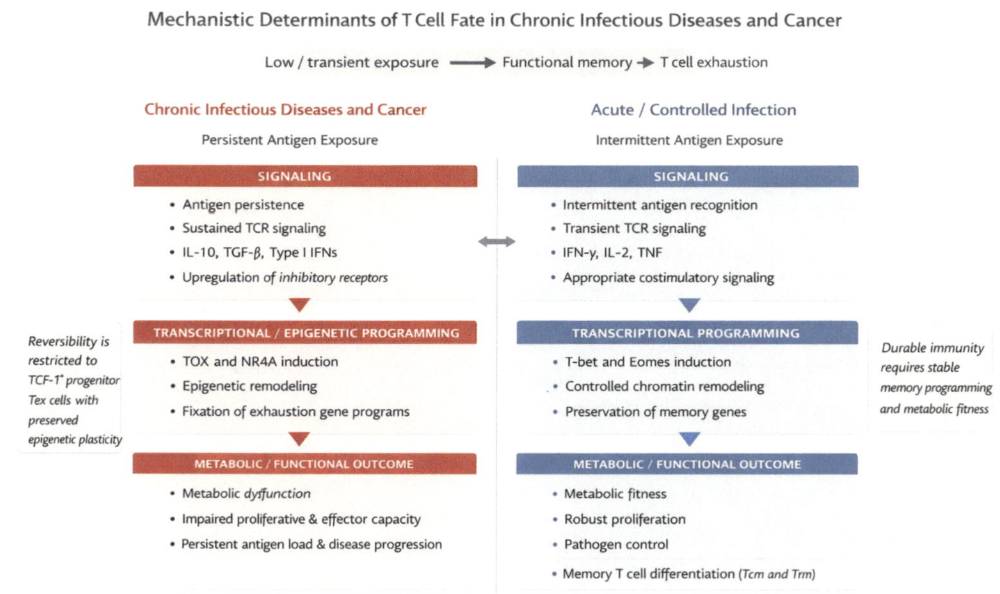

Figure 3.
Mechanistic programming of T-cell fate in chronic infectious diseases and cancer. Persistent antigen exposure in chronic infection and cancer sustains TCR signaling within an immunoregulatory cytokine milieu, driving inhibitory receptor upregulation and TOX/NR4A-dependent transcriptional reprogramming. Progressive chromatin remodeling stabilizes exhaustion-associated gene networks, while metabolic insufficiency limits proliferation and effector output, reinforcing antigen persistence and functional decline. Reversibility is primarily restricted to TCF-1⁺ progenitor-like exhausted T (TEX) cells that retain partial epigenetic plasticity. In contrast, intermittent antigen exposure during acute or controlled infection produces balanced TCR and costimulatory signaling in a proinflammatory context, enabling T-bet/Eomes-driven differentiation without exhaustion-specific epigenetic fixation. Preserved metabolic fitness and chromatin accessibility support robust effector function and pathogen clearance, followed by the formation of durable central and tissue-resident memory T-cell subsets (Tcm, Trm).

Chagas disease presents an even more striking example: although PD-1 blockade reduces *T. cruzi* burden, it simultaneously intensifies myocardial inflammation and decreases survival, demonstrating that exhaustion can serve as a physiological safeguard against tissue damage [41] (**Figure 4**).

These observations have motivated the exploration of more refined therapeutic strategies. Instead of indiscriminately reactivating exhausted cells, emerging approaches aim to modulate progenitor niches, optimize antigen presentation, and restore more favorable microenvironmental conditions. Bioenergetic flexibility, preserved in progenitor-like cells but profoundly compromised in terminally exhausted subsets, has attracted particular interest as a therapeutic entry point. Yet, strategies designed to enhance mitochondrial biogenesis, correct nutrient imbalances, or reduce oxidative stress remain in early experimental stages. Although preclinical data reveal promising biological effects, their translational potential is still uncertain and must be evaluated carefully to avoid precipitating immunopathology, especially in infections defined by fragile host–pathogen equilibria [42, 43].

Another promising direction involves selective targeting of innate pathways that reinforce deep exhaustion, particularly endosomal receptors that sustain type I interferon production. While broad inhibition of these pathways is undesirable,

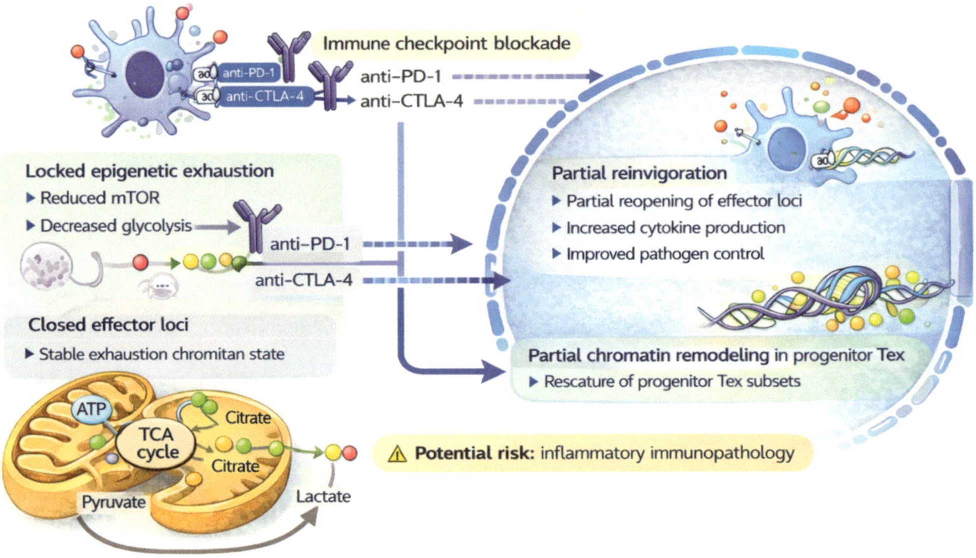

Figure 4.
Immune checkpoint blockade-mediated reinvigoration in chronic infectious diseases. Chronic antigen stimulation promotes sustained inhibitory receptor signaling, reduced mTOR activity, diminished glycolysis and stabilization of a TOX-dependent exhaustion program. This establishes a locked chromatin state with restricted accessibility at effector loci in both progenitor exhausted T cells (TCF-1⁺ TEX) and terminally exhausted T cells (terminal TEX). Checkpoint blockade with anti–PD-1 or anti–CTLA-4 interrupts suppressive signaling and preferentially reinvigorates the TCF-1⁺ progenitor exhausted T-cell subset, which retains epigenetic plasticity. Consequently, partial chromatin remodeling occurs predominantly in progenitor TEX, enabling increased cytokine production and limited reopening of effector loci. Terminally exhausted TEX, depicted in the schematic as non-responsive, exhibit minimal or no remodeling. Excessive reinvigoration may precipitate inflammatory immunopathology.

targeted modulation may reduce PD-L1 and IL-10 expression and rebalance tissue microenvironments without impairing essential antimicrobial immunity [26, 44–46]. The central challenge is to identify the therapeutic "sweet spot" at which T-cell function is sufficiently restored to enhance pathogen control, yet restrained enough to prevent irreversible tissue damage.

Looking forward, effective immunological interventions in chronic infections will likely require multilayered approaches: fine-tuning antigen presentation, implementing context-dependent metabolic modulation, applying selective and temporally controlled checkpoint blockade, and stabilizing progenitor niches. Rather than aiming for full reactivation, the strategic goal is to restore function intelligently within the most therapeutically responsive cellular compartments, aligning intervention intensity with the demands of each infected microenvironment.

In summary, as T cell exhaustion is increasingly understood as an adaptive program rather than a defect, new therapeutic possibilities emerge, not through broad reversal but through precise, proportionate modulation of immune function. Such strategies promise safer and more effective interventions that mirror the complex pathophysiology of chronic infectious diseases marked by persistent inflammation and extensive tissue remodeling.

9. Conclusion

9.1 From dysfunction to regulated adaptation

T cell exhaustion represents one of the most intricate regulatory programs shaping the pathophysiology of chronic infectious diseases. Rather than being a mere state of functional loss, exhaustion emerges as an adaptive trajectory molded by evolutionary pressures that balance pathogen control with the preservation of tissue integrity. As the transcriptional, epigenetic, and metabolic circuits sustaining this program are progressively elucidated, it becomes evident that exhaustion is as heterogeneous as the microenvironments that induce it. Liver, spleen, granulomas, mucosal surfaces, and cardiac tissues each provide distinct configurations of antigenic load, regulatory cytokines, persistent innate signaling, and bioenergetic constraints, thereby defining unique cellular trajectories and degrees of functional rigidity.

In chronic parasitic and bacterial infections, prolonged interplay among inflammation, tissue remodeling, and sustained innate activation establishes contexts in which full reversal of exhaustion is both limited and potentially detrimental. Experience from oncology has demonstrated that potent immune interventions applied without regard to tissue architecture and immunopathological risk may exacerbate pathology and compromise clinical outcomes. These observations underscore the need for therapeutic strategies guided not by indiscriminate immune reactivation but by modulation proportional to the demands of each infected microenvironment.

Emerging evidence highlights promising avenues, including stabilization of progenitor niches, restoration of metabolic competence, selective targeting of innate pathways that perpetuate dysfunctional states, and rational integration of immunotherapy with antimicrobial treatment. The future of translational approaches to chronic infections will depend on combining these strategies with spatial and temporal precision, acknowledging that exhaustion is not merely an obstacle to overcome but a fundamental component of immune equilibrium.

Ultimately, the capacity to determine when exhaustion should be preserved, attenuated, or selectively reversed may redefine therapeutic paradigms for persistent diseases, enabling interventions that are safer, biologically coherent, and aligned with the architecture of host–pathogen interaction.

Abbreviations

TLR	Toll-like receptor
IFN-I	Type I interferon
PD-1	Programmed cell death protein 1
CTLA-4	Cytotoxic T-lymphocyte-associated protein 4
TIM-3	T-cell immunoglobulin and mucin-domain-containing 3
TIGIT	T-cell immunoreceptor with Ig and ITIM domains
CD39/CD73	Ectonucleotidases regulating ATP/adenosine metabolism
TOX	Thymocyte selection–associated high-mobility group box protein
NR4A	Nuclear receptor subfamily 4, group A

BATF	Basic leucine zipper transcription factor ATF-like
TCF-1	T-cell factor 1
mTOR	Mechanistic target of rapamycin
AMPK	AMP-activated protein kinase
HIF-1α	Hypoxia-inducible factor 1 alpha

Funding

The research leading to these results received funding from the São Paulo Research Foundation (FAPESP) under grant agreement n.º 2013/08216-2 (Center for Research in Inflammatory Diseases - CRID) and a Research Project under agreement nº. 2024/04649-6.

Policies and ethical use of artificial intelligence

For the preparation of the figures in this chapter, artificial intelligence tools were used exclusively as technical support for style harmonization, visual standardization, and graphical consistency across all schematics. AI-assisted resources were applied to refine layout, color balance, element alignment, and typographic coherence, without influencing the scientific content or interpretation of the data, which remains entirely the responsibility of the author. All figures were created using *BioRender* under an active institutional license, in full compliance with the platform's terms of use and copyright policies.

Acknowledgment

The author acknowledges the use of *ChatGPT 5.2* for the language polishing of the manuscript.

Author details

Vanessa Carregaro
Department of Biochemistry and Immunology, Ribeirão Preto Medical School, University of São Paulo, Ribeirão Preto, Brazil

*Address all correspondence to: vcarregaro@usp.br; vcarregaro@fmrp.usp.br

References

[1] Wherry EJ. T cell exhaustion. Nature Immunology. 2011;**12**:492–499

[2] Wherry EJ, Kurachi M. Molecular and cellular insights into T cell exhaustion. Nature Reviews Immunology. 2015;**15**:486–499. DOI: 10.1038/nri3862

[3] McCaffrey EF, et al. The immunoregulatory landscape of human tuberculosis granulomas. Nature Immunology. 2022;**23**:318–329

[4] Gern BH, et al. TGFβ restricts expansion, survival, and function of T cells within the tuberculous granuloma. Cell Host & Microbe. 2021;**29**:594–606.e6

[5] Kagoya Y. Dissecting the heterogeneity of exhausted T cells at the molecular level. International Immunology. 2022;**34**:547–553

[6] Ando S, Araki K. CD8 T-cell heterogeneity during T-cell exhaustion and PD-1-targeted immunotherapy. International Immunology. 2022;**34**:571–577

[7] McKinney EF, Lee JC, Jayne DRW, Lyons PA, Smith KGC. T-cell exhaustion, co-stimulation and clinical outcome in autoimmunity and infection. Nature. 2015;**523**: 612–616

[8] Snell LM, McGaha TL, Brooks DG. Type I interferon in chronic virus infection and cancer. Trends in Immunology. 2017;**38**:542–557

[9] Sen DR, et al. The epigenetic landscape of T cell exhaustion. Science (1979). 2016;**354**:1165–1169

[10] Rezazadeh-Gavgani E, Majidazar R, Lotfinejad P, Kazemi T, Shamekh A. Immune Checkpoint Molecules: A Review on Pathways and Immunotherapy Implications. Immunity, Inflammation and Disease. 2025;**13**(4):e70196

[11] Saeidi A, et al. T-Cell Exhaustion in Chronic Infections: Reversing the State of Exhaustion and Reinvigorating Optimal Protective Immune Responses. Frontiers in Immunology. 2018;**9**:2569

[12] Hashimoto M, et al. CD8 T cell exhaustion in chronic infection and cancer: Opportunities for interventions. Annual Review of Medicine. 2018;**69**:301–318

[13] Belk JA, Daniel B, Satpathy AT. Epigenetic regulation of T cell exhaustion. Nature Immunology. 2022;**23**:848–860

[14] Beltra J-C, et al. Developmental Relationships of Four Exhausted CD8+ T Cell Subsets Reveals Underlying Transcriptional and Epigenetic Landscape Control Mechanisms. Immunity. 2020;**52**:825–841.e8

[15] Khan O, et al. TOX transcriptionally and epigenetically programs CD8+ T cell exhaustion. Nature. 2019;**571**:211–218

[16] Sullivan RJ, Weber JS. Immune-related toxicities of checkpoint inhibitors: Mechanisms and mitigation strategies. Nature Reviews Drug Discovery. 2022;**21**:495–508

[17] Weiss SA, et al. Epigenetic tuning of PD-1 expression improves exhausted

T cell function and viral control. Nature Immunology. 2024;**25**:1871–1883

[18] Bengsch B, et al. Bioenergetic insufficiencies due to metabolic alterations regulated by the Inhibitory Receptor PD-1 Are an Early Driver of CD8 + T Cell Exhaustion. Immunity. 2016;**45**:358–373

[19] Chen Z, Zhu Z, Hu T, Yao C, Wu T. Regulation of T cell exhaustion and stemness: Molecular mechanisms and implications for cancer immunotherapy. Cellular & Molecular Immunology. 2025;**23**:1–14

[20] Bronte V, Pittet MJ. The Spleen in Local and Systemic Regulation of Immunity. Immunity. 2013;**39**:806–818

[21] Ghosh D, Stumhofer JS. The spleen: "epicenter" in malaria infection and immunity. Journal of Leukocyte Biology. 2021;**110**:753–769

[22] Singh A, et al. Allospecific splenic Tr1 cells drive effector T cell exhaustion through up-regulated Areg-EGFR signaling to promote transplant tolerance. Science Advances. 2026;**12**: eaea0567

[23] Franco F, Jaccard A, Romero P, Yu Y-R, Ho P-C. Metabolic and epigenetic regulation of T-cell exhaustion. Nature Metabolism. 2020;**2**:1001–1012

[24] Bertoletti A. T cell fitness in the liver: How can T cells keep it up? Journal of Hepatology. 2016;**64**:1208–1210

[25] Ma S, Ming Y, Wu J, Cui G. Cellular metabolism regulates the differentiation and function of T-cell subsets. Cellular & Molecular Immunology. 2024;**21**:419–435

[26] Costa-Madeira JC, Trindade GB, Almeida PHP, Silva JS, Carregaro V. T Lymphocyte Exhaustion During Human and Experimental Visceral Leishmaniasis. Frontiers in Immunology. 2022;**13**:835711

[27] Sacramento LA, et al. Toll-Like Receptor 2 Is Required for Inflammatory Process Development during Leishmania infantum Infection. Frontiers in Microbiology. 2017;**8**:262

[28] Sacramento L, et al. Toll-Like Receptor 9 Signaling in Dendritic Cells Regulates Neutrophil Recruitment to Inflammatory Foci following Leishmania infantum Infection. Infection and Immunity. 2015;**83**:4604–4616

[29] Sacramento LA, et al. TLR4 abrogates the Th1 immune response through IRF1 and IFN-β to prevent immunopathology during L. infantum infection. PLOS Pathogens. 2020;**16**: e1008435

[30] Lima MHF, et al. Leishmania infantum Parasites Subvert the Host Inflammatory Response through the Adenosine A2A Receptor to Promote the Establishment of Infection. Frontiers in Immunology. 2017;**8**:815. DOI: 10.3389/fimmu.2017.00815

[31] Li J, et al. Reversal of the CD8+ T-Cell Exhaustion Induced by Chronic HIV-1 Infection Through Combined Blockade of the Adenosine and PD-1 Pathways. Frontiers in Immunology. 2021;**12**:687296

[32] Fonseca R, et al. Programmed Cell Death Protein 1–PDL1 Interaction Prevents Heart Damage in Chronic Trypanosoma cruzi Infection. Frontiers in Immunology. 2018;**9**:997

[33] Arana Y, Gálvez RI, Jacobs T. Role of the PD-1/PD-L1 Pathway in Experimental Trypanosoma cruzi Infection and Potential Therapeutic Options. Frontiers in Immunology. 2022;**13**:866120

[34] Lind NA, Rael VE, Pestal K, Liu B, Barton GM. Regulation of the nucleic acid-sensing Toll-like receptors. Nature Reviews Immunology. 2022;**22**:224–235

[35] Utzschneider DT, et al. T cell factor 1-expressing memory-like CD8+ T cells sustain the immune response to chronic viral infections. Immunity. 2016;**45**:415–427

[36] Zhou W, et al. Stem-like progenitor and terminally differentiated TFH-like CD4+ T cell exhaustion in the tumor microenvironment. Cell Reports. 2024;**43**:113797

[37] Zhong T, Sun S, Zhao M, Zhang B, Xiong H. The mechanisms and clinical significance of CD8+ T cell exhaustion in anti-tumor immunity. Cancer Biology & Medicine. 2025;1–21. DOI: 10.20892/j.issn.2095-3941.2024.0628

[38] Kratchmarov R, Magun AM, Reiner SL. TCF1 expression marks self-renewing human CD8+ T cells. Blood Advances. 2018;**2**:1685–1690

[39] Pauken KE, et al. Epigenetic stability of exhausted T cells limits durability of reinvigoration by PD-1 blockade. Science (1979). 2016;**354**:1160–1165

[40] Benevides L, et al. Blimp-1 signaling pathways in T lymphocytes is essential to control the Trypanosoma cruzi infection-induced inflammation. Frontiers in Immunology. 2023;**14**:1268196. DOI: 10.3389/fimmu.2023.1268196

[41] Gutierrez FRS, et al. Regulation of Trypanosoma cruzi-Induced Myocarditis by Programmed Death Cell Receptor 1. Infection and Immunity. 2011;**79**:1873–1881

[42] Wang L, et al. Regulatory T cells in homeostasis and disease: Molecular mechanisms and therapeutic potential. Signal Transduction and Targeted Therapy. 2025;**10**:345

[43] Bhatti GK, et al. Targeting mitochondrial bioenergetics as a promising therapeutic strategy in metabolic and neurodegenerative diseases. Biomedical Journal. 2022;**45**:733–748

[44] Wu H, Campillo Prados M, Vaeth M. Metabolic Regulation of T Cell Exhaustion. Immune Discovery. 2025;**1**:10005–10005

[45] Sumida TS, et al. Type I interferon transcriptional network regulates expression of coinhibitory receptors in human T cells. Nature Immunology. 2022;**23**:632–642

[46] Wu Y, et al. Revitalizing T cells: Breakthroughs and challenges in overcoming T cell exhaustion. Signal Transduction and Targeted Therapy. 2026;**11**(1):2

Chapter 6

T Cells in Disease: From Dysregulation to Therapeutic Innovation

Jinping Shu, Zaid Talal Abdulqader Al-Qadhi, Somia Shehzadi, Zhipeng Zhao and Ling Yin

Abstract

T cells play an indispensable role in resisting infections, eliminating malignant cells, and maintaining immune homeostasis as the core component of adaptive immunity. They achieve this through precise antigen-specific recognition via T cell receptors and subsequent orchestration of targeted immune responses. However, dysregulation of T cell function can lead to a series of health issues, including autoimmunity, infectious diseases and cancer, where either excessive activation or functional exhaustion disrupts the delicate balance of immune regulation. Currently, strategies targeting inhibitory signals in cancer immunotherapy have been extensively studied, immune checkpoint inhibitors such as PD-1 and CTLA-4 antibodies have been applied in the treatment of various types of cancer with remarkable clinical efficacy across multiple malignancies. Additionally, emerging therapies such as Chimeric antigen receptor T (CAR-T) cell therapy and antibody-drug conjugates (ADCs) have demonstrated their potential in enhancing anti-tumor immune responses by precisely redirecting and potentiating T cell activity against tumor cells while sparing healthy tissues. Nevertheless, defects in T cells can also result in insufficient adaptive immune defense, leading to severe consequences such as heightened vulnerability to opportunistic infections and malignancies. Primary immunodeficiencies (e.g., severe combined immunodeficiency) and secondary immunodeficiencies (e.g., immunodeficiency caused by HIV infection) are largely attributed to the loss or impairment of T cell function, often manifesting as profound and life-threatening clinical presentations from early life or progressive stages. For these immunodeficiency diseases, the development of cutting-edge therapies is advancing rapidly, including new technologies such as gene therapy and cell therapy, which are offering new hope to patients by enabling precise correction of genetic defects and restoration of functional T cell populations for sustained immune reconstitution.

Keywords: T cells, autoimmunity, cancer immunotherapy, infectious diseases, immunodeficiency

1. Introduction

T lymphocytes (T cells) are the core of the adaptive immune system, originating from the bone marrow and migrating to peripheral lymphoid tissue after thymus maturation. They recognize antigens through the T-cell receptor (TCR), directly participate in cellular immunity, and secrete cytokines to regulate global immune responses, playing a key role in the initiation, amplification, and regulation of immune responses. The specificity, memory, and self-tolerance of adaptive immunity also mainly rely on T cells – maintained by the diverse recognition and clonal expansion of TCR to form memory cells, as well as the role of thymic negative selection and regulatory T cells (Tregs). Therefore, the normal function of T cells is crucial for the body to resist infections, clear abnormal cells, and maintain internal environmental stability.

Once T-cell function is imbalanced, it can lead to various diseases. In autoimmune diseases, self-reactive T cells attack their own tissues; in infectious diseases, their insufficient function can easily cause chronic infection; in the tumor microenvironment (TME), T cells often become exhausted and unable to effectively eliminate cancer cells. With a deeper understanding of the biological mechanisms of T cells, immunotherapy targeting T cells has become an important breakthrough direction: ICIs enhance antitumor responses by releasing T-cell inhibitory signals; CAR-T therapy enhances the targeted killing ability of T cells against tumors through genetic modification; the combination of antibody–drug conjugates (ADCs) and immunosuppressants can improve the TME and enhance antigen presentation. These cutting-edge strategies provide new therapeutic hope for difficult-to-treat diseases such as tumors and autoimmune diseases [1, 2].

This chapter aims to systematically elaborate on the biological characteristics, functional classification, and mechanisms of action of T cells in the occurrence and development of diseases, and comprehensively introduce immunotherapy strategies based on T cells.

2. Biological basis of T cells

2.1 T-cell development and differentiation

T cells develop in the thymus through a process that exhibits particular features. Cells originating from the bone marrow migrate to the thymus and undergo changes in the structure of their receptors. This process generates a wide range of different receptor forms. Subsequently, through critical screening, positive selection equips them with the ability to recognize their own major histocompatibility complex (MHC) molecules (i.e., MHC restriction), while negative selection eliminates self-reactive clones to establish immune tolerance, thereby selecting mature naive T cells to enter the periphery [3, 4].

After encountering antigens in the periphery, naïve T cells are activated, proliferate, and differentiate into functional subgroups, mainly including cytotoxic T cells, helper T cells, Tregs, and long-term surviving memory cells (see **Figure 1**). This process is the cornerstone of cellular immunity; however, if disrupted, it can lead to immune deficiencies, autoimmune diseases, or tumors. The CAR-T therapy

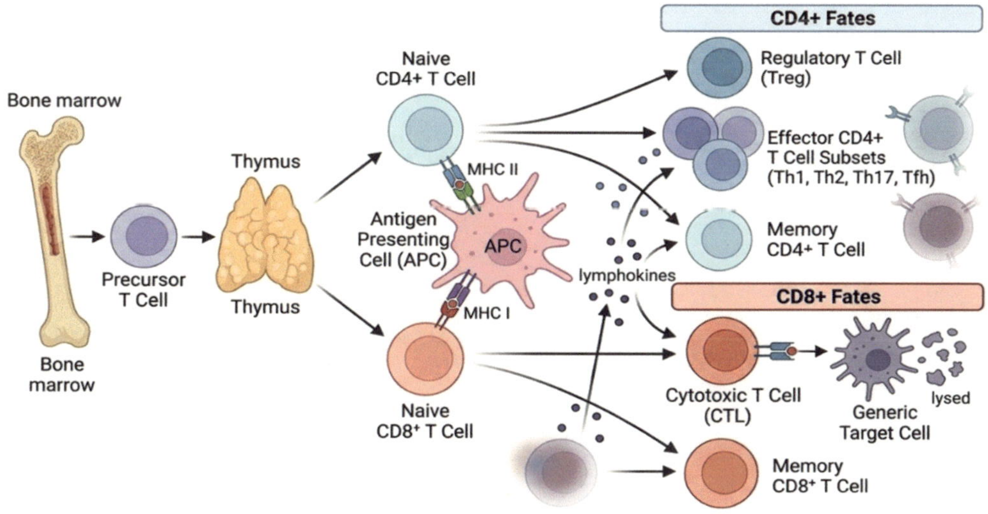

Figure 1.
Schematic overview of T-cell development and differentiation in the thymus. Multipotent hematopoietic stem cells from the bone marrow give rise to progenitor cells that migrate to the thymus. Within the thymic cortex and medulla, T-cell precursors undergo T-cell receptor gene rearrangement, generating a diverse TCR repertoire. Subsequent positive selection ensures MHC restriction, while negative selection eliminates self-reactive clones to establish central tolerance. Finally, mature naive T cells egress into the peripheral lymphoid organs. This diagram outlines the key stages in the establishment of the T-cell immune repertoire.

and ICIs, based on this biological principle, have become important treatment methods [5–7].

2.2 Subset classification and functional characteristics of T cells

The T cells can be classified according to multiple criteria: (i) differentiation status – naive, effector, and memory T cells; (ii) TCR composition – αβ T cells and γδ T cells; (iii) CD molecule expression – $CD4^+$ and $CD8^+$ T cells [8]; (iv) function – helper (Th), cytotoxic (Tc), and regulatory (Treg) T cells [9–11].

2.2.1 $CD4^+$ helper T cells

The $CD4^+$ T cells are activated upon recognition of MHC II antigen–peptide complexes on the surface of antigen-presenting cells (APCs) and differentiate into subgroups of helper T cells with diverse functions, including Th1, Th2, Th17, follicular helper T cells (Tfh), and Tregs. Each subgroup exerts different immune regulatory functions by secreting specific cytokines.

Th1 cells secrete interferon-gamma (IFN-γ), which dominates cellular immunity and fights against intracellular pathogens. The Th2 cells produce interleukin-4 (IL-4) and other cytokines, which are involved in humoral immunity, antiparasitic infections, and allergic reactions. The Th17 cells secrete IL-17, which enhances mucosal defense and is associated with autoimmune diseases. Follicular helper T cells (Tfh) are located in lymphoid follicles and assist in B-cell differentiation and antibody production through IL-21. Tregs are responsible for suppressing immune responses and maintaining self-tolerance [12].

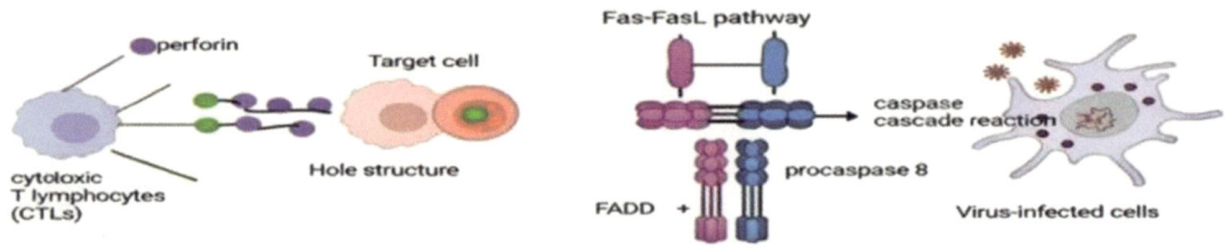

Figure 2.
Two primary mechanisms of target cell lysis by cytotoxic T lymphocytes. Pathway 1 (perforin/granzyme pathway): The CTLs release cytotoxic granules containing perforin and granzymes. Perforin forms pores in the target cell membrane, allowing granzymes to enter the cytoplasm and induce apoptosis. Pathway 2 (death receptor pathway): The Fas ligand on the CTL surface engages the Fas receptor on the target cell, triggering the intracellular caspase cascade and leading to apoptosis. These two mechanisms act in concert to efficiently eliminate virus-infected or malignant cells.

2.2.2 CD8⁺cytotoxic T cells

The CD8⁺ T cells recognize MHC I molecule antigen-peptide complexes on the surface of target cells and differentiate into cytotoxic T lymphocytes (CTLs) after activation. The CTLs kill target cells through two main mechanisms: One is to induce apoptosis of target cells by releasing perforin and granzyme; the other is to induce apoptosis of target cells through the Fas–FasL pathway (see **Figure 2**). The CD8⁺ T cells play a crucial role in clearing virus-infected cells, tumor cells, and intracellular pathogen-infected cells [8].

2.2.3 Tregs

Tregs are a crucial subset for maintaining immune tolerance and homeostasis, which mainly include cells that regulate naturally and cells that regulate through induction. These regulatory cells inhibit responses through different approaches, which include producing cytokines that inhibit, such as IL-10 and TGF-beta, removing IL-2, and directly killing cells that provide effects. When the function of regulatory cells shows problems, this can result in diseases with autoimmune features or deficiencies in the response [13–17].

2.3 TCR and signal transduction

The TCR is the molecular basis for T-cell-specific recognition of antigens, mainly composed of alpha and beta chains. Its variable region generates extremely high diversity through V(D)J gene rearrangement and can recognize a large number of antigens.

The TCR signaling transduction is a complex process involving cascade reactions of multiple signaling molecules. When TCR recognizes antigens, the ITAM motif of CD3 complex is phosphorylated, activating ZAP-70 kinase, which then transmits activation signals through downstream Ras-MAPK, PLC-γ-Ca^{2+}, and PKCθ-NF-κB signaling pathways.

T-cell activation also requires costimulatory signals, such as CD28/B7; the absence of costimulatory signals can lead to the dysfunction or apoptosis of T cells. On the contrary, inhibitory signals, such as cytotoxic T-lymphocyte–associated protein 4 (CTLA-4) and programmed cell death protein 1 (PD-1), prevent excessive responses. The dynamic balance of these two types of signals is crucial for immune homeostasis [18].

2.4 Metabolic regulation of T cells

Naive T cells are powered by oxidative phosphorylation to maintain a resting state; after activation, they quickly turn to glycolysis (Warburg effect) to rapidly synthesize biomolecules, meeting the needs of proliferation and effector functions.

T-cell subsets have different characteristic metabolic patterns: Effector T cells (such as Th1, Th17) are highly dependent on glycolysis, while memory T cells and Tregs rely on fatty acid oxidation and mitochondrial metabolism. These metabolic differences support their respective functional characteristics and become potential targets for immune regulation.

Tumor cells compete for nutrients (such as glucose) and produce metabolites, such as lactate, inhibiting the metabolic pathways of T cells and leading to their functional exhaustion in the TME. Hypoxia and malnutrition further promote T-cell metabolic reprogramming, exacerbating the formation of the exhaustion phenotype [19, 20].

3. The mechanism of T cells in autoimmune diseases

3.1 Immunological basis of autoimmune diseases

Autoimmune disease is a condition in which the immune system abnormally attacks its own tissues, leading to damage and functional impairment. Its occurrence is related to various factors, such as genetic, environmental, and immune regulatory imbalances.

Genetic factors are crucial in the development of autoimmune diseases, with the human leukocyte antigen (HLA) gene being especially important. Certain HLA alleles are strongly linked to disease risk, such as HLA-DR4 in rheumatoid arthritis (RA) and HLA-DR2 in multiple sclerosis (MS). These molecules play a key role in triggering autoimmune responses by influencing antigen presentation and T-cell recognition [21].

Environmental factors, such as infections, medications, and chemical exposures, can disrupt self-tolerance and trigger abnormal immune responses through mechanisms such as molecular mimicry and epitope spreading. Additionally, the breakdown of central and peripheral tolerance mechanisms (such as thymic negative selection and Treg function) results in the activation of self-reactive T and B cells, which then attack the body's own tissues [10, 22–26].

3.2 T-cell pathological mechanism in RA

Rheumatoid arthritis is a chronic systemic autoimmune disease primarily characterized by symmetrical polyarthritis, marked by synovial inflammation and destruction of articular cartilage and bone. T cells (mainly $CD4^+$ T cells, Ths) play a central role in the pathogenesis of RA [27].

3.2.1 Self-antigen recognition and T-cell activation

Citrullinated protein is the main self-antigen of RA. Citrullinated protein can be taken up and processed by APCs, presented to $CD4^+$ T cells through MHC II molecules, and trigger an autoimmune response.

Activated APCs in RA patients expressed costimulatory molecules and cytokines, which support $CD4^+$ T-cell activation and promote their differentiation into pathogenic effector subgroups such as Th1 and Th17.

3.2.2 Pathogenic effects of Th1 and Th17 cells

Th1 cells activate macrophages and synovial cells by secreting cytokines (IFN-γ/TNF-α), exacerbating inflammation and tissue damage. Th17 cells mainly secrete IL-17, which can recruit neutrophils and promote osteoclast differentiation, leading to bone resorption.

The IL-17 can directly stimulate synovial cells to produce various inflammatory mediators and destructive enzymes, directly participate in joint destruction, and promote B cells to produce autoantibodies, amplifying the autoimmune response [28–30].

3.2.3 Dysfunction of Tregs

Studies have shown that the proportion of Tregs in RA patients may be normal or even elevated, but their ability to suppress immune responses is significantly impaired.

The mechanisms behind Treg dysfunction include unstable Foxp3 expression, insufficient production of inhibitory cytokines, and the impact of the inflammatory microenvironment. For example, the proinflammatory cytokine IL-6 not only reduces Treg function but also promotes the differentiation of pathogenic Th17 cells, contributing to an imbalance in immune tolerance and the progression of the disease [31].

3.2.4 The role of follicular helper T cells

Follicular helper T cells (Tfh) are a subset of $CD4^+$ T cells located in lymphoid follicles that promote B-cell differentiation into plasma cells and memory B cells by secreting IL-21. There are ectopic lymphoid follicles in the synovial tissue of RA patients, which are rich in Tfh cells and B cells.

The Tfh cells drive self-reactive B cells to produce autoantibodies (such as rheumatoid factor [RF] and anticitrullinated protein antibody [ACPA]), which, in turn, form immune complexes that exacerbate inflammation and tissue damage by activating the complement system [32].

3.3 T-cell pathological mechanisms in MS

Multiple sclerosis is an inflammatory demyelinating disease of the central nervous system. T cells (especially autoreactive $CD4^+$ T cells) play a central role in the pathogenesis of MS [33].

3.3.1 Self-antigen recognition and blood–brain barrier crossing

The main self-antigens of MS are myelin proteins, including myelin basic protein (MBP), myelin-associated glycoprotein (MAG), proteolipid protein (PLP), etc. These antigens are processed by APCs in peripheral immune organs and presented to $CD4^+$ T cells through MHC II molecules [33].

Activated self-reactive T cells express adhesion molecules and chemokine receptors, enabling them to interact with endothelial cells of the blood–brain barrier and cross the barrier into the central nervous system. This process involves multiple steps, such as rolling adhesion, tight adhesion, and transendothelial migration between T cells and endothelial cells.

3.3.2 Pathogenic effects of Th1 and Th17 cells

Th1 and Th17 cells are the most important effector T-cell subsets in the pathogenesis of MS. Th1 cells activate microglia and macrophages by secreting IFN-γ, promoting inflammatory reactions and demyelination. IFN-γ can also upregulate the expression of MHC II molecules, enhance antigen presentation, and amplify autoimmune reactions. Th17 cells promote increased blood–brain barrier permeability by secreting IL-17, recruiting neutrophils and monocytes, and directly damaging oligodendrocytes and neurons [28–30].

3.3.3 Interaction between genetic and environmental factors

Genetic factors are an important basis for the onset of MS, among which the HLA-DR15 haplotype is currently the strongest known genetic risk factor. This haplotype can participate in shaping the self-reactive T-cell pool by presenting exogenous peptides and self-antigen peptides.

Among environmental factors, Epstein–Barr (EB) virus infection is a key trigger for the occurrence of MS. It can induce the production of cross-reactive T cells through mechanisms such as "molecular simulation." These cells can simultaneously recognize EB virus antigens and their own myelin antigens, thereby breaking their own tolerance and initiating autoimmune attacks [34].

3.3.4 Dysfunction of Tregs

Tregs function in MS patients is impaired, preventing the effective suppression of self-reactive T-cell activation. The mechanisms of Tregs dysfunction include lower expression of Foxp3, reduced production of inhibitory cytokines, and a diminished response to IL-2. Furthermore, the inflammatory environment in MS patients can also impact Treg function, with proinflammatory cytokines such as IL-6 hindering Treg differentiation and activity [33, 35].

3.4 The role of T cells in other autoimmune diseases

T cells are also crucial in other autoimmune diseases besides RA and MS. For example, in systemic lupus erythematosus (SLE), self-reactive T cells support B cells in producing auto antibodies against nuclear antigens, leading to the formation of immune complexes that deposit in organs and cause damage. In type 1 diabetes, autoreactive T cells attack beta cells in the pancreas, resulting in insufficient insulin production. While the mechanisms may differ, autoimmune diseases typically share the common features of abnormal activation of self-reactive T cells and dysfunction of Tregs (see **Figure 3**). This understanding provides a theoretical basis for developing T-cell–targeted therapeutic strategies [6, 32, 36].

4. The function of T cells in infectious diseases

4.1 The role of T cells in the adaptive immune response

T cells are the core of adaptive immune defense in infectious diseases. The APCs (such as dendritic cells) capture and process pathogen antigens,

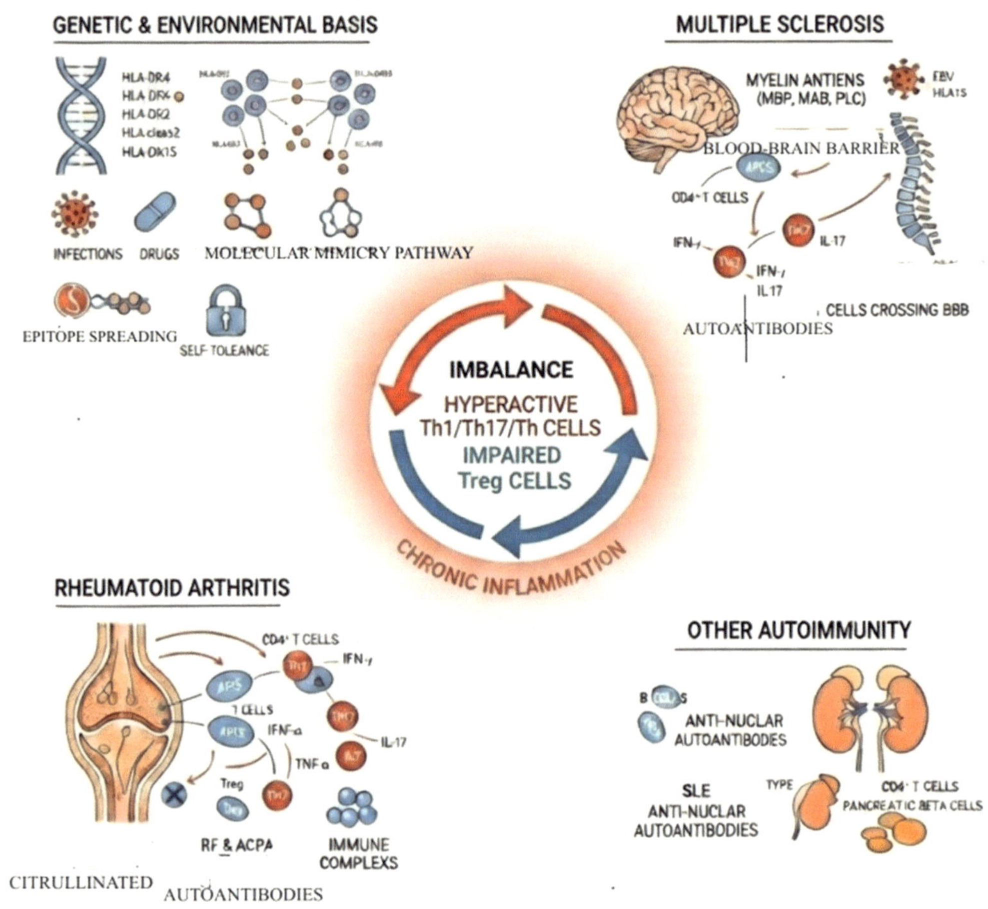

Figure 3.
The mechanism of action of T cells in autoimmune diseases: (a) Genetic and environmental basis: Human leukocyte antigen (HLA) alleles influence antigen presentation and T-cell recognition in triggering autoimmune responses. Environmental factors such as infections, medications, and chemical exposures can disrupt self-tolerance and trigger abnormal immune responses through molecular mimicry and epitope spreading. (b) RA: The citrullinated self-proteins and peptide segments are wrongly recognized, which leads to triggering abnormal autoimmune response. (c) MS: Genetic body (such as with HLA-DR15) and environmental factors (such as EBV infection) can lead to abnormal activation of T cells (mainly Th1 and Th17 cells), which can cross the blood–brain barrier and infiltrate the white matter regions of the brain and spinal cord. (d) Other autoimmune diseases: Abnormal activation of self-reactive T cells and dysfunction of tregs. In SLE, self-reactive T cells support B cells in producing autoantibodies against nuclear antigens, leading to the formation of immune complexes that deposit in organs and cause damage.

present them to T cells through MHC molecules, and initiate specific immune responses.

The CD4⁺ T cells play a crucial coordinating role and can differentiate into different functional subgroups: Th1 cells activate macrophages through IFN-γ to clear intracellular pathogens such as viruses and tuberculosis bacteria; Th2 cells fight against parasites through IL-4 and other mechanisms; Th17 cells recruit neutrophils through IL-17 to resist fungi and extracellular bacteria; Tfh cells assist B cells in producing antibodies [7].

The CD8⁺ T cells directly kill infected cells by recognizing antigen peptides presented by MHC I molecules, releasing perforin/granzyme, or inducing apoptosis of target cells through the Fas–FasL pathway, thereby clearing host cells hidden by pathogens.

4.2 T-cell response in viral infection

Viral infection can trigger a strong T-cell response, which covers the entire stage from antigen recognition, activation, and amplification to effector effects and memory formation. The response characteristics triggered by different viruses vary, reflecting the complex interactions between the virus and the host immune system.

Acute viral infections (such as influenza virus and respiratory syncytial virus) can lead to a rapid and robust T-cell response. The $CD8^+$ T cells undergo extensive expansion to directly eliminate infected cells. After the infection, most effector T cells die off, but a small subset transforms into memory T cells that provide long-term protection and can respond quickly to future infections.

Chronic viral infections (such as human immunodeficiency virus [HIV], Hepatitis C virus [HCV], Hepatitis B virus [HBV]) can cause T-cell exhaustion. Ongoing antigen stimulation depletes virus-specific T-cells, resulting in reduced function and increased expression of inhibitory receptors (such as PD-1, TIM-3, LAG-3), making it harder to effectively control the virus.

Latent viral infections (such as EBV, cytomegalovirus [CMV], herpes simplex virus [HSV]) are characterized by long-term persistence under immune control. These infections stimulate the production of numerous memory T cells, which continually monitor and clear reactivated viruses. However, this strong immune response can consume a significant amount of immune resources [37].

4.3 T-cell response in bacterial infection

T-cell response induced by bacterial infection varies depending on the bacteria type and infection site. Intracellular bacteria mainly trigger Th1-type responses, while extracellular bacteria tend to induce Th17-type responses.

Intracellular bacteria, such as Mycobacterium tuberculosis, trigger strong Th1 immunity. Activated Th1 cells secrete IFN-γ, activate macrophages to enhance their bactericidal ability, and promote granuloma formation to limit infection, but may also become lesions where bacteria remain.

Extracellular bacteria, such as Staphylococcus aureus, elicit an immune response dominated by Th17 cells. Th17 cells recruit and activate neutrophils by secreting IL-17 and enhance epithelial barrier function by utilizing IL-22, thereby playing a critical protective role in skin and mucosal infections. In addition, certain extracellular bacterial infections (such as Listeria monocytogenes) can also induce strong $CD8^+$ T-cell responses, reflecting the diversity of response mechanisms and their coevolution with pathogens [38].

4.4 Memory T-cell and vaccine design

Memory T-cell is the core to achieving long-term immune protection. Based on surface markers and tissue distribution, memory T cells can be divided into central memory T cells (Tcm, mainly located in lymphoid tissue, with strong proliferation ability), effector memory T cells (Tem, distributed in the periphery, capable of quickly functioning), and tissue-resident memory T cells (Trm, residing in specific tissues, providing local defense). These three types of memory T cells collectively provide systemic and local immune protection [39].

Next-generation vaccines, such as mRNA and viral vector vaccines, can effectively induce robust and sustained T-cell responses. For example, the COVID-19 mRNA vaccine can stimulate polyclonal $CD4^+$ and $CD8^+$ T cells that target viral proteins, offering the advantage of recognizing conserved epitopes, ensuring cross-reactivity with variants, eliminating infected cells, and providing critical protection even when antibody levels decline.

Designing effective T-cell vaccines requires careful consideration of key factors, including the selection of antigens (including incorporating multiple conserved T-cell epitopes), delivery systems (such as viral vectors or lipid nanoparticles), and adjuvants (such as TLR agonists to boost T-cell responses), all aimed at optimizing immunogenicity and protective effectiveness [40].

5. The role and challenges of T cells in tumor immunotherapy

5.1 Tumor immunoediting and T-cell response

The tumor immunoediting process involves three dynamic stages: elimination, equilibrium, and escape. In the elimination stage, the immune system detects and eliminates newly formed tumor cells, primarily through the direct attack of $CD8^+$ T cells, the coordinated action of $CD4^+$ T cells, and the involvement of other immune cells. In the equilibrium stage, the immune system and tumor cells reach a prolonged standstill, where tumor cells partially evade detection through mechanisms like antigen loss and MHC downregulation but remain under immune surveillance. In the escape phase, tumor cells create an immunosuppressive environment (e.g., by expressing immune checkpoint molecules and competing for metabolic resources) to fully suppress T-cell activity, enabling uncontrolled growth. T cells are central to both the recognition and destruction of tumor cells throughout this process, and their functional state directly influences the progression of immunoediting [23–26, 41, 42]

5.2 Tumor antigen and T-cell recognition

Tumor antigens are the molecular basis for T cells to recognize and attack tumor cells, mainly including tumor-specific antigens (such as neoantigens) produced by gene mutations and tumor-associated antigens that are abnormally highly expressed in tumors [43, 44].

Neoantigens are displayed by MHC I molecules and can be specifically detected by TCRs, triggering $CD8^+$ cytotoxic T cells to destroy tumor cells. This precise identification mechanism is the core of tumor immune surveillance and the fundamental principle behind modern immunotherapy strategies such as CAR-T therapy, TCR-T therapy, and ICIs [45, 46].

5.3 T-cell exhaustion in the TME

The TME is a complex ecosystem comprising tumor cells, immune cells, stromal cells, blood vessels, and the extracellular matrix. The TME inhibits T-cell function through multiple mechanisms, leading to T-cell exhaustion [42, 47–50].

5.3.1 Immune checkpoint molecules

Immune checkpoint molecules are regulatory receptors on the surface of T cells, which prevent excessive activation during normal immune responses. Tumor cells exploit this mechanism by overexpressing immune checkpoint ligands to inhibit T-cell function.

The PD-1/PD-L1 pathway is one of the most crucial immune checkpoint pathways. PD-1 is expressed on the surface of activated T cells, while its ligand, PD-L1, is highly expressed on the surface of tumor cells and TAMs. When PD-1 binds to PD-L1, it sends inhibitory signals that impair T-cell function (see **Figure 4**).

The CTLA-4 is an important immune checkpoint molecule that is expressed early in T-cell activation. It competes with CD28 for binding to B7 molecules, delivering inhibitory signals. CTLA-4 is also highly expressed in Tregs, where it plays a role in immune suppression.

Other immune checkpoint molecules, such as TIM-3, LAG-3, and TIGIT (which are coexpressed on exhausted T cells), also play a role in inhibiting T-cell function synergistically [51].

5.3.2 Inhibitory cells

The TME contains various inhibitory cells, such as Tregs, myeloid-derived suppressor cells (MDSCs), tumor-associated macrophages (TAMs), and others.

Tregs inhibit antitumor immunity through multiple mechanisms: secreting inhibitory cytokines (such as IL-10 and TGF-β); depleting IL-2, thereby depriving effector T cells of growth factors; directly killing effector T cells; and inhibiting the function of APCs [30, 52–54].

The MDSCs are immature myeloid cells that accumulate in the TME. The MDSCs inhibit T-cell function by producing substances such as arginase, nitric oxide (NO), and reactive oxygen species (ROS). Additionally, MDSCs can promote Treg differentiation and angiogenesis.

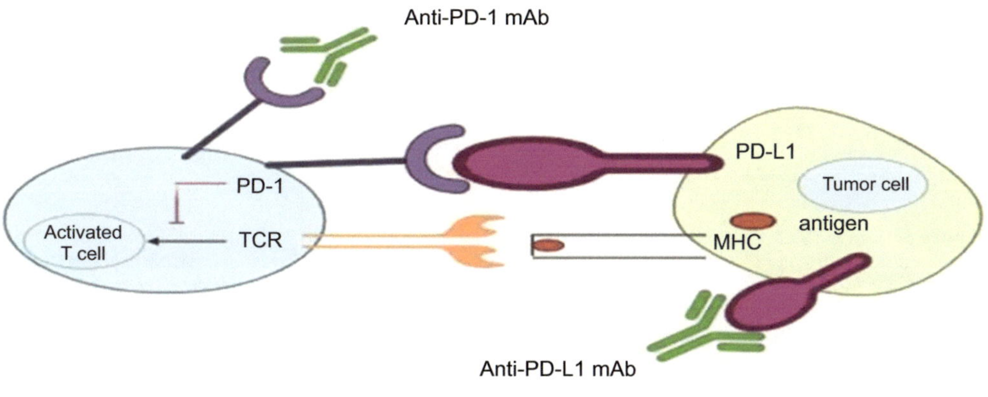

Figure 4.
The PD-1/PD-L1 immune checkpoint pathway and its inhibitory role. In the TME, tumor cells or APCs often overexpress programmed death-ligand 1. Binding of PD-L1 to the programmed death-1 receptor on activated T cells transmits an inhibitory signal, resulting in T-cell exhaustion, reduced proliferation, and diminished cytokine production, thereby facilitating immune evasion. Immune checkpoint inhibitors block this interaction, restoring T-cell antitumor activity.

The TAM usually displays an M2-like phenotype, characterized by immunosuppressive and pro-tumor activities. M2-like macrophages release inhibitory cytokines like IL-10 and TGF-β, which support angiogenesis and tissue remodeling (see **Figure 5**) [48].

5.3.3 Metabolic competition

Tumor cells and T cells compete for scarce nutrients such as glucose, amino acids, and oxygen, and evidence suggests that tumor cells generally demonstrate

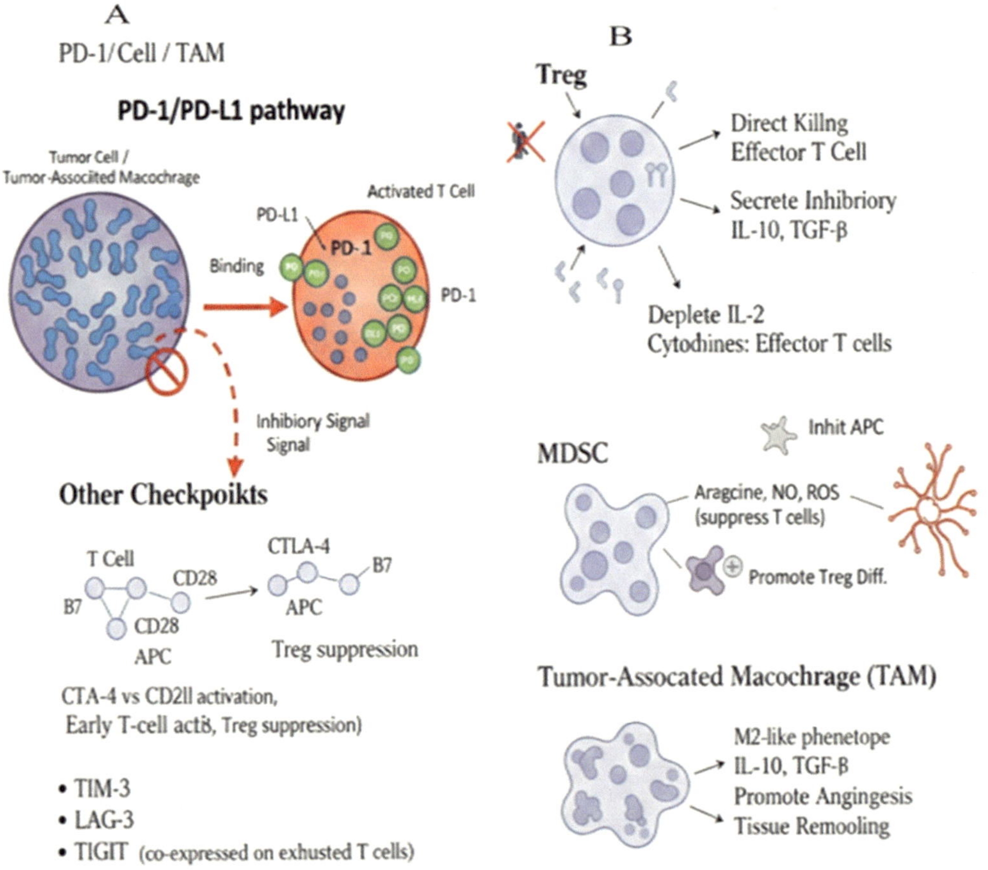

Figure 5.
Immune checkpoint molecules and their inhibitory cells. Immune checkpoint molecules are mainly expressed on the surface of T cells and are used to maintain immune tolerance. Tumor cells can utilize this mechanism by over-expressing their ligands (such as PD-L1) to continuously inhibit T-cell activation and function, leading to immune escape. (a) Immune checkpoint molecules: (1)PD-1: PD-1 of T cells binds to ligands (PD-L1/PD-L2) of tumor or immune cells, transmitting a strong inhibitory signal, which leads to T-cell exhaustion, proliferation cessation, cytokine secretion reduction, and apoptosis. (2) CTLA-4: CTLA-4 binds to the costimulatory molecules (CD80/CD86) of APCs, competitively inhibiting the complete activation of T cells. (3) Other immune checkpoint molecules: TIM-3, LAG-3, and TIGIT (coexpressed on exhausted T cells) form a complex inhibitory network and provide new targets for combination therapy. (b) Inhibitory cells (Tregs, MDSCs, TAMs): (1) Tregs: Tregs inhibit antitumor immunity through multiple mechanisms, including secreting inhibitory cytokines, killing effector T cells, and inhibiting the function of APCs. (2) MDSCs: MDSCs exert immune suppressive effects, mainly by secreting excessive reactive oxygen species (ROS) or nitric oxide (NO), leading to T-cell receptor nitrosation. (3) TAMs: M2-like macrophages release inhibitory cytokines like IL-10 and TGF-β, supporting angiogenesis and tissue remodeling.

a higher metabolic rate while proving more effective at absorbing and utilizing these critical resources.

Furthermore, glucose competition may well indicate a significant role in the metabolic suppression of T-cell function. Tumor cells engage in aerobic glycolysis by overexpressing glucose transporters, allowing them to absorb large quantities of glucose. This could demonstrate that reduced glucose levels in the TME disrupt T-cell glycolysis, thereby impairing their overall function.

Moreover, amino acid competition also appears to impact T-cell activity in important ways. Tryptophan, an essential amino acid for T-cell activation, is consumed by both tumor cells and MDSCs through the expression of indoleamine 2,3-dioxygenase (IDO), leading to the production of inhibitory metabolites such as kynurenine.

Hypoxia, a common feature of the TME, may also contribute to immune suppression. Hypoxia-inducible factor (HIF) is consistently expressed, helping tumor cells adapt to low-oxygen conditions while inhibiting T-cell function. Thus, hypoxia could promote angiogenesis and also foster epithelial–mesenchymal transition [41].

5.4 Immune checkpoint inhibitors

Immune checkpoint inhibitors restore the antitumor function of T cells by blocking inhibitory signaling pathways. These drugs have become the standard treatment for various tumors, changing the landscape of cancer therapy [51, 55, 56].

5.4.1 PD-1/PD-L1 inhibitors

PD-1 inhibitors (such as pembrolizumab and nivolumab) and PD-L1 inhibitors (such as atezolizumab and durvalumab) alleviate T-cell inhibition by blocking the PD-1/PD-L1 interaction.

The PD-1/PD-L1 inhibitors have shown efficacy in various tumors, including melanoma, nonsmall cell lung cancer, renal cell carcinoma, bladder cancer, squamous cell carcinoma of the head and neck, etc. Their efficacy is correlated with factors such as PD-L1 expression level, tumor mutational burden, and microsatellite instability.

The PD-L1 expression serves as a crucial biomarker for predicting the efficacy of PD-1/PD-L1 inhibitors. Tumors with high PD-L1 expression typically exhibit better responses, yet those with low or even no expression may also respond, highlighting the complexity of tumor immunity [57–60].

5.4.2 CTLA-4 inhibitors

The CTLA-4 inhibitors, such as ipilimumab, enhance T-cell activation by blocking the interaction between CTLA-4 and B7 molecules. The CTLA-4 primarily functions in the early stages of T-cell activation and in lymph nodes, regulating the initiation of immune responses.

The CTLA-4 inhibitors have shown significant efficacy in melanoma, extending the survival of patients with advanced disease. However, the toxicity of CTLA-4 inhibitors is higher than that of PD-1/PD-L1 inhibitors, which are more potent, and common immune-related adverse events include colitis, dermatitis, hypophysitis, etc. [43, 61].

5.4.3 Combined treatment strategy

The combination of PD-1/PD-L1 inhibitors with CTLA-4 inhibitors appears to demonstrate that these synergistic effects could substantially influence clinical outcomes. Moreover, the use of nivolumab and ipilimumab together in melanoma may indicate higher objective response rates (ORRs)[43].

Furthermore, the significant combination therapy might demonstrate longer progression-free survival than either drug alone. Given that CTLA-4 inhibitors boost T-cell activation, the mechanism behind this combination therapy may involve clonal expansion. Thus, PD-1/PD-L1 inhibitors might prevent the depletion of effector T cells in the TME. However, increased toxicity requires careful management.

Nevertheless, combination strategies include pairing ICIs with chemotherapy. Additionally, pairing with targeted therapies could demonstrate that these regimens aim to enhance antitumor immunity. Moreover, pairing with radiotherapy might work through diverse mechanisms. Notwithstanding these approaches, regimens may work together synergistically. Thus, the strategies could provide important benefits [62–65].

5.5 CAR-T cell therapy

The CAR-T therapy involves genetically engineering a patient's T cells to express a chimeric receptor capable of recognizing tumor antigens, thereby specifically killing tumor cells [66–68].

5.5.1 CAR structure and development

The basic structure of CAR includes an extracellular antigen recognition domain, a hinge region, a transmembrane region, and an intracellular signaling domain. The first generation of CAR only contained the CD3 ζ signaling domain; the second and third generations of CAR incorporated costimulatory domains (such as CD28, 4-1BB); the fourth generation of CAR (TRUCK) can also secrete cytokines or express other functional molecules.

The CD19 is the most effective target in CAR-T therapy for treating B-cell malignancies. It is uniquely expressed on the surface of B cells, both normal and cancerous. CAR-T therapy targeting CD19 has demonstrated considerable effectiveness in cases of relapsed or refractory B-cell acute lymphoblastic leukemia (B-ALL) and non-Hodgkin lymphoma [69].

Other CAR-T targets include BCMA for multiple myeloma, CD22 for B-cell malignancies, GD2 for neuroblastoma, and mesothelin for mesothelioma and pancreatic cancers [70, 71].

5.5.2 Clinical application and challenges

The CAR-T therapy has made significant advancements in the treatment of hematological malignancies. The complete remission rate (CRR) for CD19 CAR-T therapy can reach 80–90% in B-ALL, while the overall response rate (ORR) for diffuse large B-cell lymphoma is approximately 50–80% [68].

The CAR-T therapy, however, encounters several challenges, including limited effectiveness in solid tumors, tumor antigen diversity, suppression by the TME, cytokine release syndrome (CRS), and immune effector cell–associated neurotoxic syndrome (ICANS) [19, 72].

The limited effectiveness of CAR-T therapy in solid tumors is attributed to several factors, including the absence of optimal tumor-specific antigens, physical and immune barriers within the TME, inadequate T-cell infiltration, and the presence of an immunosuppressive microenvironment [17, 73–78].

5.5.3 Innovation strategy

Researchers have developed various innovative strategies: improving targeting accuracy and safety by designing bispecific CARs; constructing armored CARs to enhance T-cell proliferation, killing function, and *in vivo* persistence; developing controllable CARs to achieve on-demand control of therapeutic activity and enhance safety; using gene editing technology to prepare universal CAR-T cells to reduce immune rejection and achieve "spot" supply; and exploring the technological pathway for directly generating CAR-T cells in the body, thereby greatly simplifying the treatment process. These strategies collectively drive the development of CAR-T therapy toward safer, more effective, and more accessible directions [18, 79–82].

5.6 Combination therapy of antibody–drug conjugate and ICIs

The combination of ADCs and ICIs is an emerging cancer treatment strategy that boosts antitumor immunity through its synergistic effects.

5.6.1 Mechanism of ADC

The ADC is composed of three components: antibodies that target tumor antigens, cytotoxic payloads, and linkers. The ADC selectively binds to tumor cells via the antibodies, enters the cells, and releases the cytotoxic drugs to kill the tumor cells.

The mechanisms of action vary depending on the type of payload in the ADC: microtubule inhibitors (like MMAE, DM1) disrupt cell division; DNA-damaging agents (such as kanamycin, pyrrolobenzodiazepine [PBD] dimer) induce DNA breakage; and topoisomerase I inhibitors (e.g., SN-38, DXd) prevent DNA replication.

5.6.2 Immune synergy mechanism

The mechanism of the synergistic effect between ADC and ICI includes the following:

(1) Immunogenic cell death (ICD): The ADC induces ICD in tumor cells, releasing damage-associated molecular patterns (DAMPs) such as adenosine triphosphate (ATP), high mobility group box 1 (HMGB1), and calprotectin. These molecules activate dendritic cells and enhance antigen presentation and T-cell activation.

(2) Tumor antigen release: The ADC kills tumor cells and releases a large amount of tumor antigens, including neoantigens and shared antigens. These antigens are taken up and presented by APCs, expanding the breadth and depth of T-cell responses.

(3) TME remodeling: The ADCs can reduce tumor burden and alter the immunosuppressive properties of the TME. Some ADC payloads can also directly kill immunosuppressive cells (such as Tregs, MDSCs).

(4) Boost antigen presentation: Some ADCs, like Enfortumab Vedotin, can increase the expression of MHC molecules on tumor cells, improving their recognition by T cells.

5.6.3 Clinical progress

The combination therapy of ADC and ICI holds promising potential across various tumor types.

In urothelial carcinoma, the combination of enfortumab vedotin (which targets Nectin-4) and pembrolizumab as a first-line treatment showed significant survival benefits in the EV-302/KEYNOTE-A39 phase III trial (median overall survival: 31.5 months compared to 16.1 months in the chemotherapy group) [83].

In nonsmall cell lung cancer, first-line treatment with the ADC targeting TROP2 (sacituzumab govitecan) in combination with the PD-1 inhibitor, tagitanlimab, resulted in an ORR of 66.7%, regardless of PD-L1 expression levels [44].

In gastric cancer, a phase II clinical trial investigating the HER2 ADC (Vedotin) in combination with the PD-1/CTLA-4 bispecific antibody Cabozantinib is currently ongoing, with a strong theoretical basis and the potential for synergistic effects.

5.7 Tumor vaccines and T-cell immunity

Tumor vaccine is a therapeutic vaccine aimed at activating the patient's own T cells to specifically attack the tumor, mainly including the following types:

- Peptide/protein vaccine: Direct delivery of antigen fragments or intact proteins.

- Nucleic acid vaccines (DNA/RNA): Express and induce immune responses *in vivo* by encoding tumor antigens.

- Virus vector vaccine: Use a recombinant virus to deliver antigen genes.

- Dendritic cell vaccine: Loaded with antigens *in vitro* and transfused to efficiently activate T-cells.

Among them, the new antigen vaccine is designed based on individualized patient tumor mutations, with strong specificity, the ability to simultaneously stimulate $CD4^+$ and $CD8^+$ T-cell responses, and the advantage of reducing immune evasion. It has shown potential in some clinical trials [43, 84, 85].

Currently, tumor vaccines still face many challenges, such as TME suppression, antigen loss, individual differences, and high production costs. The future development direction includes developing universal neoantigen vaccines, optimizing delivery systems, and combining other therapies, such as ICIs, to enhance efficacy [86]. Key clinical outcomes and representative agents of these T cell–targeted immunotherapies are summarized in **Table 1**.

6. T-cell deficiency–related immunodeficiency diseases

6.1 Primary immunodeficiencies

Primary immunodeficiencies (PID) is an immune system deficiency caused by genetic factors, which leads to a decrease in the body's ability to resist infections, making it prone to recurrent infections, autoimmune diseases, and malignant tumors [87].

Treatment technique type	Representative drug/therapy	Target/ modification method	Indications	Key experiment	Core clinical data
Immune checkpoint inhibitors (PD-1 inhibitors)	Pembrolizumab	PD-1	Metastatic melanoma	KEYNOTE-006	OS was 34.2%, ORR was 33.7%
Immune checkpoint inhibitors (CTLA-4 inhibitors)	Ipilimumab	CTLA-4	Advanced melanoma	CheckMate 067	The 10-year OS in the combination nivolumab group was 52%, while it was 26% in the single-agent ipilimumab group; PFS was extended to 11.5 months
CAR-T cell therapy	Akarinis	CD19	Recurrent/ refractory diffuse large B-cell lymphoma	ZUMA-1	ORR was 83%, and OS reached 42.6%
CAR-T cell therapy	Sidakilorense Ciltacabtagene autoleucel (Carvykti)	BCMA	Refractory/ recurrent Multiple Myeloma	CARTITUDE-1	ORR was 98%, and the 4-year PFS was 55%
TCR-T therapy	Tebentafusp	Targeted gp100 peptide-HLA-A*02:01 complex	Metastatic uveal melanoma	IMCgp100-202	The median OS was 21.7 months, and the 1-year OS rate was 73.2%
TIL therapy	LN-145	Ex vivo expansion of tumor-infiltrating lymphocytes	Recurrent/ refractory cervical cancer	C-145-04	ORR was 44%, CR was 11%, and the median DOR reached 10.3 months

Note: PFS: progression-free survival, OS: overall survival, ORR: objective response rate, CRR: complete response rate, DOR: duration of response, SCID: severe combined immunodeficiency disease.

Table 1.
Key clinical trial data on T-cell-targeted tumor immunotherapy.

6.1.1 Classification and epidemiology

According to the 2014 International Federation of Immunological Societies (IUIS) classification, PID encompasses nine significantly distinct categories: the combined immunodeficiency disorders, the immunodeficiency conditions primarily attributed to antibody deficiency, other well-defined immunodeficiency syndromes, the immune regulation disorders, the defects in phagocytic cell count or function, the innate immunodeficiency disorders, the autoimmune diseases, the complement deficiencies, and the pseudophenotypes.

Moreover, the overall incidence of primary immunodeficiency may be approximately 1 in 10,000 individuals. Nevertheless, the incidence varies significantly across conditions. However, the incidence of severe combined immunodeficiency (SCID) may range from 1 in 50,000 to 1 in 100,000. Given that common variable immunodeficiency represents a distinct entity, its incidence appears to be estimated at 1 in 25,000 to 1 in 50,000 individuals.

6.1.2 PID dominated by T-cell defects

DiGeorge syndrome is a typical T-cell deficiency disease caused by the absence of 22q11.2, leading to thymic hypoplasia. The clinical manifestations are diverse, including congenital heart disease, facial deformities, hypocalcemia, immunodeficiency, and more. The degree of immune deficiency is related to the degree of thymic hypoplasia, ranging from complete loss to partial dysfunction.

Severe combined immunodeficiency is a group of diseases characterized by severe defects in T cells, often accompanied by defects in B cells and/or natural killer cells. The SCID is caused by various gene mutations, including IL2RG, JAK3, ADA, RAG1/2, etc. Children with severe infections develop symptoms within a few months after birth and often die within one year if left untreated.

Other T-cell deficiency diseases include Wiskott–Aldrich syndrome (WAS), high IgM syndrome, and Omenn syndrome.

6.2 Secondary immunodeficiencies

Secondary immunodeficiencies are immune system dysfunctions caused by nongenetic factors, including infections, drugs, malignant tumors, and malnutrition.

6.2.1 Human immunodeficiency virus/acquired immune deficiency syndrome

Acquired immune deficiency syndrome (AIDS) is a typical secondary T-cell deficiency disease caused by HIV infection. The HIV mainly infects $CD4^+$ T cells, leading to a progressive decrease in $CD4^+$ T-cell numbers and functional defects.

The progression of HIV infection appears to involve three broadly recognized stages: the acute phase, the chronic phase, and the AIDS phase. Given that the acute phase involves rapid viral replication, the evidence may well suggest that this could lead to a notably swift decline in $CD4^+$ T cells. However, during the chronic phase, viral replication may be somewhat controlled, and the $CD4^+$ T-cell count appears to decline more gradually. Thus, research could show that $CD4^+$ T-cell counts may drop below 200 cells/μL. Nevertheless, in the AIDS phase, findings suggest that individuals become vulnerable to opportunistic infections and cancers.

Antiretroviral therapy (ART) can effectively inhibit HIV replication, restore the number and function of CD4⁺ T cells, and reduce incidence rates and mortality. However, long-term HIV infection and ART may cause complications such as immune aging and chronic inflammation.

6.2.2 Iatrogenic immunosuppression

Immunosuppressive drugs are widely used in organ transplantation, autoimmune diseases, inflammatory diseases, and so on. These drugs inhibit T-cell function through different mechanisms.

Corticosteroids inhibit T-cell activation and cytokine production; calcium-regulated phosphatase inhibitors (such as cyclosporine and tacrolimus) inhibit IL-2 transcription; antiproliferative drugs (such as mycophenolate mofetil and azathioprine) inhibit T-cell proliferation; biological agents, such as anti-CD3 and anti-IL-2 R antibodies, directly target T cells [88].

Long-term immunosuppression increases the risk of infection and malignant tumors, requiring a balance between treatment efficacy and side effects.

6.2.3 Malignant tumor–associated immunodeficiency

Malignant tumors themselves can cause immune deficiencies, including the production of immunosuppressive factors by tumor cells; tumors consume nutrients; tumor-associated inflammation consumes immune cells; Treatment related immune suppression.

Hematological malignancies, such as leukemia and lymphoma, are often accompanied by significant immune deficiencies, as malignant cells directly originate from the immune system. Solid tumors can also suppress immune function through various mechanisms.

6.3 Diagnosis and evaluation

The diagnosis of immunodeficiency diseases requires a combination of clinical manifestations, laboratory tests, and genetic testing.

6.3.1 Clinical manifestations

Recurrent, severe, or opportunistic infections are the primary symptoms of immunodeficiency diseases. The nature of the infection depends on the specific immune component that is defective: T-cell defects are associated with viral, fungal, and intracellular bacterial infections; antibody defects lead to a higher susceptibility to extracellular bacterial infections; phagocytic defects increase the risk of bacterial and fungal infections.

Other clinical signs may include delayed growth and development, autoimmune disorders, allergies, and cancers. Some PIDs have unique features, such as facial abnormalities in DiGeorge syndrome and congenital heart disease.

6.3.2 Laboratory inspection

Preliminary screening includes complete blood count, immunoglobulin quantification, lymphocyte subset analysis, and vaccine antibody response.

The evaluation of T-cell function includes delayed-type hypersensitivity skin test, lymphocyte proliferation test, cytokine production assay, and TCR diversity analysis.

Advanced examinations include flow cytometry detection of surface markers and intracellular molecules, gene sequencing, and functional testing.

6.3.3 Genetic diagnosis

Genetic testing is an important means of diagnosing PID, especially for diseases with clear genetic patterns and known genes. The detection methods include Sanger sequencing, second-generation sequencing (whole exome, whole genome), chromosome microarray, etc.

Genetic diagnosis helps to clarify the cause, guide treatment, provide genetic counseling, and assist in prenatal diagnosis.

6.4 Treatment strategy

The treatment goals of immunodeficiency diseases are to control infections, restore immune function, and treat complications.

6.4.1 Supporting treatment

Anti-infection treatment forms the cornerstone of managing immunodeficiency diseases. This includes the preventive use of antibiotics, antiviral medications, and antifungal drugs; prompt treatment of acute infections; and regular monitoring of infection markers.

Immunoglobulin replacement therapy is prescribed for patients with antibody deficiencies and can be given either intravenously or subcutaneously. The dosage and frequency of treatment are adjusted according to the patient's clinical response and IgG trough levels [27].

6.4.2 Immune reconstruction

Hematopoietic stem cell transplantation (HSCT) is a potentially curative treatment for many severe PIDs, particularly SCID. Prior to transplantation, pretreatment (chemotherapy or radiotherapy) is necessary to eliminate the patient's hematopoietic system and create space for the engraftment of donor cells.

The success of HSCT depends on several factors, including donor compatibility, the patient's age and clinical condition, the pretreatment plan, and the management of posttransplant complications. Sibling donors typically provide the highest success rates for transplantation, but many patients do not have a suitable match.

Alternative donor sources, such as umbilical cord blood and haploidentical transplants, have broadened donor options; however, these options come with an increased risk of transplant-related complications. Posttransplant immunosuppressive therapy is essential to prevent graft-versus-host disease (GVHD).

6.4.3 Gene therapy

Gene therapy could demonstrate the use of gene transfer technology that may correct genetic defects and restore critical immune function. Moreover, unlike

HSCT, gene therapy might involve the use of the patient's own cells, reducing the risk of graft rejection and GVHD.

However, lentiviral vector-based gene therapy may demonstrate successful application in treating PIDs. Thus, the treatment process could involve collecting hematopoietic stem cells from patients, introducing normal genes into the cells using lentiviral vectors *in vitro*, and reinfusing genetically corrected cells into the patients.

Given that adenosine deaminase deficiency severe combined immunodeficiency (ADA-SCID) represents a significant early application, gene therapy might reasonably demonstrate immune function restoration following the important treatment, with long-term follow-up showing excellent safety. Additionally, Artemis SCID gene therapy may suggest promising results, particularly in restoring T- and B-cell function in patients.

Nevertheless, gene therapy approaches may show promise; investigation includes treatments for Wiskott–Aldrich syndrome (WAS), X-linked SCID, and chronic granulomatous disease [71].

6.4.4 Enzyme replacement therapy

Adenosine deaminase deficiency can be treated with enzyme replacement therapy, involving weekly injections of PEGylated ADA. The treatment can improve immune function, but it requires lifelong administration and is expensive.

Enzyme replacement therapy can be used as a bridging therapy for HSCT or gene therapy, or for patients who are not suitable for curative treatment.

6.5 Frontier therapies and prospects

6.5.1 New gene editing technologies

Gene editing technologies, such as CRISPR/Cas9, provide new tools for PID therapy. Unlike viral vector gene therapy, gene editing allows for precise correction at specific genomic loci, avoiding the risk of random integration.

Gene editing can be used to correct mutated genes, insert normal genes, regulate gene expression, and more. However, off-target effects, editing efficiency, and delivery systems are challenges in practical applications.

6.5.2 In vivo *gene therapy*

Traditional gene therapy requires *in vitro* manipulation of cells, which is complex and costly. *In vivo* gene therapy delivers therapeutic genes directly to target cells through viral or non-viral vectors, simplifying the treatment process [36, 89].

Adeno-associated virus (AAV) is a commonly used *in vivo* gene delivery vector, which has been successfully utilized for the treatment of various genetic diseases. However, AAV has limited capacity, and its immunogenicity may restrict repeat administration [64, 90].

6.5.3 Innovation in cell therapy

In addition to HSCT and gene therapy, new cell therapies are being explored: Regulatory T-cell therapy for autoimmune diseases and transplantation rejection;

virus-specific T-cell therapy for viral infections; and CAR-T therapy is used for PID-related malignant tumors.

These cell therapies need to address issues such as cell source, expansion, function, and safety. Universal cell therapy, which avoids rejection reactions through gene editing, is an important direction for future development [18, 91].

6.5.4 Precise immune regulation

With a deeper understanding of the immune system, precise immune regulation has become possible. By targeting specific pathways, cell subpopulations, cytokines, and other factors, immune function can be more accurately regulated, and side effects can be reduced.

Small molecule drugs, monoclonal antibodies, oligonucleotides, etc., are important tools for immune regulation. Individualized treatment plans are developed based on the patient's genetic background, immune status, clinical characteristics, and other factors. A comparison of primary and secondary T cell–related immunodeficiencies is summarized in **Table 2.**

7. Conclusion

T-cell functionality appears to be essential for adaptive immunity and the maintenance of overall health. A significant body of evidence suggests that T-cell malfunction could contribute to the onset and progression of various diseases, including autoimmune disorders, infections, and cancers. Thus, a thorough understanding of T-cell biology and disease mechanisms might provide a solid foundation for developing new treatment strategies.

In recent years, T-cell–based immunotherapies have demonstrated significant breakthroughs. Moreover, ICIs, CAR-T therapy, and other treatments may have

Category	Pathogenesis	Typical diseases	therapies	References
Primary immunodeficiencies	Congenital genetic defects, such as mutations in the IL-2 receptor gamma chain, RAG gene defects, and abnormalities in genes related to thymus development, etc.	Severe combined immunodeficiency disease (SCID), DiGeorge syndrome, chronic granulomatous disease	Hematopoietic stem cell transplantation, gene therapy, thymus transplantation, etc.	[92–100]
Secondary immunodeficiencies	Postnatal factors. Common triggers include HIV infection, chemotherapy/radiotherapy, long-term use of immunosuppressants, malignant tumors, severe malnutrition, etc.	AIDS, immune suppression after radiotherapy and chemotherapy, immune deficiency after organ transplantation	Removing the cause (such as anti-HIV treatment, adjusting the radiotherapy and chemotherapy plan), immune reconstitution, and symptomatic anti-infection treatment	[101–108]

Table 2.
Primary and secondary immunodeficiency diseases.

substantially altered the way we approach several diseases. However, challenges such as treatment resistance, managing toxicity, and addressing individual patient differences still remain. Moving forward, continued research and the development of innovative technologies could prove crucial.

It is highly likely that T-cell–based immunotherapy will become increasingly important in treating a wider variety of diseases with the continuous advancement of research and technology. However, it may require collaboration across multiple fields, involving scientists, clinicians, engineers, and policymakers to push the progress forward and realize this potential.

Additionally, T-cell immunology seems to be a rapidly developing field that not only drives medical progress but also deepens our comprehension of the fundamental aspects of life. Ranging from foundational discoveries to clinical applications, and from personalized treatments to advancements in public health, T-cell research is likely to have widespread effects at multiple levels.

Author details

Jinping Shu[1], Zaid Talal Abdulqader Al-Qadhi[2], Somia Shehzadi[3], Zhipeng Zhao[4] and Ling Yin[5,6*]

1 Department of Administration, The First Affiliated Hospital of Anhui Medical University, Hefei, China

2 Faculty of Medicine, Saba University, Marib, Yemen

3 University Institute of Medical Laboratory Technology, The University of Lahore, Lahore, Pakistan

4 Department of Rehabilitation Medicine, School of Medicine, Taizhou University, Taizhou, China

5 College of Life Sciences, Weifang Institute of Technology, Weifang, China

6 College of Medicine, University of Florida, Gainesville, USA

*Address all correspondence to: 1987.yinling@163.com

References

[1] Gao Z, Feng Y, Xu J, Liang J. T-cell exhaustion in immune-mediated inflammatory diseases: New implications for immunotherapy. Frontiers in Immunology. 2022;**13** 977394

[2] Song Y, Li J Wu Y. Evolving understanding of autoimmune mechanisms and new therapeutic strategies of autoimmune disorders. Signal Transduction and Targeted Therapy. 2024;**9**(1):263. 9th ed

[3] Zhang H, Weyand CM, Goronzy JJ. Hallmarks of the aging T-cell system. FEBS Journal. 2021;**288**(24):7123–7142

[4] Kedmi R, Littman DR. Antigen-presenting cells as specialized drivers of intestinal T cell functions. Immunity. 2024;**57**(10):2269–2279

[5] Adu-Berchie K, Obuseh FO, Mooney DJ. T cell development and function. Rejuvenation Research. 2023;**26**(4):126–138

[6] Wu C, Jiang ML, Pang T, Zhang CJ. T cell subsets and immune homeostasis. Methods in Molecular Biology. 2024;**2782**:39–63

[7] Ton Nu QC, Deka G, Park PH. $CD8^+$ T cell-based immunotherapy: promising frontier in human diseases. Biochemical Pharmacology. 2025;**237**:116909

[8] Deo AS, Sruthika SU, Karun S, Bisaria K, Sarkar K. Participation of T cells in generating immune protection against cancers. Pathology Research and Practice. 2024;**262**:155534

[9] Meitei HT, Lal G. T cell receptor signaling in the differentiation and plasticity of $CD4^+$ T cells. Cytokine and Growth Factor Reviews. 2023;**69**:14–27

[10] Song R, Jia X, Zhao J, Du P, Zhang JA. T cell receptor revision and immune repertoire changes in autoimmune diseases. International Reviews of Immunology. 2022;**41** (5):517–533

[11] Li X, Liang H, Fan J. Prospects of cytomegalovirus-specific T-Cell receptors in clinical diagnosis and therapy. Viruses. 2023;**15**(6)1334.263

[12] Zhu J, Yamane H, Paul WE. Differentiation of effector CD4 T cell populations (*). Annual Review of Immunology. 2010;**28**:445–489

[13] Owen DL, Sjaastad LE, Farrar MA. Regulatory T cell development in the thymus. The Journal of Immunology. 2019;**203**(8):2031–2041

[14] Baldwin I, Robey EA. Adjusting to self in the thymus: CD4 versus CD8 lineage commitment and regulatory T cell development. Journal of Experimental Medicine. 2024;**221**(10): e20230896

[15] Alula KM, Nguyen TT, de Zoeten EF. Regulation of intestinal regulatory T cells via stress response pathways in inflammatory bowel disease. Autoimmunity. 2026;**59** (1):2602715

[16] Dikiy S, Rudensky AY. Principles of regulatory T cell function. Immunity. 2023;**56**(2):240–255

[17] Abhishek K, Nidhi M, Chandran S, Shevkoplyas SS, Mohan C. Manufacturing regulatory T cells for

adoptive cell therapy in immune diseases: A critical appraisal. Clinical Immunology. 2023;**251**:109328

[18] Lim WA, June CH. The principles of engineering immune cells to treat cancer. Cell. 2017;**168**(4):724–740

[19] Huang M, Wang Y, Fang L, et al. T cell senescence: A new perspective on immunotherapy in lung cancer. Frontiers in Immunology. 2024;**15**:1338680

[20] Nga HT, Nguyen TL, Yi HS. T-cell senescence in human metabolic diseases. Diabetes and Metabolism Journal. 2024;**48**(5):864–881

[21] Li K, Chen R, Wang R, et al. Neuroinflammation in neurodegenerative diseases: Focusing on the mediation of T lymphocytes. Neural Regeneration Research. 2026;**21**:1864–1889

[22] Barberis M, Rojas Lopez A. T cell phenotype switching in autoimmune disorders: Clinical significance of targeting metabolism. Clinical and Translational Medicine. 2022;**12**(7):e898

[23] Sasson SC, Gordon CL, Christo SN, Klenerman P, Mackay LK. Local heroes or villains: Tissue-resident memory T cells in human health and disease. Cellular & Molecular Immunology. 2020;**17**(2):113–122

[24] Collier JL, Weiss SA, Pauken KE, Sen DR, Sharpe AH. Not-so-opposite ends of the spectrum: $CD8^+$ T cell dysfunction across chronic infection, cancer and autoimmunity. Nature Immunology. 2021;**22**(7):809–819

[25] Martin P, Sanchez-Madrid F. T cells in cardiac health and disease. The Journal of Clinical Investigation. 2025;**135**(2):e185218

[26] Molodtsov A, Turk MJ. Tissue resident CD8 memory T cell responses in cancer and autoimmunity. Frontiers in Immunology. 2018;**9**:2810

[27] Hu M, Zhou Y, Yao Z, Tang Y, Zhang Y, Liao J, Cai X, Liu L. T cell dysregulation in rheumatoid arthritis: Recent advances and natural product interventions. International Immunopharmacology. 2025;**153**:114499

[28] Hirahara K, Nakayama T. $CD4^+$ T-cell subsets in inflammatory diseases: Beyond the T h 1/T h 2 paradigm. International Immunology. 2016;**28**(4):163–171

[29] Li X, Guo D, Zou IX, Zhao L, Yang N, Liu Y. CD3($^+$)CD4(-)CD8(-) T cells: A new potential therapeutic target in treating autoimmune diseases. Frontiers in Immunology. 2025;**16**:1683418

[30] Zhu X, Zhu J. CD4 T Helper cell subsets and related human immunological disorders. International Journal of Molecular Sciences. 2020;**21**(21):8011

[31] Zhang YS, Chen YQ. Dysfunctional regulatory T cell: May be an obstacle to immunotherapy in cardiovascular diseases. Biomedicine and Pharmacotherapy. 2024;**173**:116359

[32] Dees S, Ganesan R, Singh S, Grewal IS. Regulatory T cell targeting in cancer: Emerging strategies in immunotherapy. European Journal of Immunology. 2021;**51**(2):280–291

[33] Gao Y, Lu Y, Liang X, et al. CD4($^+$) T-cell senescence in neurodegenerative disease: pathogenesis and potential therapeutic targets. Cells. 2024;**13**:749

[34] Acosta-Ampudia Y, Monsalve DM, Galeano-Sanchez D, Rojas M,

Ramirez-Santana C. Exploring the immunomodulatory effects of environmental contaminants on autoimmune patients: An in vitro approach. Journal of Translational Autoimmunity. 2026;**12**:100341

[35] Bluestone JA, McKenzie BS, Beilke J, Ramsdell F. Opportunities for Treg cell therapy for the treatment of human disease. Frontiers in Immunology. 2023;**14**:1166135

[36] Appalaneni R, Achanta N, Mohan C. Chimeric antigen receptor T-cell therapy in rheumatology: B-cell depletion 2.0. Current Opinion in Rheumatology. 2024;**36**(2):126–133

[37] Shim CH, Cho S, Shin YM, Choi JM. Emerging role of bystander T cell activation in autoimmune diseases. BMB Reports. 2022;**55**(2):57–64

[38] Shiromizu CM, Jancic CC. γδ T lymphocytes: An effector cell in autoimmunity and infection. Frontiers in Immunology. 2018;**9**:2389

[39] Barnaba V. T cell memory in infection, cancer, and autoimmunity. Frontiers in Immunology. 2021;**12**:811968

[40] O'Brien EM, Tylek T, Geisler HC, et al. Macrophage cell therapy enabled by interleukin-4 mRNA-loaded lipid nanoparticles to sustain a pro-reparative phenotype in inflammatory injuries. Biomaterials. 2026;**328**:123869

[41] Wherry EJ, Kurachi M. Molecular and cellular insights into T cell exhaustion. Nature Reviews Immunology. 2015;**15**(8):486–499

[42] Wang Z, Xing Y, Shang D, Jin X. Exploring the key functions of T cells and the regulation of the immune microenvironment in prostate cancer using single-cell RNA sequencing and bulk RNA sequencing. Autoimmunity. 2026;**59**(1):2596700

[43] Vesely MD, Schreiber RD. Cancer immunoediting: Antigens, mechanisms, and implications to cancer immunotherapy. Annals of the New York Academy of Sciences. 2013;**1284**(1):1–5

[44] Li Y, Sharma A, Schmidt-Wolf IGH. Evolving insights into the improvement of adoptive T-cell immunotherapy through PD-1/PD-L1 blockade in the clinical spectrum of lung cancer. Molecular Cancer. 2024;**23**(1):80

[45] Rodriguez-Sevilla JJ, Colla S. T-cell dysfunctions in myelodysplastic syndromes. Blood. 2024;**143**(14):1329–1343

[46] Dunn GP, Bruce AT, Ikeda H, Old LJ, Schreiber RD. Cancer immunoediting: From immunosurveillance to tumor escape. Nature Immunology. 2002;**3**(11):991–998

[47] Żyłka KA-O, Kubicki T, Gil L, Dytfeld D. T-cell exhaustion in multiple myeloma. Expert Review of Hematology. 2024;**17**(7):295–312

[48] Xie H, Xi X, Lei T, Liu H, Xia Z. CD8(+) T cell exhaustion in the tumor microenvironment of breast cancer. Frontiers in Immunology. 2024;**15**:1507283

[49] Gajewski TF, Schreiber H, Fu YX. Innate and adaptive immune cells in the tumor microenvironment. Nature Immunology. 2013;**14**(10):1014–1022

[50] Wang H, Franco F, Ho P-C. Metabolic regulation of Tregs in cancer:

Opportunities for immunotherapy. Trends in Cancer. 2017;**3**(8):583–592

[51] Duan J, Wang Y, Jiao S. Checkpoint blockade-based immunotherapy in the context of tumor microenvironment: Opportunities and challenges. Cancer Medicine. 2018;**7**(9):4517–4529

[52] Knochelmann HM, Dwyer CJ, Bailey SR, et al. When worlds collide: Th17 and Treg cells in cancer and autoimmunity. Cellular & Molecular Immunology 2018;**15**:458–469

[53] Oparaugo NC, Ouyang K, Nguyen NPN, Nelson AM, Agak GW. Human regulatory T cells: Understanding the role of tregs in select autoimmune skin diseases and post-transplant nonmelanoma skin cancers. International Journal of Molecular Sciences. 2023;**24**(2):1527

[54] Khan U, Ghazanfar H. T lymphocytes and autoimmunity. International Review of Cell and Molecular Biology. 2018;**341**:125–168

[55] Sharma P, Allison JP. The future of immune checkpoint therapy. Science. 2015;**348**(6230):56–61

[56] Charlene M, Fares EMVA, Charles G, Drake K, et al. Mechanisms of resistance to immune checkpoint blockade: Why Does checkpoint inhibitor immunotherapy not work for all patients? American Society of Clinical Oncology Educational Book. 2019;**39**:147–164

[57] Sharpe AH, Pauken KE. The diverse functions of the PD1 inhibitory pathway. Nature Reviews Immunology. 2018;**18**(3):153–167

[58] Yost KE, Satpathy AT, Wells DK, et al. Clonal replacement of tumor-specific T cells following PD-1 blockade. Nature Medicine 2019;**25**:1251–1259

[59] Chen L, Han X. Anti-PD-1/PD-L1 therapy of human cancer: Past, present, and future. The Journal of Clinical Investigation. 2015;**125**(9):3384–3391

[60] Zheng P, Dou Y, Wang Q. Immune response and treatment targets of chronic hepatitis B virus infection: Innate and adaptive immunity. Frontiers in Cellular and Infection Microbiology. 2023;**13**:1206720

[61] Ascierto PA, Kalos M, Schaer DA, Callahan MK, Wolchok JD. Biomarkers for immunostimulatory monoclonal antibodies in combination strategies for melanoma and other tumor types. Clinical Cancer Research. 2013;**19**(5):1009–1020

[62] Liu Y, Xiao L, Nie X, et al. Lenvatinib potentiates the antitumor efficacy of combined radiotherapy and PD-L1 blockade in lung adenocarcinoma. Cancer Biology & Therapy 2026;**27**:2610526

[63] Yin L, Zhou S, Zhang H, et al. Reprogramming the tumor microenvironment: Synergistic mechanisms of antibody-drug conjugates and immune checkpoint inhibitors. Antibody Therapeutics 2025;**8**:262–274

[64] Yin L, Keeler GD, Zhang Y, et al. AAV3-miRNA vectors for growth suppression of human hepatocellular carcinoma cells in vitro and human liver tumors in a murine xenograft model in vivo. Gene Therapy 2021;**28**:422–434

[65] Sadelain M, Riviere I, Riddell S. Therapeutic T cell engineering. Nature. 2017;**545**(7655):423–431

[66] Tang Y, Q E, Ma L, et al. Oncolytic virus OVV-03 enhances CAR-T cell therapy against glioblastoma via immune modulation and specific HER2 upregulation. Oncoimmunology 2026;**15**:2612377

[67] June CH, O'Connor RS, Kawalekar OU, Ghassemi S, Milone MC. CAR T cell immunotherapy for human cancer. Science. 2018;**359**(6382): 1361–1365

[68] Globerson Levin A, Riviere I, Eshhar Z, Sadelain M. CAR T cells: Building on the CD19 paradigm. European Journal of Immunology. 2021;**51**(9):2151–2163

[69] Żyłka K, Kubicki T, Gil L, Dytfeld D. T-cell exhaustion in multiple myeloma. Expert Review of Hematology. 2024;**17**(7):295–312

[70] Mazzanti N, Tamot N, Francese A, et al. Fine-tuning affinity and spacer design enhances T cell potency in DLL3 and BCMA CAR T cells. MAbs 2026;**18**:2602989

[71] Labanieh L, Majzner RG, Mackall CL. Programming CAR-T cells to kill cancer. Nature Biomedical Engineering. 2018;**2**(6):377–391

[72] Lim M, Jung SE, Koh CH, Jeong H, Moon Y, Seo H. The LXRβ/NF-κB axis reprograms CAR-T cells to resist exhaustion in the tumor microenvironment. Oncoimmunology. 2026;**15**(1):2611615

[73] Ullrich F, Bröckelmann PJ, Turki AT, et al. Impact of immunological aging on T cell-mediated therapies in older adults with multiple myeloma and lymphoma. Journal for ImmunoTherapy of Cancer. 2024;**12**(12):e009462

[74] Dagher OK, Schwab RD, Brookens SK, Posey Jr AD. Advances in cancer immunotherapies. Cell. 2023;**186**(8):1814–1814e1811

[75] Arabi F, Torabi-Rahvar M, Shariati A, Ahmadbeigi N, Naderi M. Antigenic targets of CAR T Cell Therapy. A retrospective view on clinical trials. Experimental Cell Research. 2018;**369**(1):1–10

[76] Maude SL, Laetsch TW, Buechner J, et al. Tisagenlecleucel in children and young adults with B-cell lymphoblastic leukemia. The New England Journal of Medicine 2018;**378**:439–448

[77] Cui K, He W, Huang N, Zhu S, Jiang D, Yang W, Zeng Y, Farooq MA, Xu G. The challenges and progress of CAR-T cell therapy in the treatment of solid tumors. Molecular and Cellular Biochemistry. 2025;**480**(10):5345–5367

[78] Dickinson K, Yee EJ, Vigil I, Schulick RD, Zhu Y. GPCRs: Emerging targets for novel T cell immune checkpoint therapy. Cancer Immunology, Immunotherapy. 2024;**73**(12):253

[79] Lewis L, Valvi D, Gedaly R, Marti F. Mitochondrial unfolded protein response in regulatory T cell function: A protective mechanism in immune aging. Frontiers in Immunology. 2025;**16**:1621759

[80] Topalian SL, Drake CG, Pardoll DM. Immune checkpoint blockade: A common denominator approach to cancer therapy. Cancer Cell. 2015;**27**(4):450–461

[81] Sadreddini S, Baradaran B, Aghebati-Maleki A, Sadreddini S,

Shanehbandi D, A-ml FA. Immune checkpoint blockade opens a new way to cancer immunotherapy. Journal of Cellular Physiology. 2019;**234**(6): 8541–8549

[82] Shen R, Kapnick SM, Edwards C, et al. Co-localization of lymph node therapeutics enhances T cell activation and anti-tumor response. Biomaterials. 2026;**328**:123786

[83] Neelapu SS, Locke FL, Bartlett NL, et al. Axicabtagene ciloleucel CAR T-cell therapy in refractory large B-cell lymphoma. The New England Journal of Medicine. 2017;**377**:2531–2544

[84] Holder KA, Ings DP, Hatfield KM, et al. Predictive markers of SARS-CoV-2 spike-specific cytotoxic T cell activity following omicron breakthrough infection. Emerging Microbes & Infections 2026;**15**:2602317

[85] Surowka M, Darowski D, Hutter-Karakoc I, et al. P329G-engager: A universal mix & match antibody-based adaptor platform for cancer immunotherapy. MAbs. 2026;**18**:2602993

[86] Zhang Z, Lu M, Qin Y, et al. Neoantigen: A new breakthrough in tumor immunotherapy. Frontiers in Immunology. 2021;**12**:672356

[87] Rojas M, Acosta-Ampudia Y, Heuer LS, Zang W, Monsalve DM, Ramírez-Santana C, Anaya JM, Ridgway WM, Ansari AA, Gershwin ME. Antigen-specific T cells and autoimmunity. Journal of Autoimmunity. 2024;**148**:103303

[88] Pol JG, Caudana P, Paillet J, Piaggio E, Kroemer G. Effects of interleukin-2 in immunostimulation and immunosuppression. Journal of Experimental Medicine. 2020;**217**(1): e20191247

[89] Klesmith JR, Su L, Wu L, Schrack IA, Dufort FJ, Birt A, Ambrose C, Hackel BJ, Lobb RR, Rennert PD. Retargeting CD19 chimeric antigen receptor T cells via engineered CD19-fusion proteins. Molecular Pharmaceutics. 2019;**16**(8):3544–3558

[90] Keeler AM, Zhan W, Ram S, Fitzgerald KA, Gao G. The curious case of AAV immunology. Molecular Therapy. 2025;**33**(5):1946–1965

[91] Rosenberg SA, Restifo NP. Adoptive cell transfer as personalized immunotherapy for human cancer. Science. 2015;**348**(6230):62–68

[92] Walter JE, Ayala IA, Milojevic D. Autoimmunity as a continuum in primary immunodeficiency. Current Opinion in Pediatrics. 2019;**31**(6):851–862

[93] Ballow M, Sánchez-Ramón S, Walter JE. Secondary immune deficiency and primary immune deficiency crossovers: Hematological malignancies and autoimmune diseases. Frontiers in Immunology. 2022;**13** 928062

[94] Devonshire AL, Makhija M, Approach to Primary Immunodeficiency. Allergy and Asthma Proceedings. 2019;**40**(6):465–469

[95] Klangkalya N, Fleisher TA, Rosenzweig SD. Diagnostic tests for primary immunodeficiency disorders: Classic and genetic testing. Allergy and Asthma Proceedings. 2024;**45**(5):355–363

[96] Nelson CS, Baloh CH. Immunodeficiency: Overview of

primary immune regulatory disorders (PIRDs). Allergy and Asthma Proceedings. 2024;**45**(5):332–339

[97] Rai R, Thrasher AJ, Cavazza A. Gene Editing for the Treatment of Primary Immunodeficiency Diseases. Human Gene Therapy. 2021;**32**(1–2):43–51

[98] Regina J, Doms J, Kampouri E et al. Immunodeficiencies in adults: Key considerations for diagnosis and management. Clinical Reviews in Allergy and Immunology. 2025;**68**(1):92

[99] Szabolcs P, Cavazzana-Calvo M, Fischer A, Veys P. Bone marrow transplantation for primary immunodeficiency diseases. Pediatric Clinics of North America. 2010;**57**(1):207–237

[100] Stray-Pedersen A, Sorte HS, Samarakoon P et al. Primary immunodeficiency diseases: Genomic approaches delineate heterogeneous Mendelian disorders. Journal of Allergy and Clinical Immunology. 2017;**139**(1):232–245

[101] Allegra A, Tonacci A, Musolino C, Pioggia G, Gangemi S. Secondary Immunodeficiency in Hematological Malignancies: Focus on Multiple Myeloma and Chronic Lymphocytic Leukemia. Frontiers in Immunology. 2021;**12**:738915

[102] Blincoe A, Labrosse R, Abraham RS. Acquired B-cell deficiency secondary to B-cell-depleting therapies. Journal of Immunological Methods. 2022;**511**:113385

[103] Pourshahnazari P, Betschel SD, Kim VHD, Waserman S, Zhu R, Kim H. Secondary Immunodeficiency. Allergy, Asthma & Clinical Immunology. 2025;**20**(Suppl 3):80

[104] Arts RJW, Janssen NAF, van de Veerdonk FL, Barcenas-Morales G. Anticytokine Autoantibodies in Infectious Diseases: A Practical Overview. International Journal of Molecular Sciences. 2023;**25**(1):515

[105] Chan SCW, Lau CS. Systemic Lupus Erythematosus and Immunodeficiency. Rheumatology and Immunology Research. 2021;**2**(3):131–138

[106] Friman V, Winqvist O, Blimark C, Langerbeins P, Chapel H, Dhalla F. Secondary immunodeficiency in lymphoproliferative malignancies. Hematology and Oncology. 2016;**34**(3):121–132

[107] Rivière JG, Cantenys-Saba R, Carot-Sans G et al. Current perspectives and challenges of using artificial intelligence in immunodeficiencies. Journal of Allergy and Clinical Immunology. 2025;**156**(4):878–888

[108] Herman KE, Tuttle KL, Chinen J. Overview of secondary immunodeficiency. Allergy and Asthma Proceedings. 2024;**45**(5):347–354

Chapter 7

Tissue-Resident Memory T Cells in Diseases: Pathogenic Mechanisms and Emerging Therapeutic Strategies

Daoyuan Xie, Yu Tian, Jie Zhang, Miao He, Lianying Wu and Guanting Lu

Abstract

Tissue-resident memory T (T_{RM}) cells are a distinct lineage of memory T cells that establish long-term residence in nonlymphoid tissues and provide rapid, localized immune protection. Their strategic positioning supports frontline defense against recurrent infections and contributes to antitumor surveillance, yet the same persistence can sustain chronic inflammation and autoimmunity when resident programs become pathogenic. This chapter synthesizes current concepts of T_{RM} differentiation, retention, and microenvironmental adaptation, and compares T_{RM}-associated mechanisms across infection, cancer, and immune-mediated inflammatory diseases. We further highlight emerging translational opportunities to therapeutically modulate T_{RM} cells or their niches – including cytokine/signaling manipulation, checkpoint-based approaches, metabolic and microenvironmental interventions, and tissue-directed vaccination – while emphasizing key challenges for tissue-specific precision immunology.

Keywords: tissue-resident memory T cells, T_{RM} cells, immune surveillance, cancer immunity, tissue microenvironment, immunotherapy

1. Introduction

The immune system's capacity to remember prior antigen exposure and respond more efficiently upon reencounter is a cornerstone of adaptive immunity. This phenomenon, known as immunological memory, is largely mediated by T lymphocytes, which not only expand during primary immune responses but also generate long-lived progeny that persist after antigen clearance. For decades, memory T (T_{MEM}) cells were primarily conceptualized as circulating populations that patrol the blood, lymph, and secondary lymphoid organs, thereby enabling rapid systemic recall responses [1, 2]. Within this classical framework, circulating memory T cells are subdivided into central memory T (T_{CM}) cells, which preferentially home to lymphoid tissues and exhibit strong proliferative potential, and effector memory T (T_{EM}) cells, which circulate through peripheral sites and can rapidly execute effector functions [3, 4]. This circulation-centered view provided a powerful explanation for systemic protection but could not fully account for the speed and anatomical localization of many real-world recall responses, particularly at barrier sites where pathogens first invade. The recognition that memory can be stored directly within tissues – rather than relying solely on continual recirculation – has reshaped the conceptual landscape of T cell immunology and introduced tissue residency as a fundamental dimension of immune memory [5, 6].

Tissue-resident memory T (T_{RM}) cells represent a distinct subset of memory T cells that establish durable residence within nonlymphoid tissues and typically do not recirculate through the blood or lymphatic system [7, 8]. They have been identified across a wide range of anatomical sites, including barrier tissues such as the skin, gastrointestinal tract, respiratory tract, and urogenital tract, as well as nonbarrier organs such as the brain and liver [9–17]. Their widespread distribution underscores their strategic role as "sentinels" positioned at sites of frequent antigen exposure. Phenotypically, T_{RM} cells are commonly defined by the expression of residency-associated molecules that reinforce tissue retention and spatial organization, including CD69, CD103, and CD49a [18, 19]. These markers are not merely descriptive; they correspond to functional retention mechanisms: CD69 suppresses sphingosine-1-phosphate receptor 1 (S1P1)-driven egress signals and thereby limits tissue egress; CD103 (integrin $\alpha E\beta 7$) binds epithelial E-cadherin to promote epithelial anchoring and stable positioning; and CD49a (integrin $\alpha 1$) interacts with collagen-rich structures, supporting localization within basement-membrane niches and reinforcing cytotoxic capacity [20, 21]. The clinical relevance of T_{RM} cells stems from their ability to generate rapid, localized immune responses precisely where disease processes unfold. On the protective side, T_{RM} cells provide frontline defense against reinfection by previously encountered pathogens and contribute to antitumor immunity through swift cytokine release, cytotoxic effector activity, and orchestration of local tissue immune networks [22, 23]. Their tissue anchoring makes them particularly attractive targets for strategies aimed at strengthening mucosal or organ-specific immunity, including vaccines designed to induce protective resident memory or immunotherapies intended to amplify local tumor surveillance [24]. Conversely, this same persistence and rapid reactivity can become maladaptive. When activation is dysregulated or antigens are self-derived, T_{RM} cells may sustain chronic inflammation, amplify tissue injury, and contribute to autoimmune or inflammatory diseases [25]. These dual roles – protection versus pathology – highlight both the promise and complexity of therapeutically manipulating T_{RM} cell biology. Translationally, the central challenge is achieving tissue-specific modulation that suppresses pathogenic resident programs while preserving systemic immune competence and protective memory.

In this chapter, we provide a structured overview of T_{RM} cell biology and its disease relevance, emphasizing the mechanistic principles that govern tissue residency, functional specialization, and microenvironmental adaptation. We then synthesize evidence linking T_{RM} cells to major disease categories – including autoimmunity and chronic inflammatory disorders, cancer immune surveillance and evasion, and chronic or recurrent infections – and highlight their context-dependent protective and pathogenic roles. Finally, we discuss emerging therapeutic strategies that target T_{RM} cells or their tissue niches, including immune modulation, checkpoint-based approaches, metabolic interventions, and tissue-directed vaccination, with a focus on translational opportunities and key challenges for precision immunology.

2. Core biology of T_{RM} cells

2.1 Developmental cues and lineage commitment

T_{RM} cells constitute a distinct lineage of memory T cells that long-term reside within nonlymphoid tissues and provide rapid, localized immune protection. T_{RM} cell differentiation is a progressive and context-dependent process, shaped by tissue-derived cytokine signals and stabilized by transcriptional programs associated with tissue residency [26]. This process integrates environmental signals such as TGF-β, IL-15, and IL-7 with transcriptional regulators, including Hobit, Blimp-1, and RUNX3 to establish stable tissue residency.

Within peripheral tissues, locally available cytokines provide core instructive signals that regulate T_{RM} cell differentiation and maintenance, particularly in $CD8^+$ T_{RM} cell subsets [27]. TGF-β, especially in epithelial and barrier sites, cooperates with TCR signaling to induce CD103 and drive SMAD-dependent transcriptional programs that support long-term residency; it also helps repress egress-associated genes such as S1PR1 and KLF2, thereby limiting tissue exit [28–31]. In parallel, interleukin-15 (IL-15) supports T_{RM} cell survival and effector competence via JAK–STAT signaling, promotes antiapoptotic and metabolic programs, and has been implicated in maintaining functional heterogeneity, inducing residency-associated transcriptional features (including HOBIT/ZNF683 in some contexts), and sustaining mitochondrial fatty-acid oxidation (FAO) [32–35]. In certain tissues, interleukin-7 (IL-7) further complements IL-15–mediated signals by engaging its receptor CD127 and activating downstream STAT5 pathways, thereby promoting T_{RM} cell longevity and homeostatic stability [36, 37].

Beyond cytokine instruction, durable commitment requires transcriptional "locking" mechanisms that convert transient niche signals into stable residency programs. RUNX3 acts as a gatekeeper of epithelial-type residency by enabling a TGF-β–responsive transcriptional network that promotes core residency features in $CD8^+$ T cells [38]. Hobit (ZNF683) and Blimp-1 (PRDM1) then consolidate retention by repressing recirculation programs, effectively stabilizing the resident state [39].

Conceptually, this RUNX3–Hobit/Blimp-1 axis functions as a two-layer control system, linking tissue-derived cues to long-term positioning and rapid local protective capacity in nonlymphoid tissues.

2.2 Molecular signatures of tissue residency

2.2.1 CD69-S1PR1 axis

CD69, a member of the C-type lectin family, plays an important role in promoting the retention of T_{RM} cells within peripheral tissues. Although CD69 is widely used as a phenotypic marker for identifying T_{RM} cells under homeostatic conditions, its expression is highly dynamic and can be rapidly induced by a variety of activating signals [40, 41]. Functionally, CD69 antagonizes S1P1, thereby limiting

T cell responsiveness to sphingosine-1-phosphate (S1P) gradients and restricting cellular egress from tissues [20, 42]. Through this mechanism, CD69 contributes to the maintenance of tissue residency by preventing T cell exit into the circulation. Although CD69 is recognized as an important contributor to T_{RM} cell biology, its precise role in regulating intratissue positioning and tissue-specific immune function remains incompletely defined [43].

2.2.2 CD103–E-cadherin interaction

CD103 (αEβ7 integrin) is a defining surface molecule of T_{RM} cells and plays an important role in tissue retention and local immune surveillance. Its expression on T_{RM} cells is regulated by specific transcriptional programs, with RUNX family members – particularly RUNX2 and RUNX3 – contributing to CD103 induction and stabilization [44]. Functionally, CD103 binds to E-cadherin expressed on epithelial cells, promoting the localization and prolonged retention of T_{RM} cells within epithelial tissues and epithelial tumor niches, often in close proximity to target cells [21, 45, 46]. Although CD103 is widely regarded as a hallmark marker of T_{RM} cells, its expression is highly tissue-dependent. CD103 is prominently expressed by T_{RM} cells in mucosal and epithelial tissues – including the reproductive tract, skin, lungs, small intestine, and salivary glands – where it is closely associated with effective tissue retention and immunosurveillance [47–49]. In contrast, T_{RM} cells in nonepithelial compartments frequently lack CD103 expression and instead rely on alternative adhesion and retention pathways, such as VLA-1 (α1β1) and LFA-1 (αLβ2), to maintain tissue residency [13]. Collectively, these findings highlight the context-dependent utilization of CD103–E-cadherin interactions and underscore the adaptability of T_{RM} cells to distinct tissue environments.

2.2.3 CD49a–collagen anchoring

CD49a, the α1 subunit of integrin α1β1, has emerged as an important regulator of T_{RM} cell retention and function, although its role has historically been less well characterized than that of other T_{RM} cell-associated molecules. Upon binding to collagen I and IV within the extracellular matrix (ECM), CD49a promotes integrin redistribution toward focal adhesion sites, thereby strengthening T cell attachment to the ECM and triggering downstream effector responses, including cytotoxic activity and IFN-γ production [15, 50, 51]. Consistent with these functions, CD49a contributes to the retention of T cells in multiple tissues, including the lung, skin, and liver, and is particularly prominent on epidermal T_{RM} cells [52–54].

2.2.4 CXCR6–CXCL16-mediated retention

CXCR6, a chemokine receptor for CXCL16, has emerged as a distinctive molecular marker of T_{RM} cells and plays an important role in local immunosurveillance. Within tumor microenvironments, CXCR6 mediates interactions between T_{RM} cells and specialized subsets of dendritic cells (DCs), promoting the proliferation and maintenance of $CXCR6^{+}$ T_{RM} cell populations [55]. These interactions have been shown to be critical for effective antitumor vaccination and have been proposed, based on mechanistic insights from T_{RM} cell studies, as a potential strategy to enhance intratumoral retention of adoptively transferred

T cells, including CAR-T cells [55, 56]. Accordingly, CXCR6 expression on T_{RM} cells has been associated with improved responsiveness to immunotherapy, underscoring its value as a biomarker for T_{RM} cell involvement in cancer immune responses.

2.3 Metabolic adaptation in tissue niches

To persist long-term within nonlymphoid tissues, T_{RM} cells must adapt to a range of environmental constraints, including nutrient limitation, hypoxia, and metabolic stress. These challenges are met through specialized metabolic adaptation programs that optimize energy utilization and support cellular survival [57]. A defining feature of T_{RM} cell metabolism is the preferential reliance on FAO. Multiple studies have demonstrated that, under nutrient-restricted conditions in which glucose and amino acids are limited, T_{RM} cells depend on CPT1a-mediated transport of fatty acids into mitochondria to sustain β-oxidation and energy production [58, 59]. Given that T_{RM} cells frequently occupy nutrient-poor tissue niches, lipid metabolism represents a major energy source supporting their long-term functional competence [60].

Beyond lipid utilization, the availability of key nutrients such as glucose and amino acids can differentially shape tissue-resident versus circulating memory T-cell programs [59]. In many tissues, T_{RM} cells develop within microenvironments where nutrients fluctuate and competition is high (e.g., inflamed mucosa or tumors), creating selective pressure for metabolic flexibility rather than reliance on a single substrate [27, 61]. Compared with recirculating effector-like T cells that often depend on glucose-driven glycolysis to sustain rapid proliferation and short-term effector output, T_{RM} cells appear more adapted to nutrient-limited niches by tuning nutrient uptake, maintaining mitochondrial fitness, and balancing anabolic demands with long-term survival [58]. Amino-acid availability (e.g., glutamine and branched-chain amino acids) can further influence mTOR-dependent anabolic signaling and thereby bias the balance between durable residency-associated maintenance programs and highly proliferative circulating effector states [62].

Hypoxia is a common feature of many tissue environments and influences T_{RM} cell development and maintenance [63]. Under low oxygen tension, hypoxia-inducible factor-1α (HIF-1α) becomes stabilized and transcriptionally active, initiating adaptive gene expression programs that enable cellular survival [64]. HIF-1α induces glycolytic enzymes and also modulates mitochondrial function and FAO, contributing to metabolic reprogramming and energy homeostasis in T_{RM} cells [65–67]. Through enhanced glucose uptake and lactate production, HIF-1α signaling partially compensates for energy deficits under hypoxic conditions. In parallel, its coordinated regulation with FAO supports T_{RM} cell survival in environments characterized by both oxygen and nutrient limitation [64]. Beyond metabolic control, HIF-1α has been implicated in the regulation of ECM remodeling and adhesion molecule expression, providing additional structural and metabolic support for stable tissue residency under hypoxic stress [68, 69]. Collectively, these adaptations enable T_{RM} cells to integrate metabolic, environmental, and signaling inputs into a coherent survival strategy within tissue niches [70].

The development and maintenance of T_{RM} cells, therefore, rely on the synergistic integration of local cytokine signaling, adhesion-mediated interactions, and metabolic adaptation mechanisms, which together form a tightly interconnected immunoregulatory network [30, 71]. Among these, TGF-β acts as a central regulator by inducing CD103 expression to reinforce epithelial adhesion while concurrently reshaping cellular metabolism, including activation of FAO pathways, thereby supporting energy homeostasis in hypoxic and nutrient-restricted tissues [27, 72]. IL-15 and IL-7 further complement this process by activating antiapoptotic pathways such as PI3K–AKT signaling, extending T_{RM} cells' lifespan and functional persistence [73]. In addition, adhesion molecules such as integrin αEβ7 not only provide structural anchorage but also transmit mechanotransductive signals that influence metabolic gene expression and reinforce metabolic reprogramming [74, 75]. Through these coordinated mechanisms, T_{RM} cells acquire a metabolically adapted tissue-resident state that supports durable positioning and rapid, localized immune responses against infection or tumor dissemination within barrier tissues [76].

3. T_{RM} cells as drivers of chronic inflammation and autoimmunity

3.1 T_{RM} cells and "lesion memory"

Accumulating evidence from infectious and chronic inflammatory disease models indicates that T_{RM} cells provide a cellular basis for lesion memory, a phenomenon in which previously affected tissue sites remain immunologically primed long after the apparent resolution of disease. A defining feature of lesion memory is the persistence of T_{RM} cells following clinical remission. In multiple neurotropic viral infection models, including MuPyV, cytomegalovirus (CMV), herpes simplex virus (HSV), and West Nile virus (WNV) infection, $CD8^+$ T_{RM} cells persist within the central nervous system (CNS) parenchyma after viral clearance and contribute to long-term local immune surveillance [77–80]. Notably, maintenance of these T_{RM} cell populations can occur independently of IL-15, indicating a tissue-adapted homeostatic mechanism distinct from that of circulating memory T cells [81].

Beyond long-term persistence, T_{RM} cells exhibit a pronounced capacity for rapid local recall responses, which underlies site-specific disease relapse. Upon antigen reencounter, T_{RM} cells rapidly proliferate and produce effector cytokines such as IFN-γ and TNF-α, amplifying immune responses directly within affected tissues [80]. In respiratory viral infection models, including influenza virus infection, T_{RM} cell-mediated recall responses provide effective localized protection against reinfection [82–84]. In chronic inflammatory and autoimmune diseases, reactivation of T_{RM} cells is closely associated with lesion activity and tissue pathology.

The long-term persistence of T_{RM} cells after clinical remission, and their ability to mount rapid, localized recall responses, establish a form of tissue-intrinsic immune memory that links prior inflammatory or infectious events to future site-specific disease relapse [85–87].

3.2 Disease-specific pathogenic mechanisms

Accumulating evidence indicates that T_{RM} cells, while essential for host protection, also play pathogenic roles in autoimmune and inflammatory diseases. In disorders such as rheumatoid arthritis (RA) and systemic lupus erythematosus (SLE), tissue-localized T_{RM} cells secrete proinflammatory cytokines and chemokines that sustain local inflammation and drive progressive tissue damage, fibrosis, and organ dysfunction [88–90].

3.2.1 T_{RM} cells – mediated pathogenic mechanisms in rheumatoid arthritis

In RA synovium, T_{RM} cells are enriched within inflamed joints and engage in close interactions with synovial fibroblasts, forming a pathogenic immune–stromal niche [91]. Upon local antigen recognition, synovial T_{RM} cells undergo clonal expansion and secrete inflammatory mediators such as GM-CSF, which promotes fibroblast activation and drives macrophage and osteoclast precursor differentiation, thereby accelerating bone erosion [92, 93]. In parallel, T_{RM} cell-derived IL-17 amplifies synovial inflammation by inducing fibroblast production of IL-6, CXCL12, and RANKL, a key driver of osteoclastogenesis [94]. Together, these cytokine circuits establish a self-reinforcing inflammatory loop that sustains chronic synovitis and joint destruction [94]. Beyond joints, T_{RM} cells also contribute to extraarticular RA manifestations. In RA-associated interstitial lung disease, pulmonary T_{RM} cells act as local inflammatory initiators, producing IL-17 and GM-CSF in response to environmental or autoantigenic cues. These cytokines activate fibroblasts and promote profibrotic signaling, linking T_{RM} cell activity to progressive pulmonary inflammation and fibrosis [95–97].

3.2.2 T_{RM} cells-mediated pathogenic mechanisms in systemic lupus erythematosus

In SLE, particularly cutaneous lupus erythematosus, skin-resident T_{RM} cells, characterized by CD69 and CD103 expression, persist long-term and maintain local immune activation [90, 98]. Upon ultraviolet or inflammatory stimulation, these T_{RM} cells produce type I interferons, notably IFN-α, which enhance antigen presentation and induce keratinocyte-derived inflammatory mediators, forming a self-sustaining inflammatory network that underlies lesion persistence and relapse [99]. In lupus nephritis, renal T_{RM} cells participate directly in local autoantibody production. These cells form immunological synapses with B cells via CD40–CD40L interactions and secrete IL-21, promoting B-cell activation, plasma-cell differentiation, and pathogenic immunoglobulin production. This T_{RM} cell–B-cell crosstalk contributes to immune-complex deposition and correlates with the severity of glomerular injury [100–102].

3.2.3 T_{RM} cell-mediated pathogenic mechanisms in systemic sclerosis

Systemic sclerosis (SSc) is characterized by progressive fibrosis and vasculopathy. Emerging evidence suggests that aberrantly activated T_{RM} cells contribute to fibrogenesis through the secretion of profibrotic mediators, particularly TGF-β [103]. TGF-β drives fibroblast activation, myofibroblast differentiation, and excessive ECM deposition, leading to tissue stiffening and organ dysfunction. Although direct evidence of T_{RM} cell-derived TGF-β in human SSc remains limited, inflammatory lesion environments and parallels with other autoimmune diseases support a contributory role for T_{RM} cells in local fibrotic circuits [104]. Epigenetic dysregulation is increasingly recognized as a mechanism that reinforces aberrant T_{RM} cell activation in SSc. Studies of T cells from patients with SSc have revealed widespread alterations in DNA methylation patterns, leading to dysregulated expression of immune regulatory genes and a persistently activated T_{RM} cell-like state [105, 106]. In parallel, abnormalities in histone modifications further disrupt transcriptional control, predisposing T_{RM} cells to exaggerated inflammatory responses [107]. As a consequence of these epigenetic changes, T_{RM} cells exhibit sustained production of proinflammatory and profibrotic cytokines, including TGF-β, which promotes fibroblast activation, ECM deposition, and endothelial dysfunction [108, 109].

3.2.4 T_{RM} cells-mediated pathogenic mechanisms in primary Sjögren's syndrome

In primary Sjögren's syndrome, T_{RM} cells residing in salivary glands persist long-term and contribute to glandular dysfunction [110]. Upon activation, these T_{RM} cells secrete lymphotoxin-α, establishing an early proinflammatory microenvironment that disrupts acinar integrity and impairs secretion, even before overt lymphocytic infiltration occurs [111–113]. Sustained T_{RM} cell activity progressively damages glandular architecture, leading to irreversible loss of salivary function and clinical xerostomia [114, 115].

Collectively, T_{RM} cells underlie the pathogenesis of multiple autoimmune disorders through disease-specific cellular and molecular mechanisms, as summarized in **Figure 1**.

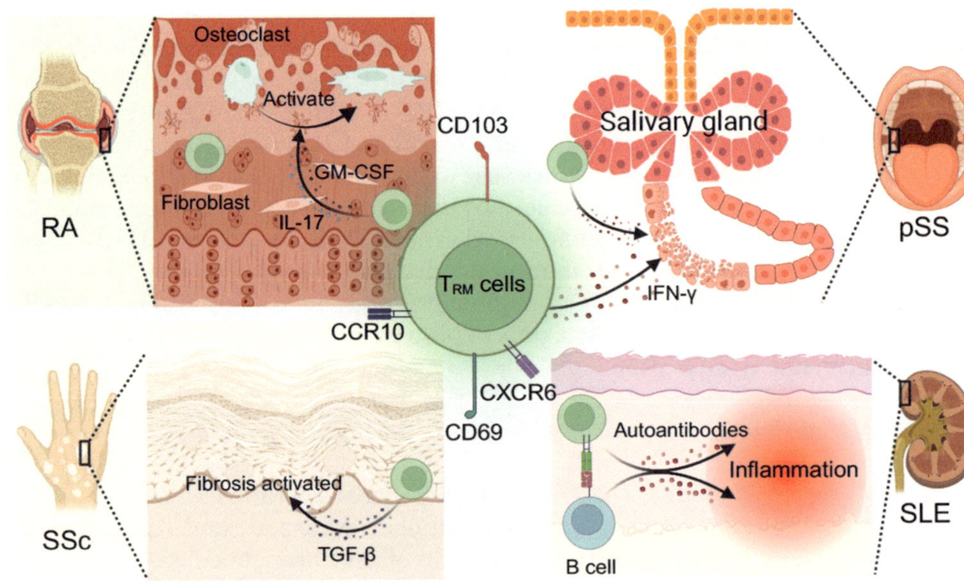

Figure 1.
Mechanistic overview of T_{RM} cells and their pathogenic roles across autoimmune diseases. T_{RM} cell markers include CD69, CD103, CXCR6, and CCR10, maintained by Cytokine signaling through transforming growth factor-β (TGF-β), Interleukin-15 (IL-15), and Interleukin-7 (IL-7). In rheumatoid arthritis (RA), synovial T_{RM} cells interact with fibroblasts, secrete granulocyte–macrophage colony-stimulating factor (GM-CSF), and promote osteoclast activation, contributing to joint erosion. In primary Sjögren's Syndrome (pSS), $CD8^+$ T_{RM} cells in the salivary glands release cytotoxic mediators that damage glandular epithelium. In systemic sclerosis (SSc), T_{RM} cell-derived TGF-β drives fibroblast activation and tissue fibrosis, accompanied by epigenetic reprogramming of local immune cells. In systemic lupus erythematosus (SLE), T_{RM} cells in the skin and kidney produce type I interferons and form immune synapses with B cells, facilitating autoantibody production. Together, these findings highlight T_{RM} cells as critical mediators of tissue inflammation, fibrotic remodeling, and disease-specific "inflammatory memory." (Adopted from Tian et al. [25]).

4. T_{RM} cells in tumor immunity and immune evasion

The TME exhibits highly complex heterogeneity among different types of tumors, and there is a variety of immune cells in tumors [116, 117]. $CD8^+$ T_{RM} cells play a crucial role in tumor immune surveillance and immunotherapy, and their intratumoral infiltration is closely related to favorable prognostic outcomes in patients with cancer [118–120]. Tumor-localizing $CD8^+$ T_{RM} cells in solid tumors are frequently defined by the following characteristics: expression of CD103, CD69, and/or VLA-1 (CD49) [121–124].

4.1 Antitumor surveillance by T_{RM} cells

Substantial evidence proves that a greater density of $CD103^+CD8^+$ T_{RM} cells in the TME is associated with a better response to immunotherapy and a better survival outcome for patients with cancers [125]. Beyond direct cytotoxic killing, T_{RM} cells exert potent antitumor effects by releasing significant amounts of cytokines and chemokines, particularly IFN-γ and TNF-α, which activate other immune cells within the TME. IFN-γ produced by T_{RM} cells promotes the production of chemokines and antimicrobial molecules in the TME and recruits circulating central memory T (TCM) cells, which have been shown to differentiate into T_{RM} cells in tumor models [126, 127]. Concurrently, TNF-α released by T_{RM} cells promotes the rapid maturation of DCs. Furthermore, studies in viral infection models indicate that IL-2 produced by T_{RM} cells can upregulate granzyme B (GZMB) in natural killer (NK) cells, suggesting a role in coordinating innate and adaptive immunity [128].

Recent strategies have focused on harnessing preexisting antiviral T_{RM} cells to fight tumors. Virus-specific T_{RM} cells ($CD103^+CD69^+$) for influenza A virus (IAV), Epstein-Barr virus (EBV), and/or cCMV populate the mouse and human glioblastoma (GBM) microenvironment [129]. Similarly, hepatitis B virus-specific $CD8^+$ T_{RM} cells in hepatocellular carcinoma (HCC) tissues can be reactivated by viral peptides [130]. Local injection of these peptides triggers rapid proliferation of T_{RM} cells and the production of IFN-γ, TNF-α, and IL-2. This reactivation induces a robust antitumor immune response, characterized by the accumulation of $CD8^+$ T cells, NK cells, and DCs within tumors, the activation of DCs in draining lymph nodes, and, ultimately, the limitation of tumor growth [23, 131].

4.2 T_{RM} cells in the tumor microenvironment

Substantial evidence indicates that a high density of $CD103^+CD8^+$ T_{RM} cells in the TME correlates with a better response to immunotherapy and improved survival outcomes for cancer patients [44, 132, 133]. However, these cells also commonly express a suite of inhibitory immune checkpoint molecules, indicating a regulated or exhausted state within the TME.

In NSCLC patients, the density of T_{RM} cells ($CD103^+CD8^+$) shows a significant positive correlation with the expression of PD-1, Tim-3, and GZMB, and a negative association with tumor angiogenesis [134, 135]. Cytokine production profiles are also heterogeneous: $CD103^+CD4^+$ PD-1 low TILs produce the most TNF-α and IFN-γ, while $CD103^+CD4^+PD\text{-}1^+$ and $CD69^+CD4^+PD\text{-}1^+$ TILs produce CXCL13 [136]. In gastric cancer (GC), PD-(L)1 blockade can increase the proportion of $CD8^+CD103^+$ T_{RM} cells both in vivo and in vitro and restore their cytolytic capacity by upregulating fatty acid-binding protein 4 and 5 expression [137]. Single-cell sequencing reveals that $CD8^+$ T_{RM} cells in GC simultaneously exhibit an effector memory phenotype (expressing CD103, CD49α, GZMB, CXCL13) and exhaustion markers (expressing CTLA-4, TIM-3, PD-1, and TIGIT) [138]. Notably, the function of these $CD103^+CD69^+CD8^+$ T_{RM} cells can be suppressed by the gastric microbiome, particularly *Methylobacterium*, leading to tumor immune escape and a poor prognosis [138]. In colorectal cancer (CRC) and CRC liver metastasis patients, antiangiogenic therapy can enhance the infiltration and IFN-γ secretion of T_{RM} cells, and reinfusing $CD103^+CD8^+$ T_{RM} cells achieves better antitumor effects [139]. Research has identified zinc finger protein 683 (ZNF683) expression as a candidate marker for cancer-specific T_{RM} cells in CRC, suggesting it is a promising new target for regulating cancer immunity [140]. In triple-negative breast cancer (TNBC), a typically immunologically "cold" tumor, $CD8^+CD103^+$ T_{RM} cell-like cells are particularly significant for immunotherapy and tend to express higher levels of immune checkpoint molecules such as PD-1, CTLA-4, TIM-3, and LAG-3 [141]. Furthermore, clonal overlap between T_{RM} cells in breast cancer tissue and those in the urogenital tract has been observed, potentially indicating a shared immune response mechanism where T_{RM} cells traffic between tissues, contributing to a coordinated systemic defense against malignancies [21, 142].

These findings suggest that $CD8^+$ T_{RM} cells are a prognostic biomarker for survival outcomes in patients with solid tumors. Furthermore, the inhibitory immune checkpoint molecules expressed on T_{RM} cells, such as PD-1 and CTLA-4, may serve as potential targets for cancer immunotherapy.

4.3 The complexity of T_{RM} cells: Insights from organ-specific tumor contexts

The role of T_{RM} cells in the TME is not universally beneficial; their function is highly context-dependent and organ-specific. Under certain conditions, T_{RM} cells can exhibit immunosuppressive functions that may promote tumor progression. Cutaneous squamous cell carcinoma (cSCC) serves as a prime example of this "double-edged sword" nature. In cSCC, $CD8^+CD103^+$ T_{RM} cells display an immunosuppressive phenotype associated with a poor prognosis [143]. These cells highly express inhibitory markers like CD39, CTLA-4, and PD-1 and produce increased IL-10, thereby inhibiting antitumor immune responses and promoting tumor growth and metastasis. Notably, these immunosuppressive T_{RM} cells are more abundant in cSCC tissue than in normal skin and blood, highlighting their active role in tumor immune modulation.

In summary, T_{RM} cells constitute a functionally diverse and dynamic population within the tumor immune microenvironment. A comprehensive understanding of their complex roles across different organs, tumor types, and specific TME conditions is crucial for developing precise and effective T_{RM} cell-targeted therapeutic strategies.

5. T_{RM} cells in infection and tissue-specific host defense

T_{RM} cells are critical sentinels in peripheral tissues, providing rapid and localized defense against recurrent infections. Their function represents a double-edged sword, offering essential protection while potentially contributing to immunopathology and chronic inflammation if dysregulated.

5.1 Rapid recall responses to reinfection

T_{RM} cells are essential for mediating swift and effective immune responses upon reexposure to pathogens. In neurotropic viral infections – such as those caused by mouse polyomavirus (MuPyV), CMV, HSV, and WNV – antigen-specific $CD8^+$ T_{RM} cells persist within the CNS parenchyma long after clearance [78–80]. Upon rechallenge, these cells promptly secrete effector molecules like granzymes, perforin, and IFN-γ to control viral replication. The CXCL10/CXCR3 chemokine axis is crucial in shaping this protective T_{RM} cell immunity, as demonstrated in models of recurrent HSV-1 infection [80]. During IAV infection, $CD8^+$ T_{RM} cells are recruited to the airways via the CXCR6/CXCL16 signaling axis for ectopic defense, where they confer protection against reinfection through cytokine (IFN-γ, TNF-α) and cytolytic molecule (perforin, GZMB) production [82, 84].

$CD4^+$ T_{RM} cells also contribute directly and indirectly; for instance, lung $CD4^+$ resident helper T (TRH) cells secrete IFN-γ to promote the development of protective $CD103^+CD8^+$ T_{RM} cells during IAV infection [144]. In mucosal tissues, such as the female reproductive tract after HSV-2 infection, both $CD4^+$ and $CD8^+$ T_{RM} cells are maintained and can respond rapidly, primarily via cytokine secretion, like IFN-γ, to limit viral spread [145, 146]. This principle extends to bacterial contexts, where prior lung infection with *Streptococcus pneumoniae* seeds $CD4^+$ T_{RM} cells that, upon heterotypic rechallenge, produce IL-17A to recruit neutrophils swiftly [147]. This is also exemplified in urinary tract infections (UTIs), where uropathogenic *E. coli* (UPEC)-specific T_{RM} cells are generated and retained in the bladder mucosa after primary infection. Upon secondary challenge, they rapidly activate, secreting interferon-gamma (IFN-γ) to recruit neutrophils and initiate a swift defensive cascade [148].

5.2 Balance between protection and immunopathology

While T_{RM} cells are indispensable for host defense, their reactivation can sometimes induce excessive inflammation and tissue damage, highlighting a delicate balance between protection and pathology. In the urogenital tract, the same T_{RM} cells that protect against recurrent UTIs can, through their persistent activation and cytokine production, contribute to bladder inflammation and tissue damage, potentially exacerbating symptoms [149, 150]. In the CNS, antigen-specific reactivation of $CD8^+$ T_{RM} cells can lead to significant neuroinflammation, neuropathology, and even cognitive decline, largely mediated through IFN-γ stimulation of microglia [87, 151]. In bacterial infections, the same IL-17A produced by lung $CD4^+$ T_{RM} cells that clears *Streptococcus pneumoniae* or *Staphylococcus aureus* can contribute to inflammatory pathology if unregulated [147, 152]. Similarly, in the context of *Helicobacter pylori* colonization, $CD8^+$ T_{RM} cells infiltrating the gastric mucosa contribute to both pathogen control and immunopathological damage [153]. In chronic inflammatory diseases, this balance is often tipped toward pathology. For example, in Crohn's disease, a population of $CD103^+CD161^+CCR5^+CD4^+$ T_{RM} cells produces substantial amounts of type 1 inflammatory cytokines, orchestrating local inflammation [154]. In primary biliary cholangitis, highly activated $CD8^+$ T_{RM} cells mediate bile duct damage via production of IL-17 and IL-22 [155, 156]. This dichotomy underscores the need for precise immune regulation to harness the protective functions of T_{RM} cells while minimizing collateral tissue damage.

5.3 Chronic infection and recurrent inflammation

T_{RM} cells are pivotal players in the dynamics of chronic infections and are often linked to the recurrence and persistence of inflammatory diseases. Their long-term residency can sustain low-grade inflammation or drive disease flares.

In chronic urogenital infections, T_{RM} cells underpin both recurrent disease and latency. In recurrent UTIs, the very persistence of UPEC-specific T_{RM} cells defines the immunological memory of the bladder, yet their failure to prevent recurrence highlights a need for more effective vaccine strategies aimed at boosting their function [148, 157]. In chronic HSV-2 infection, the density and maintenance of genital T_{RM} cells, which persist via IL-15-independent mechanisms, influence disease severity and recurrence [81]. Furthermore, T_{RM} cells surveil latent viruses like CMV and EBV in the urogenital tract, poised to respond if reactivation occurs [13].

During chronic *Helicobacter pylori* infection, vaccine-induced $CD4^+$ T_{RM} cells ($CD69^+CD103^-$) can proliferate and differentiate in situ upon challenge, contributing to ongoing gastric immunity and inflammation [158]. In parasitic infections, such as chronic *Toxoplasma gondii* infection, $CD8^+$ T_{RM} cells that accumulate in the brain continuously produce IFN-γ and TNF-α to control the parasite, sustaining a neuroinflammatory environment [159]. In autoimmune and inflammatory diseases, T_{RM} cells are major drivers of chronicity. In multiple sclerosis (MS) lesions, $CD69^+CD103^+CD49a^+PD\text{-}1^+$ T_{RM} cells are enriched and correlate with active demyelination; these cells, which may include EBV-specific clones with impaired viral control, persist as local inflammatory reservoirs [16, 160]. In the skin of patients with psoriasis or atopic dermatitis, IL-17-producing $CD8^+$ T_{RM} cells contribute to disease relapse through persistent cytokine production [161, 162]. Furthermore, in chronic liver diseases (e.g., autoimmune hepatitis, steatohepatitis) and lupus nephritis, the expansion and cytokine-driven activation of T_{RM} cells heightens organ-specific inflammation [163–167].

The persistence of T_{RM} cells across diverse tissues – brain, gut, liver, skin – underscores their central role in the cycle of recurrent inflammation and suggests that targeting T_{RM} cell maintenance or their proinflammatory cytokines (e.g., IL-17, IFN-γ) could be a therapeutic strategy to achieve long-term remission.

6. Therapeutic strategies targeting T_{RM} cells

T_{RM} cells are distributed across multiple organs and can rapidly trigger potent local immune responses, providing durable protection against infections and malignant transformation. Their enrichment is frequently associated with favorable clinical outcomes, and their tissue positioning enables early control of viral exposure, limiting local replication and dissemination. Therefore, therapeutic strategies may aim to promote T_{RM} cell generation, reinvigorate suppressed T_{RM} cell functions, or attenuate pathogenic T_{RM} cell programs in chronic inflammation and autoimmunity (**Figure 2**, **Table 1**).

6.1 Cytokine and signaling pathway modulation

The survival and proliferation of T_{RM} cells depend substantially on IL-15 signaling, which activates downstream effectors via the JAK–STAT pathway – particularly

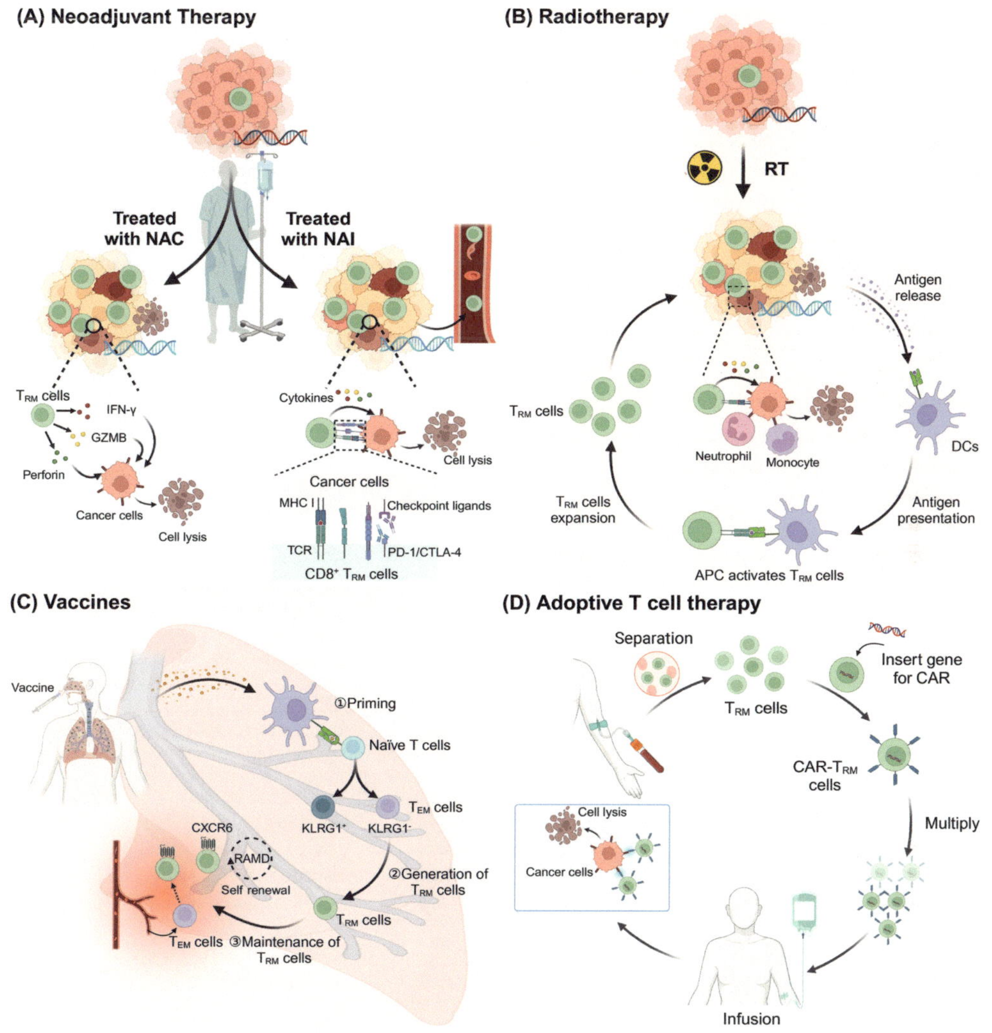

Figure 2.

Multimodal strategies to enhance protective T_{RM} cells in cancers. (a) Neoadjuvant therapy: 1) Neoadjuvant chemotherapy (NAC): Tumors treated with NAC can induce DNA chain breaks, leading to cell apoptosis. T_{RM} cells secrete IFN-γ, GZMB, and perforin to kill tumor cells. 2) Neoadjuvant immunotherapy (NAI): Anti-PD-1/anti-CTLA-4 antibodies are used to block immune checkpoints and restore exhausted T_{RM} cells. Additionally, NAI can facilitate the exit of T_{RM} cells from tumors into the circulation, thereby promoting systemic tumor immunity. (b) Radiotherapy: T_{RM} cells exhibit strong radiation resistance and proliferate extensively when stimulated by tumor antigens. They secrete cytokines such as TGF-β, which recruit neutrophils and monocytes into the TME, thereby promoting an antitumor immune response. (c) Vaccines: Vaccines induce the formation of pathogen-specific T_{RM} cells in the lungs. The maintenance of lung CD8+ T_{RM} cells relies on replenishment from circulating CD8+ T_{EM} cells or on the local proliferation of lung CD8+ T_{RM} cells in repair-associated memory depots (RAMDs). (d) Adoptive T-cell therapy: T_{RM} cells from patients are collected and engineered to express a specific antigen on their surface, creating CAR-T_{RM} cells. These CAR-T_{RM} cells are then multiplied in large quantities in vitro and infused back into the patient's body to target and eliminate blood tumors. This figure was designed using BioRender (https://biorender.com/). (Adopted from Xie et al. [19]).

STAT5 – to support T_{RM} cell maintenance and function [168]. Consequently, JAK inhibitors can effectively block IL-15 signal transduction, reducing T_{RM} cell survival and dampening the secretion of proinflammatory cytokines, with clinically meaningful benefits reported in inflammatory skin diseases such as vitiligo and psoriasis [169]. Beyond decreasing baseline survival signals, JAK inhibition may also blunt antigen-triggered local inflammatory recall responses, providing a foundation for rational combination strategies [170, 171].

TGF-β is a critical tissue-derived cue that promotes T_{RM} cell differentiation/retention in epithelial contexts and also serves as a major immunoregulatory and

Therapeutic strategies	Disease types	Treatment strategies	Mechanistic rationale	References
Cytokine and signaling pathway modulation	Inflammatory skin diseases (vitiligo, psoriasis)	JAK inhibitors	Block IL-15 signaling; reduce T_{RM} cell survival and proinflammatory cytokine secretion	[166–169]
	Tumors	TGF-β–targeted modulation	TGF-β contributes to intratumoral T-cell reprogramming and may support T_{RM} cell-associated radioresistance	[170]
	Fibrotic disease (systemic sclerosis)	Target αv-integrin–mediated latent TGF-β activation	Reduce/interrupte TGF-β activation	[171]
	Psoriasis and other Th17-mediated diseases	Anti-IL-23 antibodies (e.g., risankizumab); anti-IL-17 antibodies (e.g., secukinumab)	Durable remission, partly via indirect disruption of T_{RM} cell-driven cytokine feedback loops, addresses the IL-23/IL-17 "inflammatory memory pool"	[172–175]
Immune checkpoint–based strategies	Tumors	ICIs targeting CTLA-4 and PD-1/PD–L1; neoadjuvant immunotherapy (NAI)	Anti-PD-1 preventive treatment increases $CD8^+$ T_{RM} cell infiltration and long-term benefit; anti-PD-1 + anti-CTLA-4 expands $CD69^+CD103^+CD8^+$ T_{RM} cells and enhances cytotoxicity	[135, 178–180]
		Combination regimens to convert cold→hot: chemotherapy, radiotherapy, or CRT + ICIs	Cold tumors lack intratumoral T cells, limiting ICI efficacy; combinations increase T-cell infiltration and reshape the TME, improving ICI sensitivity; CRT-exposed TME is enriched in $CD103^+CD8^+$ T_{RM} cells	[192–195]

Therapeutic strategies	**Disease types**	**Treatment strategies**	**Mechanistic rationale**	**References**
Metabolic and microenvironmental interventions	Tumors	Target FAO dependence (e.g., CPT1a pathway)	$CD8^+CD103^+$ T_{RM} cells depend on FAO; metabolic rewiring prolongs T_{RM} cell lifespan and enhances antitumor immunity	[196]
	Rheumatic models; SLE	Metformin (AMPK activation; mTORC1 inhibition)	Broad immune-metabolic modulation may influence the Th17/Treg balance, is associated with reduced relapse risk and steroid-sparing trends, and shows improved PROs in SLE.	[219–221]
	Tumors/ inflamed tissues	Hypoxia/tissue-stress niche modulation	Hypoxia and stress shape T-cell fate; evidence in irradiated tumors suggests TGF-β regulates T-cell reprogramming and contributes to T_{RM} cell-associated radioresistance → supports niche-focused modulation to restore T_{RM} cell function (cancer) or reduce persistence (autoimmunity).	[170]
	Rheumatic disease (RA)	Smart nanoparticle delivery of siRNA (e.g., macrophage-targeted polymersomes; MMP-2/ pH-responsive platform delivering triptolide/ metformin)	Silences pathogenic genes; reverses glucocorticoid resistance and yields synergistic antiinflammatory/joint-protective effects (CIA model); platform limits inflammatory infiltration and remodels vascular–immune–inflammatory milieu.	[197, 198]
		Synthetic-biology engineering of fibroblasts (FLS)	Reprogram local fibroblasts as in situ "drug factories" to reshape the joint microenvironment; a niche-directed paradigm potentially synergistic with systemic therapies and destabilizing T_{RM} cell-supportive circuits.	[199–201]

Therapeutic strategies	Disease types	Treatment strategies	Mechanistic rationale	References
Vaccines and tissue-directed immunotherapy	Infection prevention and tumor immunotherapy	Mucosal vaccination (e.g., intranasal LAIV; adenoviral vector + IL-1β; antibody-targeted vaccination to DCs; intranasal ChAd-SARS-CoV-2; Shiga toxin B subunit vector; H. pylori vaccine)	Route-dependent induction of protective T_{RM} cells: mucosal routes elicit lung or gastric T_{RM} cells, whereas systemic routes may not.	[203, 205, 222, 223]
	Smallpox/vaccinia-related models	Epidermal disruption/ skin scarification (MVA)	Elicits strong T-cell responses, including T_{RM} /T_{CM} cells; MVA via scarification increases lung antigen-specific $CD8^+$ T_{RM} cells and protects against lethal respiratory challenge.	[202, 206, 207]
	Tumors	Adjuvants and combinations: carbomer nanoemulsion + CpG/ GLA; topical CpG; neoantigen peptide vaccine (NeoVAC) + α-PD -1	Induce systemic or mucosal lung $CD4^+$ T_{RM} cells; enhance T_{RM} cell generation; NeoVAC + α-PD-1 increases $CD8^+$ T_{RM} cell infiltration and establishes long-term antitumor immune memory in HCC.	[208–210]
		NAC; radiotherapy; radioimmunotherapy designs	NAC: increases intratumoral T_{RM} cells and enhances antitumor immunity. Radiotherapy: RT + therapeutic vaccine increases T_{RM} cells; T_{RM} cells contribute to tumor control via motility/IFN-γ; RT releases DAMPs, recruiting myeloid cells.	[125, 170, 211–213, 215]
		Adoptive immunotherapy/engineered cells: ACT; T_{RM} cells-programming; CAR-T with T_{RM} cell-like phenotype induction (TGF-β, IL-15)	Runx3 loss prevents T-cell accumulation in tumors; Runx3 overexpression increases T_{RM} cell-like populations and improves survival; CAR-T cells inducing a T_{RM} cell-like phenotype may improve retention/ durability.	[44, 216, 217]

Table 1.
Potential therapeutic strategies based on T_{RM} cells.

profibrotic mediator in several diseases. In tumors, transcriptomic analyses suggest that TGF-β contributes to the reprogramming of intratumoral T cells and may support T_{RM} cell-associated radioresistance, motivating interest in TGF-β–targeted modulation within the TME [172]. In fibrotic settings such as SSc, multiple αv integrins (αvβ1/β3/β5/β6/β8) participate in latent TGF-β activation; accordingly, targeting αv-integrin–mediated TGF-β activation is considered a particularly promising antifibrotic approach [173].

IL-17 and IL-23 are pivotal in sustaining T_{RM} cells' effector function and maintaining a proinflammatory microenvironment [174]. In psoriasis, T_{RM} cells represent a key source of IL-17, whereas IL-23 provides essential survival and functional support; the IL-23/IL-17 axis relies on a local "inflammatory memory pool" formed by T_{RM} cells to drive relapse [175]. Clinically, anti-IL-23 antibodies (e.g., risankizumab) and anti-IL-17 antibodies (e.g., secukinumab) achieve significant efficacy in psoriasis and other Th17-mediated diseases, and part of their durable remission likely reflects indirect disruption of T_{RM} cell-driven cytokine feedback loops [176, 177].

6.2 Immune checkpoint–based strategies

Immune checkpoint inhibitor (ICI) therapy has demonstrated remarkable clinical efficacy, with monoclonal antibodies targeting CTLA-4 and PD-1/PD–L1 increasingly used across tumor types [178]. Neoadjuvant immunotherapies (NAIs) using ICIs have achieved clinical success in multiple cancers, and accumulating evidence suggests that these benefits are closely linked to intratumoral T_{RM} cells [179]. For example, anti-PD-1 preventive treatment increased $CD8^+$ T_{RM} cell infiltration over prolonged periods and provided long-term benefits to patients with ESCC [137, 180]. Combination anti-PD-1 and anti-CTLA-4 therapy expanded intratumoral $CD69^+CD103^+CD8^+$ T_{RM} cells, enhanced cytotoxic capacity in TNBC, and provided local immune protection against tumor rechallenge [181]. In preclinical models, anti-PD-1 therapy similarly increased intratumoral T_{RM} cell populations and delayed tumor progression compared with T cell therapy alone [182]. Comparable associations between T_{RM} cell enrichment and therapeutic response have been reported in melanoma, MIBC, HNSC, NSCLC, LUAD, cervical cancer, gastrointestinal cancers, and nonmetastatic clear cell renal cell carcinoma [183–191].

Mechanistically, T_{RM} cell-rich tumors may respond well to PD-1/PD–L1 blockade [192, 193]. Preexisting resident T cells can act as an intratumoral effector reservoir. They can rapidly produce cytokines and execute cytotoxic functions. They may also promote antigen spreading through interactions with local DCs. Together, these effects can amplify endogenous antitumor immunity. In contrast, "cold" tumors often show limited baseline T-cell infiltration. In this setting, combination regimens may be required to improve ICI responsiveness [194, 195]. Such regimens can first recruit T cells into the tumor. They can then imprint or reinforce residency programs. Examples include radiotherapy or chemotherapy, oncolytic approaches, and vaccine-based priming [196, 197]. Niche-shaping cytokine or chemokine cues may further support a TRM-permissive microenvironment. Ultimately, these strategies may convert the tumor microenvironment into a state that is more responsive to PD-1/PD–L1 blockade [180].

A key limitation is that ICIs are most effective in "hot" tumors with substantial immune infiltration; in contrast, "cold" tumors often lack sufficient intratumoral T cells, constraining ICI efficacy [194, 195]. Thus, clinical strategies increasingly emphasize combination regimens that increase T cell infiltration and reshape the TME to improve ICI sensitivity, including chemotherapy, radiotherapy, or chemoradiotherapy (CRT) plus ICIs [196, 198–200]. Notably, in early-stage TNBC, the presence of T_{RM} cells within breast tissue correlates with improved long-term survival after chemotherapy combined with anti-PD-1 therapy [181]. CRT-exposed TMEs are also highly enriched in $CD103^{+}CD8^{+}$ T_{RM} cells in both CRC patients and CT26-bearing mice, supporting T_{RM} cells as a functional substrate for combined modality immunotherapy [196].

6.3 Metabolic and microenvironmental interventions

6.3.1 Metabolic interventions

T_{RM} cells often exhibit heightened bioenergetic demands for long-term survival and effector competence, with a notable reliance on FAO. In gastric adenocarcinoma, $CD8^{+}CD103^{+}$ T_{RM} cells undergo metabolic reprogramming and depend on FAO, with CPT1a acting as a rate-limiting enzyme; metabolic rewiring can prolong T_{RM} cells' lifespan and enhance antitumor immunity [61]. These observations suggest that FAO pathways (e.g., CPT1a) may serve as metabolic handles to either support beneficial T_{RM} cell function in cancer or restrain pathogenic tissue-resident programs in chronic inflammation, depending on the therapeutic goal.

6.3.2 Hypoxia modulation

Within tumors and inflamed tissues, hypoxia and stress-associated metabolic constraints shape T-cell fate and function. Transcriptomic evidence in irradiated tumors indicates that TGF-β may act as a regulator of T-cell reprogramming within the TME and contribute to T_{RM} cell-associated radioresistance [172]. This aligns with a broader view that hypoxia-related programs and tissue stress responses can be therapeutically manipulated – either to restore T_{RM} cells' effector capacity in cancer or to reduce the persistence of pathogenic T_{RM} cells in autoimmune lesions – through niche-focused modulation.

6.3.3 Nanotechnology-assisted delivery

T_{RM} cell persistence depends on ECM, chemokines, stromal, and immune interactions. Therefore, remodeling lesion microenvironments to weaken T_{RM} cell-supportive circuits is attractive.

Functionalized nanocarriers can deliver siRNAs to targeted cells within lesions, silencing pathogenic genes and perturbing inflammatory circuits that sustain T_{RM} cell survival and function. For example, macrophage-targeted polymeric polymersomes that sequentially deliver TNF-α siRNA (siTNFα), followed by dexamethasone, reverse glucocorticoid resistance in the collagen-induced arthritis model, achieving synergistic antiinflammatory and joint-protective effects [201]. Another microenvironment-driven deformable nanoplatform responds to elevated MMP-2 and acidic pH in RA joints, forms a physical barrier limiting inflammatory infiltration, and releases payloads (e.g., triptolide, metformin) to remodel the vascular–immune–inflammatory milieu; preclinical studies demonstrate specificity and safety for local gene and drug delivery [202].

An emerging strategy is to reprogram local fibroblasts using synthetic-biology tools to create in situ "drug factories" that continuously secrete therapeutic proteins. In rheumatic diseases – particularly RA – engineering fibroblast-like synoviocytes (FLS) to reshape the joint microenvironment offers a niche-directed paradigm that could synergize with systemic therapies and potentially destabilize T_{RM} cell-supportive circuits [203–205].

6.4 Vaccines and tissue-directed immunotherapy

6.4.1 Vaccines to induce protective T_{RM} cells

T_{RM} cells are central to vaccine-induced protective immunity and have become a major focus in vaccine development for infection prevention and tumor immunotherapy. Evidence from animal models indicates that the route of immunization is a key determinant of T_{RM} cell formation: intramuscular immunization generally elicits weaker T_{RM} cell responses than mucosal or epidermal routes, likely because muscle contains relatively few DCs [206]. Accordingly, mucosal and epidermal vaccination strategies are particularly relevant for generating robust tissue immunity.

Mucosal vaccines can induce pathogen-specific T_{RM} cells at portals of entry. Intranasal administration of live attenuated influenza virus induces both $CD4^+$ and $CD8^+$ T_{RM} cells in the lung, whereas systemic immunization does not [207]. Coexpression of IL-1β can enhance the mucosal immunogenicity of adenoviral vector influenza vaccines [208]. "Antibody-targeted vaccination" strategies that deliver antigens to respiratory DCs can generate lung $CD8^+$ T_{RM} cells with high GZMB and IFN-γ, conferring strong protection against lethal influenza infection [209]. Collectively, these studies support mucosal vaccination as a direct route to establish protective T_{RM} cells at barrier surfaces.

Epidermal disruption is also highly effective in eliciting strong T cell responses, including T_{RM} and T_{CM} cells, contributing historically to successful vaccination (e.g.,vaccinia-based smallpox vaccination) [206, 210]. When administered via skin scarification, modified vaccinia virus Ankara (MVA) immunization produces greater numbers of lung antigen-specific $CD8^+$ T_{RM} cells and protects against lethal respiratory challenges [211].

Vaccine adjuvants further enhance T_{RM} cell responses. Carbomer-based nanoemulsion systems incorporating TLR9 agonist CpG or TLR4 agonist GLA can drive systemic or mucosal lung $CD4^+$ T_{RM} cell responses and provide protection even in the absence of detectable neutralizing antibodies [212]. Topical CpG during subcutaneous immunization can enhance T_{RM} cell generation [213]. In tumor settings, a neoantigen peptide vaccine combined with α-PD-1 can elicit robust antitumor responses and establish long-term immune memory in HCC by increasing $CD8^+$ T_{RM} cell infiltration [214].

6.4.2 Tissue-directed immunotherapy: Chemotherapy/radiotherapy combinations and adoptive approaches

To address "cold" tumors, multimodal regimens enrich intratumoral T_{RM} cells and improve ICI responsiveness [195, 196, 198–200]. Neoadjuvant chemotherapy (NAC) with platinum agents induces DNA damage and apoptosis and benefits T_{RM}

cell-enriched tumors; enriched $CD8^+CD103^+$ T_{RM} cells predict higher pathologic complete response rates with platinum-containing NAC [127, 215, 216]. NAC is also associated with increased intratumoral T_{RM} cells and enhanced antitumor immunity [182].

Radiotherapy intersects with T_{RM} cell biology: high $CD103^+$ T_{RM} cell infiltration is associated with improved prognosis in cervical cancer receiving radiotherapy, and therapeutic vaccination plus radiotherapy increases intratumoral $CD103^+CD8^+$ T_{RM} cells in preclinical models [113]. T_{RM} cells may be more radioresistant than circulating T cells, and surviving intratumoral T cells show increased motility and IFN-γ production, supporting tumor control [172, 217]. CD103–E-cadherin adhesion can trigger outside-in signaling (Pyk2, paxillin), promoting migration and effector function after irradiation [218]. Radiotherapy also releases DAMPs and recruits neutrophils/monocytes, supporting radioimmunotherapy designs [219].

Adoptive T cell therapy can be viewed as infusing tumor-experienced T cells with T_{RM} cell-like programs. In murine melanoma, Runx3 deficiency impairs intratumoral accumulation and worsens outcomes, whereas Runx3 overexpression increases T_{RM} cell-like populations and improves survival [44]. CAR-T is effective in hematologic malignancies but is limited in solid tumors by trafficking/infiltration barriers [220]. Inducing a T_{RM} cell-like phenotype using TGF-β and IL-15 may improve tissue retention and durability [221]. PD-1-targeting CAR-T can selectively deplete liver $CD8^+$ T_{RM} cells and alleviate autoimmune cholangitis in a disease model [155].

6.4.3 Disease-context caution: Suppressing pathogenic T_{RM} cells in autoimmunity

While T_{RM} cells are desirable for infection control and tumor surveillance, they can be pathogenic in autoimmune diseases such as vitiligo and psoriasis. In this context, strategies that prevent the formation of new T_{RM} cells or reduce the survival of established T_{RM} cell populations may provide therapeutic benefit. Notably, short-term anti-CD122 (IL-15 signaling inhibition) suppresses T_{RM} cells' production of IFN-γ, whereas long-term treatment can eliminate T_{RM} cells from skin lesions in vitiligo [222].

7. Conclusion(s)

T_{RM} cells redefine immunological memory by establishing a durable, strategically positioned immune layer within nonlymphoid tissues, enabling rapid in situ recall responses against reinfection and malignant transformation. Yet, the same persistence that underlies protection can also sustain "lesion memory," promoting relapse, chronic inflammation, and tissue damage when antigenic or inflammatory cues are dysregulated. Translationally, T_{RM} cell biology supports a context-dependent therapeutic logic: amplify or reinvigorate protective T_{RM} cell responses in infection and cancer (tissue-directed vaccination, checkpoint-based strategies), while restraining pathogenic T_{RM} cell circuits in autoimmunity and chronic inflammatory disease through pathway, niche, or metabolic interventions. Future progress will depend on integrating spatial and single-cell profiling to match T_{RM} cell states with tissue- and disease-specific interventions for durable control with minimal systemic cost.

Acknowledgments

This research was funded by the Chronic Disease Management Research Project of the National Health Commission Capacity Building and Continuing Education Center (GWJJMB202510025060), National Natural Science Foundation of China (32500813), Postdoctoral Fellowship Program of CPSF (GZC20251503), China Postdoctoral Science Foundation (2025M781899), Sichuan Science and Technology Program (2024ZYD0149; 2026NSFSC1940), Special Research Foundation for the Postdoctoral Program of Sichuan Province (TB2024017), Key Research and Development Project of Deyang Science and Technology Bureau (2024SZY016, 2025SYCX061), and Special Fund for Incubation Projects of Deyang People's Hospital (FRH202501, FHT202501). The authors acknowledge the use of ChatGPT for the language polishing of the manuscript.

Conflict of Interest

The authors declare no conflict of interest.

Author details

Daoyuan Xie[1,2†], Yu Tian[2†], Jie Zhang[3], Miao He[1], Lianying Wu[2] and Guanting Lu[2*]

1 Cancer Center, Deyang People's Hospital of Chengdu University of Traditional Chinese Medicine, Deyang, China

2 Laboratory of Translational Medicine Research, Deyang People's Hospital of Chengdu University of Traditional Chinese Medicine, Deyang, China

3 Department of Rheumatology and Immunology, Deyang People's Hospital, Chengdu University of Traditional Chinese Medicine, Deyang, China

† These authors contributed equally to this work

*Address all correspondence to: guantlv@126.com

References

[1] Omilusik KD, Goldrath AW. Remembering to remember: T cell memory maintenance and plasticity. Current Opinion in Immunology. 2019;**58**:89–97. DOI: 10.1016/j.coi.2019.04.009

[2] Mueller SN, Gebhardt T, Carbone FR, Heath WR. Memory T cell subsets, migration patterns, and tissue residence. Annual Review of Immunology. 2013;**31**:137–161. DOI: 10.1146/annurev-immunol-032712-095954

[3] Sallusto F, Geginat J, Lanzavecchia A. Central memory and effector memory T cell subsets: Function, generation, and maintenance. Annual Review of Immunology. 2004;**22**:745–763. DOI: 10.1146/annurev.immunol.22.012703.104702

[4] Masopust D, Soerens AG. Tissue-resident T Cells and other resident leukocytes. Annual Review of Immunology. 2019;**37**:521–546. DOI: 10.1146/annurev-immunol-042617-053214

[5] Kok L, Masopust D, Schumacher TN. The precursors of CD8 (+) tissue resident memory T cells: From lymphoid organs to infected tissues. Nature Reviews Immunology. 2022;**22**(5):283–293. DOI: 10.1038/s41577-021-00590-3

[6] Yenyuwadee S, Sanchez-Trincado Lopez JL, Shah R, Rosato PC, Boussiotis VA. The evolving role of tissue-resident memory T cells in infections and cancer. Science Advances. 2022;**8**(33):eabo5871. DOI: 10.1126/sciadv.abo5871

[7] Mueller SN, Mackay LK. Tissue-resident memory T cells: Local specialists in immune defence. Nature Reviews Immunology. 2016;**16**(2):79–89. DOI: 10.1038/nri.2015.3

[8] Park CO, Kupper TS. The emerging role of resident memory T cells in protective immunity and inflammatory disease. Nature Medicine. 2015;**21**(7):688–697. DOI: 10.1038/nm.3883

[9] Li L, Liu P, Chen C, Yan B, Chen X, Li J, et al. Advancements in the characterization of tissue resident memory T cells in skin disease. Clinical Immunology. 2022;**245**:109183

[10] Liu G, Wang Z, Li S. Heterogeneity and plasticity of tissue-resident memory T cells in skin diseases and homeostasis: A review. Frontiers in Immunology. 2024;**15**:1378359. DOI: 10.3389/fimmu.2024.1378359

[11] FitzPatrick MEB, Provine NM, Garner LC, Powell K, Amini A, Irwin SL, et al. Human intestinal tissue-resident memory T cells comprise transcriptionally and functionally distinct subsets. Cell Reports. 2021;**34**(3):108661. DOI: 10.1016/j.celrep.2020.108661

[12] Carbone FR. Unique properties of tissue-resident memory T cells in the lungs: Implications for COVID-19 and other respiratory diseases. Nature Reviews Immunology. 2023;**23**(5):329–335. DOI: 10.1038/s41577-022-00815-z

[13] Parga-Vidal L, van Aalderen MC, Stark R, van Gisbergen K. Tissue-resident memory T cells in the urogenital tract. Nature Reviews Nephrology. 2022;**18**(4):209–223. DOI: 10.1038/s41581-021-00525-0

[14] Poon MML, Caron DP, Wang Z, Wells SB, Chen D, Meng W, et al. Tissue adaptation and clonal segregation of human memory T cells in barrier sites. Nature Immunology. 2023;**24**(2):309–319. DOI: 10.1038/s41590-022-01395-9

[15] Szabo PA, Miron M, Farber DL. Location, location, location: Tissue resident memory T cells in mice and humans. Science Immunology. 2019;**4**(34):eaas9673. DOI: 10.1126/sciimmunol.aas9673

[16] Fransen NL, Hsiao CC, van der Poel M, Engelenburg HJ, Verdaasdonk K, Vincenten MCJ, et al. Tissue-resident memory T cells invade the brain parenchyma in multiple sclerosis white matter lesions. Brain. 2020;**143**(6):1714–1730. DOI: 10.1093/brain/awaa117

[17] Li Y, You Z, Tang R, Ma X. Tissue-resident memory T cells in chronic liver diseases: Phenotype, development and function. Frontiers in Immunology. 2022;**13**:967055. DOI: 10.3389/fimmu.2022.967055

[18] Chen L, Shen Z. Tissue-resident memory T cells and their biological characteristics in the recurrence of inflammatory skin disorders. Cellular & Molecular Immunology. 2020;**17**(1):64–75. DOI: 10.1038/s41423-019-0291-4

[19] Xie D, Lu G, Mai G, Guo Q, Xu G. Tissue-resident memory T cells in diseases and therapeutic strategies. MedComm (2020). 2025;**6**(1):e70053. DOI: 10.1002/mco2.70053

[20] Shiow LR, Rosen DB, Brdickova N, Xu Y, An J, Lanier LL, et al. CD69 acts downstream of interferon-alpha/beta to inhibit S1P1 and lymphocyte egress from lymphoid organs. Nature. 2006;**440**(7083):540–544. DOI: 10.1038/nature04606

[21] Duhen T, Duhen R, Montler R, Moses J, Moudgil T, de Miranda NF, et al. Co-expression of CD39 and CD103 identifies tumor-reactive CD8 T cells in human solid tumors. Nature Communications. 2018;**9**(1):2724. DOI: 10.1038/s41467-018-05072-0

[22] Gebhardt T, Palendira U, Tscharke DC, Bedoui S. Tissue-resident memory T cells in tissue homeostasis, persistent infection, and cancer surveillance. Immunological Reviews. 2018;**283**(1):54–76. DOI: 10.1111/imr.12650

[23] Menares E, Galvez-Cancino F, Caceres-Morgado P, Ghorani E, Lopez E, Diaz X, et al. Tissue-resident memory CD8(+) T cells amplify anti-tumor immunity by triggering antigen spreading through dendritic cells. Nature Communications. 2019;**10**(1):4401. DOI: 10.1038/s41467-019-12319-x

[24] Gavil NV, Cheng K, Masopust D. Resident memory T cells and cancer. Immunity. 2024;**57**(8):1734–1751. DOI: 10.1016/j.immuni.2024.06.017

[25] Tian Y, Zhang J, Wu L, Zhang C, Zheng F, Yang Y, et al. Tissue-Resident Memory T Cells in Rheumatoid Immune Diseases: Pathogenic Mechanisms and Therapeutic Strategies. Biomedicines. 2025;**13**(12):2945. DOI: 10.3390/biomedicines13122945

[26] Christo SN, Park SL, Mueller SN, Mackay LK. The Multifaceted Role of Tissue-Resident Memory T Cells. Annual Review of Immunology. 2024;**42**(1):317–345. DOI: 10.1146/annurev-immunol-101320-020220

[27] Hasan F, Chiu Y, Shaw RM, Wang J, Yee C. Hypoxia acts as an environmental cue for the human tissue-resident memory T cell differentiation program. JCI Insight. 2021;**6**(10):e138970. DOI: 10.1172/jci.insight.138970

[28] Corgnac S, Boutet M, Kfoury M, Naltet C, Mami-Chouaib F. The Emerging Role of CD8+ Tissue Resident Memory T (TRM) Cells in Antitumor Immunity: A Unique Functional Contribution of the CD103 Integrin. Frontiers In Immunology. 2018;**9**:1904. DOI: 10.3389/fimmu.2018.01904

[29] Zhang N, Bevan MJ. Transforming growth factor-β signaling controls the formation and maintenance of gut-resident memory T cells by regulating migration and retention. Immunity. 2013;**39**(4):687–696. DOI: 10.1016/j.immuni.2013.08.019

[30] Qiu Z, Chu TH, Sheridan BS. TGF-β: Many Paths to CD103+ CD8 T Cell Residency. Cells. 2021;**10**(5):989. DOI: 10.3390/cells10050989

[31] Milner JJ, Goldrath AW. Transcriptional programming of tissue-resident memory CD8+ T cells. Current Opinion in Immunology. 2018;**51**:162–169. DOI: 10.1016/j.coi.2018.03.017

[32] Li X, Deng J, Liu X, Zhou Y, Bi T, Chen J, et al. Tissue-resident immune cells in cervical cancer: Emerging roles and therapeutic implications. Frontiers In Immunology. 2025;**16**:1541950

[33] Man K, Duarte da Silva VA, Potemkin N, Gabriel SS, Mason T, Elmzzahi T, et al. Stem-like tissue-resident memory T cells control functional heterogeneity and reactivation of T cell memory in the intestine. Science Immunology. 2025;**10**(112):eadw1992. DOI: 10.1126/sciimmunol.adw1992

[34] Jarjour NN, Wanhainen KM, Peng C, Gavil NV, Maurice NJ, Borges da Silva H, et al. Responsiveness to interleukin-15 therapy is shared between tissue-resident and circulating memory CD8+ T cell subsets. Proceedings of the National Academy of Sciences of the United States of America. 2022;**119**(43):e2209021119. DOI: 10.1073/pnas.2209021119

[35] Xu A, Bhanumathy KK, Wu J, Ye Z, Freywald A, Leary SC, et al. IL-15 signaling promotes adoptive effector T-cell survival and memory formation in irradiation-induced lymphopenia. Cell & Bioscience. 2016;**6**:30

[36] Choi H, Kim Y, Jung YW. The Function of Memory CD8+ T Cells in Immunotherapy for Human Diseases. Immune Network. 2023;**23**(1):e10. DOI: 10.4110/in.2023.23.e10

[37] Chen D, Tang T-X, Deng H, Yang X-P, Tang Z-H. Interleukin-7 Biology and Its Effects on Immune Cells: Mediator of Generation, Differentiation, Survival, and Homeostasis. Frontiers In Immunology. 2021;**12**:747324. DOI: 10.3389/fimmu.2021.747324

[38] Fonseca R, Burn TN, Gandolfo LC, Devi S, Park SL, Obers A, et al. Runx3 drives a CD8+ T cell tissue residency program that is absent in CD4+ T cells. Nature Immunology. 2022;**23**(8):1236–1245. DOI: 10.1038/s41590-022-01273-4

[39] Mackay LK, Minnich M, Kragten NAM, Liao Y, Nota B, Seillet C, et al. Hobit and Blimp1 instruct a universal transcriptional program of tissue residency in lymphocytes.

Science. 2016;**352**(6284):459–463. DOI: 10.1126/science.aad2035

[40] Povoleri GAM, Durham LE, Gray EH, Lalnunhlimi S, Kannambath S, Pitcher MJ, et al. Psoriatic and rheumatoid arthritis joints differ in the composition of CD8+ tissue-resident memory T cell subsets. Cell Reports. 2023;**42**(5):112514. DOI: 10.1016/j.celrep.2023.112514

[41] Siracusa F, Durek P, McGrath MA, Sercan-Alp O, Rao A, Du W, et al. CD69 (+) memory T lymphocytes of the bone marrow and spleen express the signature transcripts of tissue-resident memory T lymphocytes. European Journal of Immunology. 2019;**49** (6):966–968. DOI: 10.1002/eji.201847982

[42] Notario L, Alari-Pahissa E, Albentosa A, Leiva M, Sabio G, Lauzurica P. Anti-CD69 therapy induces rapid mobilization and high proliferation of HSPCs through S1P and mTOR. Leukemia. 2018;**32**(6):1445–1457. DOI: 10.1038/s41375-018-0052-x

[43] Cibrian D, Sanchez-Madrid F. CD69: From activation marker to metabolic gatekeeper. European Journal of Immunology. 2017;**47**(6):946–953. DOI: 10.1002/eji.201646837

[44] Milner JJ, Toma C, Yu BF, Zhang K, Omilusik K, Phan AT, et al. Runx3 programs CD8+ T cell residency in non-lymphoid tissues and tumours. Nature. 2017;**552**(7684):253–257. DOI: 10.1038/nature24993

[45] Oliveira G, Egloff AM, Afeyan AB, Wolff JO, Zeng Z, Chernock RD, et al. Preexisting tumor-resident T cells with cytotoxic potential associate with response to neoadjuvant anti-PD-1 in head and neck cancer. Science Immunology. 2023;**8**(87):eadf4968. DOI: 10.1126/sciimmunol.adf4968

[46] van Hooren L, Handgraaf SM, Kloosterman DJ, Karimi E, van Mil LWHG, Gassama AA, et al. CD103+ regulatory T cells underlie resistance to radio-immunotherapy and impair CD8+ T cell activation in glioblastoma. Nature Cancer. 2023;**4**(5):665–681. DOI: 10.1038/s43018-023-00547-6

[47] Mackay LK, Rahimpour A, Ma JZ, Collins N, Stock AT, Hafon ML, et al. The developmental pathway for CD103 (+)CD8+ tissue-resident memory T cells of skin. Nature Immunology. 2013;**14** (12):1294–1301. DOI: 10.1038/ni.2744

[48] Sheridan BS, Pham QM, Lee YT, Cauley LS, Puddington L, Lefrancois L. Oral infection drives a distinct population of intestinal resident memory CD8(+) T cells with enhanced protective function. Immunity. 2014;**40** (5):747–757. DOI: 10.1016/j.immuni.2014.03.007

[49] Casey KA, Fraser KA, Schenkel JM, Moran A, Abt MC, Beura LK, et al. Antigen-independent differentiation and maintenance of effector-like resident memory T cells in tissues. Journal of Immunology. 2012;**188** (10):4866–4875. DOI: 10.4049/jimmunol.1200402

[50] Eckert IN, Ribechini E, Jarick KJ, Strozniak S, Potter SJ, Beilhack A, et al. VLA-1 Binding to Collagen IV Controls Effector T Cell Suppression by Myeloid-Derived Suppressor Cells in the Splenic Red Pulp. Frontiers in Immunology. 2021;**11**:616531

[51] Cheuk S, Schlums H, Serezal IG, Martini E, Chiang SC, Marquardt N, et al. CD49a Expression Defines Tissue-Resident CD8+ T Cells Poised for

Cytotoxic Function in Human Skin. Immunity. 2017;**46**(2):287–300. DOI: 10.1016/j.immuni.2017.01.009

[52] Cooper GE, Mayall J, Donovan C, Haw TJ, Budden KF, Hansbro NG, et al. Antiviral Responses of Tissue-resident CD49a+ Lung Natural Killer Cells Are Dysregulated in Chronic Obstructive Pulmonary Disease Am. Journal of Respiratory and Critical Care Medicine. 2023;**207**(5):553–565. DOI: 10.1164/rccm.202205-0848OC

[53] Zitti B, Hoffer E, Zheng W, Pandey RV, Schlums H, Perinetti Casoni G, et al. Human skin-resident CD8+ T cells require RUNX2 and RUNX3 for induction of cytotoxicity and expression of the integrin CD49a. Immunity. 2023;**56**(6):1285–1302.e7. DOI: 10.1016/j.immuni.2023.05.003

[54] Bai L, Vienne M, Tang L, Kerdiles Y, Etiennot M, Escaliere B, et al. Liver type 1 innate lymphoid cells develop locally via an interferon-γ-dependent loop. Science. 2021;**371**(6536):eaba4177. DOI: 10.1126/science.aba4177

[55] Di Pilato M, Kfuri-Rubens R, Pruessmann JN, Ozga AJ, Messemaker M, Cadilha BL, et al. CXCR6 positions cytotoxic T cells to receive critical survival signals in the tumor microenvironment. Cell. 2021;**184**(17):4512–4530.e22. DOI: 10.1016/j.cell.2021.07.015

[56] Wang T, Shen Y, Luyten S, Yang Y, Jiang X. Tissue-resident memory CD8+ T cells in cancer immunology and immunotherapy. Pharmacological Research. 2020;**159**:104876. DOI: 10.1016/j.phrs.2020.104876

[57] van der Gracht ETI, Behr FM, Arens R. Functional Heterogeneity and Therapeutic Targeting of Tissue-Resident Memory T Cells. Cells. 2021;**10**(1):164. DOI: 10.3390/cells10010164

[58] Pan Y, Tian T, Park CO, Lofftus SY, Mei S, Liu X, et al. Survival of tissue-resident memory T cells requires exogenous lipid uptake and metabolism. Nature. 2017;**543**(7644):252–256. DOI: 10.1038/nature21379

[59] Varanasi SK, Kumar SV, Rouse BT. Determinants of Tissue-Specific Metabolic Adaptation of T Cells. Cell Metabolism. 2020;**32**(6):908–919. DOI: 10.1016/j.cmet.2020.10.013

[60] Han S-J, Glatman Zaretsky A, Andrade-Oliveira V, Collins N, Dzutsev A, Shaik J, et al. White Adipose Tissue Is a Reservoir for Memory T Cells and Promotes Protective Memory Responses to Infection. Immunity. 2017;**47**(6):1154–1168.e6. DOI: 10.1016/j.immuni.2017.11.009

[61] Lin R, Zhang H, Yuan Y, He Q, Zhou J, Li S, et al. Fatty Acid Oxidation Controls CD8(+) Tissue-Resident Memory T-cell Survival in Gastric Adenocarcinoma. Cancer Immunology Research. 2020;**8**(4):479–492. DOI: 10.1158/2326-6066.CIR-19-0702

[62] Sinclair LV, Rolf J, Emslie E, Shi YB, Taylor PM, Cantrell DA. Control of amino-acid transport by antigen receptors coordinates the metabolic reprogramming essential for T cell differentiation. Nature Immunology. 2013;**14**(5):500–508. DOI: 10.1038/ni.2556

[63] Liikanen I, Lauhan C, Quon S, Omilusik K, Phan AT, Bartrolí LB, et al. Hypoxia-inducible factor activity promotes antitumor effector function

and tissue residency by CD8+ T cells. Journal of Clinical Investigation. 2021;**131**(7):e143729. DOI: 10.1172/JCI143729

[64] Yfantis A, Mylonis I, Chachami G, Nikolaidis M, Amoutzias GD, Paraskeva E, et al. Transcriptional Response to Hypoxia: The Role of HIF-1-Associated Co-Regulators. Cells. 2023;**12**(5):798. DOI: 10.3390/cells12050798

[65] Salmond RJ. Regulation of T Cell Activation and Metabolism by Transforming Growth Factor-Beta. Biology (Basel). 2023;**12**(2):297. DOI: 10.3390/biology12020297

[66] Shen H, Ojo OA, Ding H, Mullen LJ, Xing C, Hossain MI, et al. HIF1α-regulated glycolysis promotes activation-induced cell death and IFN-γ induction in hypoxic T cells. Nature Communications. 2024;**15**(1):9394. DOI: 10.1038/s41467-024-53593-8

[67] Huang X, Zhao L, Peng R. Hypoxia-Inducible Factor 1 and Mitochondria: An Intimate Connection. Biomolecules. 2022;**13**(1):50. DOI: 10.3390/biom13010050

[68] Gilkes DM, Bajpai S, Chaturvedi P, Wirtz D, Semenza GL. Withdrawal: Hypoxia-inducible factor 1 (HIF-1) promotes extracellular matrix remodeling under hypoxic conditions by inducing P4HA1, P4HA2, and PLOD2 expression in fibroblasts. Journal of Biological Chemistry. 2023;**299**(9):105144. DOI: 10.1016/j.jbc.2023.105144

[69] Hanumegowda C, Mohan ME. Hypoxia Inducible Factor-1α in Pulmonary Fibrosis: A Promising Therapeutic Target. European Journal of Medical and Health Sciences. 2025;**7**(2):27–31. DOI: 10.24018/ejmed.2025.7.2.2256

[70] Chen Z, Dudek J, Maack C, Hofmann U. Pharmacological inhibition of GLUT1 as a new immunotherapeutic approach after myocardial infarction. Biochemical Pharmacology. 2021;**190**:114597. DOI: 10.1016/j.bcp.2021.114597

[71] Osman M, Park SL, Mackay LK. Tissue-resident memory T (TRM) cells: Front-line workers of the immune system. European Journal of Immunology. 2023;**53**(11):e2250060. DOI: 10.1002/eji.202250060

[72] Liu H, Chen Y-G. The Interplay Between TGF-β Signaling and Cell Metabolism. Frontiers in Cell and Developmental Biology. 2022;**10**:846723. DOI: 10.3389/fcell.2022.846723

[73] Dijkgraaf FE, Kok L, Schumacher TNM. Formation of Tissue-Resident CD8+ T-Cell Memory. Cold Spring Harbor Perspectives in Biology. 2021;**13**(8):a038117. DOI: 10.1101/cshperspect.a038117

[74] Harjunpää H, Somermäki R, Saldo Rubio G, Fusciello M, Feola S, Faisal I, et al. Loss of β2-integrin function results in metabolic reprogramming of dendritic cells, leading to increased dendritic cell functionality and anti-tumor responses. Oncoimmunology. 2024;**13**(1):2369373. DOI: 10.1080/2162402X.2024.2369373

[75] Splitt RL, DeMali KA. Metabolic reprogramming in response to cell mechanics. Biology of the Cell. 2023;**115**(5):e202200108. DOI: 10.1111/boc.202200108

[76] Barros L, Ferreira C, Veldhoen M. The fellowship of regulatory and tissue-resident memory cells. Mucosal Immunology. 2022;**15**(1):64–73. DOI: 10.1038/s41385-021-00456-w

[77] Mockus TE, Shwetank Lauver MD, HM R, CS N, Salameh T, et al. CD4 T cells control development and maintenance of brain-resident CD8 T cells during polyomavirus infection. PLoS Pathogens. 2018;**14**(10):e1007365. DOI: 10.1371/journal.ppat.1007365

[78] Brizic I, Susak B, Arapovic M, Huszthy PC, Hirsl L, Kvestak D, et al. Brain-resident memory CD8(+) T cells induced by congenital CMV infection prevent brain pathology and virus reactivation. European Journal of Immunology. 2018;**48**(6):950–964. DOI: 10.1002/eji.201847526

[79] Shrestha B, Samuel MA, Diamond MS. CD8+ T cells require perforin to clear West Nile virus from infected neurons. Journal of Virology. 2006;**80**(1):119–129. DOI: 10.1128/JVI.80.1.119-129.2006

[80] Srivastava R, Khan AA, Chilukuri S, Syed SA, Tran TT, Furness J, et al. CXCL10/CXCR3-Dependent Mobilization of Herpes Simplex Virus-Specific CD8(+) T(EM) and CD8(+) T(RM) Cells within Infected Tissues Allows Efficient Protection against Recurrent Herpesvirus Infection and Disease. Journal of Virology. 2017;**91**(14): e00278–17. DOI: 10.1128/JVI.00278-17

[81] Schenkel JM, Fraser KA, Casey KA, Beura LK, Pauken KE, Vezys V, et al. IL-15-Independent Maintenance of Tissue-Resident and Boosted Effector Memory CD8 T Cells. Journal of Immunology. 2016;**196**(9):3920–3926. DOI: 10.4049/jimmunol.1502337

[82] Wein AN, McMaster SR, Takamura S, Dunbar PR, Cartwright EK, Hayward SL, et al. CXCR6 regulates localization of tissue-resident memory CD8 T cells to the airways. Journal of Experimental Medicine. 2019;**216**(12):2748–2762. DOI: 10.1084/jem.20181308

[83] McMaster SR, Wilson JJ, Wang H, Kohlmeier JE. Airway-Resident Memory CD8 T Cells Provide Antigen-Specific Protection against Respiratory Virus Challenge through Rapid IFN-gamma Production. Journal of Immunology. 2015;**195**(1):203–209. DOI: 10.4049/jimmunol.1402975

[84] Wu X, Wu P, Shen Y, Jiang X, Xu F. CD8(+) Resident Memory T Cells and Viral Infection. Frontiers in Immunology. 2018;**9**:2093. DOI: 10.3389/fimmu.2018.02093

[85] Vincenti I, Page N, Steinbach K, Yermanos A, Lemeille S, Nunez N, et al. Tissue-resident memory CD8(+) T cells cooperate with CD4(+) T cells to drive compartmentalized immunopathology in the CNS. Science Translational Medicine. 2022;**14**(640):eabl6058. DOI: 10.1126/scitranslmed.abl6058

[86] Frieser D, Pignata A, Khajavi L, Shlesinger D, Gonzalez-Fierro C, Nguyen XH, et al. Tissue-resident CD8 (+) T cells drive compartmentalized and chronic autoimmune damage against CNS neurons. Science Translational Medicine. 2022;**14**(640):eabl6157. DOI: 10.1126/scitranslmed.abl6157

[87] Ayasoufi K, Wolf DM, Namen SL, Jin F, Tritz ZP, Pfaller CK, et al. Brain resident memory T cells rapidly expand and initiate neuroinflammatory responses following CNS viral infection. Brain, Behavior, and Immunity. 2023;**112**:51–76

[88] LW WH, Li Q, et al. Pathogenic role of tissue-resident memory T cells in autoimmune diseases. Autoimmunity Reviews. 2018;**17**(9):906–911. DOI: 10.1016/j.autrev.2018.03.014

[89] Gao A, Zhao W, Wu R, Su R, Jin R, Luo J, et al. Tissue-resident memory T cells: The key frontier in local synovitis memory of rheumatoid arthritis. Journal of Autoimmunity. 2022;**133**:102950

[90] Ryan GE, Harris JE, Richmond JM. Resident Memory T Cells in Autoimmune Skin Diseases. Frontiers In Immunology. 2021;**12**:652191. DOI: 10.3389/fimmu.2021.652191

[91] Alivernini S, Tolusso B, Ferraccioli G, Gremese E, Kurowska-Stolarska M, McInnes IB. Driving chronicity in rheumatoid arthritis: Perpetuating role of myeloid cells. Clinical and Experimental Immunology. 2018;**193**(1):13–23. DOI: 10.1111/cei.13098

[92] McInnes IB, Schett G. Pathogenetic insights from the treatment of rheumatoid arthritis. Lancet. 2017;**389** (10086):2328–2337. DOI: 10.1016/S0140-6736(17)31472-1

[93] Firestein GS. The immunopathogenesis of rheumatoid arthritis. Current Opinion in Rheumatology. 1991;**3**(3):398–406. DOI: 10.1097/00002281-199106000-00012

[94] Kondo N, Kuroda T, Kobayashi D. Cytokine Networks in the Pathogenesis of Rheumatoid Arthritis. International Journal of Molecular Sciences. 2021;**22** (20):10922. DOI: 10.3390/ijms222010922

[95] Lin Y-J, Anzaghe M, Schülke S. Update on the Pathomechanism, Diagnosis, and Treatment Options for Rheumatoid Arthritis. Cells. 2020;**9** (4):880. DOI: 10.3390/cells9040880

[96] Kadura S, Raghu G. Rheumatoid arthritis-interstitial lung disease: Manifestations and current concepts in pathogenesis and management. European Respiratory Review. 2021;**30** (160):210011. DOI: 10.1183/16000617.0011-2021

[97] Manfredi A, Cassone G, Luppi F, Atienza-Mateo B, Cavazza A, Sverzellati N, et al. Rheumatoid arthritis related interstitial lung disease. Expert Review of Clinical Immunology. 2021;**17** (5):485–497. DOI: 10.1080/1744666X.2021.1905524

[98] Gu H-J, Song S, Roh JY, Jung Y, Kim HJ. Expression pattern of tissue-resident memory T cells in cutaneous lupus erythematosus. Lupus. 2021;**30**(9):1427–1437. DOI: 10.1177/09612033211017218

[99] Tian J, Shi L, Zhang D, Yao X, Zhao M, Kumari S, et al. Dysregulation in keratinocytes drives systemic lupus erythematosus onset. Cellular & Molecular Immunology. 2025;**22**(1):83–96. DOI: 10.1038/s41423-024-01240-z

[100] Vincent FB, Figgett WA, Hibbs ML. Hallmark of Systemic Lupus Erythematosus: Role of B Cell Hyperactivity. In Hoi A, editor. Pathogenesis of Systemic Lupus Erythematosus: Insights from Translational Research. Cham: Springer International Publishing; 2021. p. 9–36

[101] Bocharnikov AV, Keegan J, Wacleche VS, Cao Y, Fonseka CY, Wang G, et al. PD-1hiCXCR5–T peripheral helper cells promote B cell responses in lupus via MAF and IL-21. JCI Insight. 2019;**4**(20):

e130062. DOI: 10.1172/jci.insight.130062

[102] Ramanujam M, Steffgen J, Visvanathan S, Mohan C, Fine JS, Putterman C. Phoenix from the flames: Rediscovering the role of the CD40-CD40L pathway in systemic lupus erythematosus and lupus nephritis. Autoimmunity Reviews. 2020;**19**(11):102668. DOI: 10.1016/j.autrev.2020.102668

[103] Altorok N, Kahaleh B. Epigenetics and systemic sclerosis. Seminars in Immunopathology. 2015;**37**(5):453–462. DOI: 10.1007/s00281-015-0504-6

[104] Gaydosik AM, Tabib T, Domsic R, Khanna D, Lafyatis R, Fuschiotti P. Single-cell transcriptome analysis identifies skin-specific T-cell responses in systemic sclerosis. Annals of the Rheumatic Diseases. 2021;**80**(11):1453–1460. DOI: 10.1136/annrheumdis-2021-220209

[105] Yu J, Tang R, Ding K. Epigenetic Modifications in the Pathogenesis of Systemic Sclerosis. International Journal of General Medicine. 2022;**15**:3155–3166. DOI: 10.2147/ijgm.S356877

[106] Li T, Ortiz-Fernández L, Andrés-León E, Ciudad L, Javierre BM, López-Isac E, et al. Epigenomics and transcriptomics of systemic sclerosis CD4+ T cells reveal long-range dysregulation of key inflammatory pathways mediated by disease-associated susceptibility loci. Genome Medicine. 2020;**12**(1):81. DOI: 10.1186/s13073-020-00779-6

[107] Dees C, Pötter S, Zhang Y, Bergmann C, Zhou X, Luber M, et al. TGF-β-induced epigenetic deregulation of SOCS3 facilitates STAT3 signaling to promote fibrosis. Journal of Clinical Investigation. 2020;**130**(5):2347–2363. DOI: 10.1172/jci122462

[108] Volkmann ER, Andréasson K, Smith V. Systemic sclerosis. Lancet. 2023;**401**(10373):304–318. DOI: 10.1016/s0140-6736(22)01692-0

[109] Denton CP, Khanna D. Systemic sclerosis. Lancet. 2017;**390**(10103):1685–1699. DOI: 10.1016/s0140-6736(17)30933-9

[110] Ambudkar I. Calcium signaling defects underlying salivary gland dysfunction. Biochimica et Biophysica Acta (BBA). Molecular Cell Research. 2018;**1865**(11, Part B):1771–1777. DOI: 10.1016/j.bbamcr.2018.07.002

[111] Srivastava A, Makarenkova HP. Innate Immunity and Biological Therapies for the Treatment of Sjögren's Syndrome. International Journal of Molecular Sciences. 2020;**21**(23):9172

[112] Shen L, Suresh L, Wu J, Xuan J, Li H, Zhang C, et al. A role for lymphotoxin in primary Sjogren's disease. Journal of Immunology. 2010;**185**(10):6355–6363. DOI: 10.4049/jimmunol.1001520

[113] Sharma R, Chaudhari KS, Kurien BT, Grundahl K, Radfar L, Lewis DM, et al. Sjögren Syndrome without Focal Lymphocytic Infiltration of the Salivary Glands. The Journal of Rheumatology. 2020;**47**(3):394–399. DOI: 10.3899/jrheum.181443

[114] Mauro D, Lin X, Pontarini E, Wehr P, Guggino G, Tang Y, et al. CD8+ tissue-resident memory T cells are expanded in primary Sjögren's disease and can be therapeutically targeted by CD103 blockade. Annals of the Rheumatic Diseases. 2024;**83**(10):1345–1357. DOI: 10.1136/ard-2023-225069

[115] Yura Y, Hamada M. Outline of Salivary Gland Pathogenesis of Sjögren's Syndrome and Current Therapeutic Approaches. International Journal of Molecular Sciences. 2023;**24**(13):11179. DOI: 10.3390/ijms241311179

[116] Ferro S, Huber V, Rivoltini L. Mechanisms of tumor immunotherapy, with a focus on thoracic cancers. Journal of Thoracic Disease. 2018;**10**(7):4619–4631. DOI: 10.21037/jtd.2018.07.30

[117] Hinshaw DC, Shevde LA. The Tumor Microenvironment Innately Modulates Cancer Progression. Cancer Research. 2019;**79**(18):4557–4566. DOI: 10.1158/0008-5472.CAN-18-3962

[118] Galon J, Angell HK, Bedognetti D, Marincola FM. The continuum of cancer immunosurveillance: Prognostic, predictive, and mechanistic signatures. Immunity. 2013;**39**(1):11–26. DOI: 10.1016/j.immuni.2013.07.008

[119] Peske JD, Woods AB, Engelhard VH. Control of CD8 T-Cell Infiltration into Tumors by Vasculature and Microenvironment. Advances in Cancer Research. 2015;**128**:263–307. DOI: 10.1016/bs.acr.2015.05.001

[120] Fu Q, Chen N, Ge C, Li R, Li Z, Zeng B, et al. Prognostic value of tumor-infiltrating lymphocytes in melanoma: A systematic review and meta-analysis. Oncoimmunology. 2019;**8**(7):1593806. DOI: 10.1080/2162402X.2019.1593806

[121] Boddupalli CS, Bar N, Kadaveru K, Krauthammer M, Pornputtapong N, Mai Z, et al. Interlesional diversity of T cell receptors in melanoma with immune checkpoints enriched in tissue-resident memory T cells. JCI Insight. 2016;**1**(21):e88955. DOI: 10.1172/jci.insight.88955

[122] Djenidi F, Adam J, Goubar A, Durgeau A, Meurice G, de Montpreville V, et al. CD8+CD103+ tumor-infiltrating lymphocytes are tumor-specific tissue-resident memory T cells and a prognostic factor for survival in lung cancer patients. Journal of Immunology. 2015;**194**(7):3475–3486. DOI: 10.4049/jimmunol.1402711

[123] Murray T, Fuertes Marraco SA, Baumgaertner P, Bordry N, Cagnon L, Donda A, et al. Very Late Antigen-1 Marks Functional Tumor-Resident CD8 T Cells and Correlates with Survival of Melanoma Patients. Frontiers in Immunology. 2016;**7**:573

[124] Webb JR, Milne K, Nelson BH. PD-1 and CD103 Are Widely Coexpressed on Prognostically Favorable Intraepithelial CD8 T Cells in Human Ovarian Cancer. Cancer Immunology Research. 2015;**3**(8):926–935. DOI: 10.1158/2326-6066.CIR-14-0239

[125] La Manna MP, Di Liberto D, Lo Pizzo M, Mohammadnezhad L, Shekarkar Azgomi M, Salamone V, et al. The Abundance of Tumor-Infiltrating CD8(+) Tissue Resident Memory T Lymphocytes Correlates with Patient Survival in Glioblastoma. Biomedicines. 2022;**10**(10):2454. DOI: 10.3390/biomedicines10102454

[126] Ariotti S, Hogenbirk MA, Dijkgraaf FE, Visser LL, Hoekstra ME, Song JY, et al. T cell memory. Skin-resident memory CD8(+) T cells trigger a state of tissue-wide pathogen alert. Science. 2014;**346**(6205):101–105. DOI: 10.1126/science.1254803

[127] Savas P, Virassamy B, Ye C, Salim A, Mintoff CP, Caramia F, et al. Single-cell profiling of breast cancer T cells reveals a tissue-resident memory

subset associated with improved prognosis. Nature Medicine. 2018;**24**(7):986–993. DOI: 10.1038/s41591-018-0078-7

[128] Schenkel JM, Fraser KA, Beura LK, Pauken KE, Vezys V, Masopust D. T cell memory. Resident memory CD8 T cells trigger protective innate and adaptive immune responses. Science. 2014;**346**(6205):98–101. DOI: 10.1126/science.1254536

[129] Ning J, Gavil NV, Wu S, Wijeyesinghe S, Weyu E, Ma J, et al. Functional virus-specific memory T cells survey glioblastoma. Cancer Immunology, Immunotherapy. 2022;**71**(8):1863–1875. DOI: 10.1007/s00262-021-03125-w

[130] Cheng Y, Gunasegaran B, Singh HD, Dutertre CA, Loh CY, Lim JQ, et al. Non-terminally exhausted tumor-resident memory HBV-specific T cell responses correlate with relapse-free survival in hepatocellular carcinoma. Immunity. 2021;**54**(8):1825–1840e7. DOI: 10.1016/j.immuni.2021.06.013

[131] Rosato PC, Wijeyesinghe S, Stolley JM, Nelson CE, Davis RL, Manlove LS, et al. Virus-specific memory T cells populate tumors and can be repurposed for tumor immunotherapy. Nature Communications. 2019;**10**(1):567. DOI: 10.1038/s41467-019-08534-1

[132] Corgnac S, Malenica I, Mezquita L, Auclin E, Voilin E, Kacher J, et al. CD103(+)CD8(+) T(RM) Cells Accumulate in Tumors of Anti-PD-1-Responder Lung Cancer Patients and Are Tumor-Reactive Lymphocytes Enriched with Tc17. Cell Reports Medicine. 2020;**1**(7):100127. DOI: 10.1016/j.xcrm.2020.100127

[133] Byrne A, Savas P, Sant S, Li R, Virassamy B, Luen SJ, et al. Tissue-resident memory T cells in breast cancer control and immunotherapy responses. Nature Reviews Clinical Oncology. 2020;**17**(6):341–348. DOI: 10.1038/s41571-020-0333-y

[134] Yang G, Cai S, Hu M, Li C, Yang L, Zhang W, et al. Spatial features of specific $CD103^{+}CD8^{+}$ tissue-resident memory T cell subsets define the prognosis in patients with non-small cell lung cancer. Journal of Translational Medicine. 2024;**22**(1):27. DOI: 10.1186/s12967-023-04839-4

[135] van der Leun AM, Thommen DS, Schumacher TN. CD8(+) T cell states in human cancer: Insights from single-cell analysis. Nature Reviews Cancer. 2020;**20**(4):218–232. DOI: 10.1038/s41568-019-0235-4

[136] Oja AE, Piet B, van der Zwan D, Blaauwgeers H, Mensink M, de Kivit S, et al. Functional Heterogeneity of CD4(+) Tumor-Infiltrating Lymphocytes With a Resident Memory Phenotype in NSCLC. Frontiers in Immunology. 2018;**9**:2654

[137] Nose Y, Saito T, Yamamoto K, Yamashita K, Tanaka K, Yamamoto K, et al. The tissue-resident marker CD103 on peripheral blood T cells predicts responses to anti-PD-1 therapy in gastric cancer. Cancer Immunology, Immunotherapy. 2023;**72**(1):169–181. DOI: 10.1007/s00262-022-03240-2

[138] Peng R, Liu S, You W, Huang Y, Hu C, Gao Y, et al. Gastric Microbiome Alterations Are Associated with Decreased CD8+ Tissue-Resident Memory T Cells in the Tumor Microenvironment of Gastric Cancer. Cancer Immunology Research. 2022;**10**

(10):1224–1240. DOI: 10.1158/2326-6066.CIR-22-0107

[139] Liu S, Wang P, Wang P, Zhao Z, Zhang X, Pan Y, et al. Tissue-resident memory CD103⁺CD8⁺ T cells in colorectal cancer: Its implication as a prognostic and predictive liver metastasis biomarker. Cancer Immunology, Immunotherapy. 2024;**73**(9):176. DOI: 10.1007/s00262-024-03709-2

[140] Kitakaze M, Uemura M, Hara T, Chijimatsu R, Motooka D, Hirai T, et al. Cancer-specific tissue-resident memory T-cells express ZNF683 in colorectal cancer. British Journal of Cancer. 2023;**128**(10):1828–1837. DOI: 10.1038/s41416-023-02202-4

[141] Pal B, Chen Y, Vaillant F, Capaldo BD, Joyce R, Song X, et al. A single-cell RNA expression atlas of normal, preneoplastic and tumorigenic states in the human breast. The EMBO Journal. 2021;**40**(11):e107333. DOI: 10.15252/embj.2020107333

[142] Moesta AK, Li XY, Smyth MJ. Targeting CD39 in cancer. Nature Reviews Immunology. 2020;**20**(12):739–755. DOI: 10.1038/s41577-020-0376-4

[143] Lai C, Coltart G, Shapanis A, Healy C, Alabdulkareem A, Selvendran S, et al. CD8⁺CD103⁺ tissue-resident memory T cells convey reduced protective immunity in cutaneous squamous cell carcinoma. Journal for Immunotherapy of Cancer. 2021;**9**(1):e001807. DOI: 10.1136/jitc-2020-001807

[144] Laidlaw BJ, Zhang N, Marshall HD, Staron MM, Guan T, Hu Y, et al. CD4+ T cell help guides formation of CD103+ lung-resident memory CD8+ T cells during influenza viral infection. Immunity. 2014;**41**(4):633–645. DOI: 10.1016/j.immuni.2014.09.007

[145] Peng T, Phasouk K, Bossard E, Klock A, Jin L, Laing KJ, et al. Distinct populations of antigen-specific tissue-resident CD8+ T cells in human cervix mucosa. JCI Insight. 2021;**6**(15):e149950. DOI: 10.1172/jci.insight.149950

[146] Posavad CM, Zhao L, Dong L, Jin L, Stevens CE, Magaret AS, et al. Enrichment of herpes simplex virus type 2 (HSV-2) reactive mucosal T cells in the human female genital tract. Mucosal Immunology. 2017;**10**(5):1259–1269. DOI: 10.1038/mi.2016.118

[147] Shenoy AT, Wasserman GA, Arafa EI, Wooten AK, Smith NMS, Martin IMC, et al. Lung CD4(+) resident memory T cells remodel epithelial responses to accelerate neutrophil recruitment during pneumonia. Mucosal Immunology. 2020;**13**(2):334–343. DOI: 10.1038/s41385-019-0229-2

[148] Rousseau M, Lacerda Mariano L, Canton T, Ingersoll MA. Tissue-resident memory T cells mediate mucosal immunity to recurrent urinary tract infection. Science Immunology. 2023;**8**(83):eabn4332. DOI: 10.1126/sciimmunol.abn4332

[149] Mora-Bau G, Platt AM, van Rooijen N, Randolph GJ, Albert ML, Ingersoll MA. Macrophages subvert adaptive immunity to urinary tract infection. PLoS Pathogens. 2015;**11**(7):e1005044. DOI: 10.1371/journal.ppat.1005044

[150] Lacerda Mariano L, Rousseau M, Varet H, Legendre R, Gentek R, Saenz

Coronilla J, et al. Functionally distinct resident macrophage subsets differentially shape responses to infection in the bladder. Science Advances. 2020;**6**(48):eabc5739. DOI: 10.1126/sciadv.abc5739

[151] Garber C, Soung A, Vollmer LL, Kanmogne M, Last A, Brown J, et al. T cells promote microglia-mediated synaptic elimination and cognitive dysfunction during recovery from neuropathogenic flaviviruses. Nature Neuroscience. 2019;**22**(8):1276–1288. DOI: 10.1038/s41593-019-0427-y

[152] Hendriks A, Mnich ME, Clemente B, Cruz AR, Tavarini S, Bagnoli F, et al. Staphylococcus aureus-specific tissue-resident memory CD4$^+$ T Cells are abundant in healthy human skin. Frontiers in Immunology. 2021;**12**:642711

[153] Koch MRA, Gong R, Friedrich V, Engelsberger V, Kretschmer L, Wanisch A, et al. CagA-specific Gastric CD8(+) Tissue-Resident T Cells control Helicobacter pylori during the early infection phase. Gastroenterology. 2023;**164**(4):550–566. DOI: 10.1053/j.gastro.2022.12.016

[154] Yokoi T, Murakami M, Kihara T, Seno S, Arase M, Wing JB, et al. Identification of a unique subset of tissue-resident memory CD4(+) T cells in Crohn's disease. Proceedings of the National Academy of Sciences of the United States of America. 2023;**120**(1): e2204269120. DOI: 10.1073/pnas.2204269120

[155] Zhu HX, Yang SH, Gao CY, Bian ZH, Chen XM, Huang RR, et al. Targeting pathogenic CD8$^+$ tissue-resident T cells with chimeric antigen receptor therapy in murine autoimmune cholangitis. Nature Communications. 2024;**15**(1):2936. DOI: 10.1038/s41467-024-46654-5

[156] Zimmer CL, von Seth E, Buggert M, Strauss O, Hertwig L, Nguyen S, et al. A biliary immune landscape map of primary sclerosing cholangitis reveals a dominant network of neutrophils and tissue-resident T cells. Science Translational Medicine. 2021;**13**(599):eabb3107. DOI: 10.1126/scitranslmed.abb3107

[157] Saz-Leal P, Ligon MM, Diez-Rivero CM, Garcia-Ayuso D, Mohanty S, Vinuela M, et al. MV140 mucosal vaccine induces targeted immune response for enhanced clearance of Uropathogenic E. coli in experimental urinary tract infection. Vaccines (Basel). 2024;**12** (5):535. DOI: 10.3390/vaccines12050535

[158] Xu N, Ruan G, Liu W, Hu C, Huang A, Zeng Z, et al. Vaccine-induced gastric CD4(+) tissue-resident memory T cells proliferate in situ to amplify immune response against Helicobacter pylori insult. Helicobacter. 2019;**24**(5): e12652. DOI: 10.1111/hel.12652

[159] Landrith TA, Sureshchandra S, Rivera A, Jang JC, Rais M, Nair MG, et al. CD103(+) CD8 T Cells in the Toxoplasma-Infected brain exhibit a tissue-resident memory transcriptional profile. Frontiers in Immunology. 2017;**8**:335

[160] Serafini B, Rosicarelli B, Veroni C, Aloisi F. Tissue-resident memory T cells in the multiple sclerosis brain and their relationship to Epstein-Barr virus infected B cells. Journal of Neuroimmunology. 2023;**376**:578036. DOI: 10.1016/j.jneuroim.2023.578036

[161] Bangert C, Rindler K, Krausgruber T, Alkon N, Thaler FM, Kurz H, et al. Persistence of mature dendritic cells, T_H2A, and Tc2 cells characterize clinically resolved atopic dermatitis under IL-4Rα blockade. Science Immunology. 2021;**6**(55): eabe2749. DOI: 10.1126/sciimmunol.abe2749

[162] Steel KJA, Srenathan U, Ridley M, Durham LE, Wu SY, Ryan SE, et al. Polyfunctional, proinflammatory, tissue-resident memory phenotype and function of synovial interleukin-17A +CD8+ T Cells in Psoriatic Arthritis. Arthritis & Rheumatology. 2020;**72**(3):435–447. DOI: 10.1002/art.41156

[163] Han JW, Shin EC. Liver-Resident Memory CD8(+) T Cells: Possible Roles in Chronic HBV Infection. International Journal of Molecular Sciences. 2020;**22**(1):283. DOI: 10.3390/ijms22010283

[164] Rodrigues A, Claro M, Alexandre-Pires G, Santos-Mateus D, Martins C, Valerio-Bolas A, et al. Leishmania infantum antigens modulate memory cell subsets of liver resident T lymphocyte. Immunobiology. 2017;**222**(2):409–422. DOI: 10.1016/j.imbio.2016.08.009

[165] Koda Y, Teratani T, Chu PS, Hagihara Y, Mikami Y, Harada Y, et al. CD8(+) tissue-resident memory T cells promote liver fibrosis resolution by inducing apoptosis of hepatic stellate cells. Nature Communications. 2021;**12**(1):4474. DOI: 10.1038/s41467-021-24734-0

[166] You Z, Li Y, Wang Q, Zhao Z, Li Y, Qian Q, et al. The clinical significance of hepatic CD69(+) CD103(+) CD8(+) resident-memory T Cells in autoimmune hepatitis. Hepatology. 2021;**74**(2):847–863. DOI: 10.1002/hep.31739

[167] Stelma F, de Niet A, Sinnige MJ, van Dort KA, van Gisbergen K, Verheij J, et al. Human intrahepatic CD69 + CD8+ T cells have a tissue resident memory T cell phenotype with reduced cytolytic capacity. Scientific Reports. 2017;7(1):6172. DOI: 10.1038/s41598-017-06352-3

[168] Blauvelt A. Resident Memory T cells in Psoriasis: Key to a Cure? Journal of Psoriasis and Psoriatic Arthritis. 2022;7(4):157–159. DOI: 10.1177/24755303221127338

[169] Su X, Liu F. Targeting the IL-15/CD122 signaling pathway: Reversing TRM cell-mediated immune memory in vitiligo. Frontiers In Immunology. 2025;**16**:1639732. DOI: 10.3389/fimmu.2025.1639732

[170] Mattsson J, Israelsson E, Björhall K, Yrlid LF, Thörn K, Thorén A, et al. Selective Janus kinase 1 inhibition resolves inflammation and restores hair growth offering a viable treatment option for alopecia areata. Skin Health and Disease. 2023;**3**(3):e209. DOI: 10.1002/ski2.209

[171] Yari S, Kikuta J, Shigyo H, Miyamoto Y, Okuzaki D, Furusawa Y, et al. JAK inhibition ameliorates bone destruction by simultaneously targeting mature osteoclasts and their precursors. Inflammation and Regeneration. 2023;**43**(1):18. DOI: 10.1186/s41232-023-00268-4

[172] Park SL, Gebhardt T, Mackay LK. Tissue-resident memory T Cells in cancer immunosurveillance. Trends in Immunology. 2019;**40**(8):735–747. DOI: 10.1016/j.it.2019.06.002

[173] Leask A, Fadl A, Naik A. A modest proposal: Targeting αv integrin-mediated activation of latent TGFbeta as a novel therapeutic approach to treat scleroderma fibrosis. Expert Opinion on Investigational Drugs. 2024;**33**(3): 279–285. DOI: 10.1080/13543784.2024.2323528

[174] Liu T, Li S, Ying S, Tang S, Ding Y, Li Y, et al. The IL-23/IL-17 pathway in inflammatory skin diseases: From bench to bedside. Frontiers in Immunology. 2020;**11**:2020

[175] Dong C, Lin L, Du J. Characteristics and sources of tissue-resident memory T cells in psoriasis relapse. Current Research in Immunology. 2023;**4**:100067. DOI: 10.1016/j.crimmu.2023.100067

[176] Huang Y-W, Tsai T-F. A drug safety evaluation of risankizumab for psoriasis. Expert Opinion on Drug Safety. 2020;**19**(4):395–402. DOI: 10.1080/14740338.2020.1736034

[177] Çelik MS, Aktaş H. The effect of IL-17 and IL-23 ınhibitors on hematological ınflammatory parameters in patients with psoriasis vulgaris. Irish Journal of Medical Science. 2025;**194**(4):1329–1334. DOI: 10.1007/s11845-025-03969-6

[178] Markham MJ, Wachter K, Agarwal N, Bertagnolli MM, Chang SM, Dale W, et al. Clinical Cancer Advances 2020: Annual Report on progress against cancer from the American Society of Clinical Oncology. Journal of Clinical Oncology. 2020;**38**(10):1081. DOI: 10.1200/JCO.19.03141

[179] Blanc C, Hans S, Tran T, Granier C, Saldman A, Anson M, et al. Targeting resident memory T Cells for cancer immunotherapy. Frontiers in Immunology. 2018;**9**:1722

[180] Xiao Z, Yan R, Liu H, Huang X, Liang Z, An G, et al. Preventive treatment with PD-1 antibody increases tissue-resident memory T Cells Infiltration and delays Esophageal Carcinogenesis. Cancer Prevention Research (Philadelphia). 2023;**16**(12):669–679. DOI: 10.1158/1940-6207.CAPR-23-0196

[181] Virassamy B, Caramia F, Savas P, Sant S, Wang J, Christo SN, et al. Intratumoral CD8(+) T cells with a tissue-resident memory phenotype mediate local immunity and immune checkpoint responses in breast cancer. Cancer Cell. 2023;**41**(3):585–601e8. DOI: 10.1016/j.ccell.2023.01.004

[182] Enamorado M, Iborra S, Priego E, Cueto FJ, Quintana JA, Martinez-Cano S, et al. Enhanced anti-tumour immunity requires the interplay between resident and circulating memory CD8(+) T cells. Nature Communications. 2017;**8**:16073

[183] Ribas A, Shin DS, Zaretsky J, Frederiksen J, Cornish A, Avramis E, et al. PD-1 blockade expands intratumoral memory T Cells. Cancer Immunology Research. 2016;**4**(3):194–203. DOI: 10.1158/2326-6066.CIR-15-0210

[184] Pizzolla A, Keam SP, Vergara IA, Caramia F, Thio N, Wang M, et al. Tissue-resident memory T cells from a metastatic vaginal melanoma patient are tumor-responsive T cells and increase after anti-PD-1 treatment. Journal for Immunotherapy of Cancer. 2022;**10**(5):e004574. DOI: 10.1136/jitc-2022-004574

[185] Jin K, Yu Y, Zeng H, Liu Z, You R, Zhang H, et al. $CD103^{+}CD8^{+}$

tissue-resident memory T cell infiltration predicts clinical outcome and adjuvant therapeutic benefit in muscle-invasive bladder cancer. British Journal of Cancer. 2022;**126**(11):1581–1588. DOI: 10.1038/s41416-022-01725-6

[186] Sievers C, Craveiro M, Friedman J, Robbins Y, Yang X, Bai K, et al. Phenotypic plasticity and reduced tissue retention of exhausted tumor-infiltrating T cells following neoadjuvant immunotherapy in head and neck cancer. Cancer Cell. 2023;**41**(5):887–902e5. DOI: 10.1016/j.ccell.2023.03.014

[187] Marceaux C, Weeden CE, Gordon CL, Asselin-Labat ML. Holding our breath: The promise of tissue-resident memory T cells in lung cancer. Translational Lung Cancer Research. 2021;**10**(6):2819–2829. DOI: 10.21037/tlcr-20-819

[188] Zhang C, Yin K, Liu SY, Yan LX, Su J, Wu YL, et al. Multiomics analysis reveals a distinct response mechanism in multiple primary lung adenocarcinoma after neoadjuvant immunotherapy. Journal for Immunotherapy of Cancer. 2021;**9**(4):e002312. DOI: 10.1136/jitc-2020-002312

[189] Wang F, Yue S, Huang Q, Lei T, Li X, Wang C, et al. Cellular heterogeneity and key subsets of tissue-resident memory T cells in cervical cancer. NPJ Precision Oncology. 2024;**8**(1):145. DOI: 10.1038/s41698-024-00637-3

[190] Sato H, Meng S, Hara T, Tsuji Y, Arao Y, Sasaki K, et al. Tissue-resident memory T Cells in gastrointestinal cancers: Prognostic significance and therapeutic implications. Biomedicines. 2024;**12**(6):1342. DOI: 10.3390/biomedicines12061342

[191] Singla N, Nirschl TR, Obradovic AZ, Shenderov E, Lombardo K, Liu X, et al. Immunomodulatory response to neoadjuvant nivolumab in non-metastatic clear cell renal cell carcinoma. Scientific Reports. 2024;**14**(1):1458. DOI: 10.1038/s41598-024-51889-9

[192] Damei I, Caidi A, Auclin E, Adam J, Mella S, Hasan M, et al. Different tumour-resident memory T-cell subsets regulate responses to anti-PD-1 and anti-CTLA-4 cancer immunotherapies. Nature Communications. 2025;**16**(1):5588. DOI: 10.1038/s41467-025-60657-w

[193] Weeden CE, Gayevskiy V, Marceaux C, Batey D, Tan T, Yokote K, et al. Early immune pressure initiated by tissue-resident memory T cells sculpts tumor evolution in non-small cell lung cancer. Cancer Cell. 2023;**41**(5):837–852e6. DOI: 10.1016/j.ccell.2023.03.019

[194] Bonaventura P, Shekarian T, Alcazer V, Valladeau-Guilemond J, Valsesia-Wittmann S, Amigorena S, et al. Cold Tumors: A therapeutic challenge for immunotherapy. Frontiers in Immunology. 2019;**10**:168

[195] Khosravi GR, Mostafavi S, Bastan S, Ebrahimi N, Gharibvand RS, Eskandari N. Immunologic tumor microenvironment modulators for turning cold tumors hot. Cancer Communications (London). 2024;**44**(5):521–553. DOI: 10.1002/cac2.12539

[196] E LMJ, Kirilovsky A, Lecoester B, El Sissy C, Boullerot L, Rangan L, et al. Chemoradiation triggers antitumor Th1 and tissue resident memory-polarized immune responses to improve immune checkpoint inhibitors therapy. Journal for Immunotherapy of Cancer. 2021;**9**

(7):e002256. DOI: 10.1136/jitc-2020-002256

[197] Nizard M, Roussel H, Diniz MO, Karaki S, Tran T, Voron T, et al. Induction of resident memory T cells enhances the efficacy of cancer vaccine. Nature Communications. 2017;**8**:15221

[198] Rivera Vargas T, Apetoh L. Can immunogenic chemotherapies relieve cancer cell resistance to immune checkpoint inhibitors? Frontiers in Immunology. 2019;**10**:1181. DOI: 10.3389/fimmu.2019.01181

[199] Zappasodi R, Merghoub T, Wolchok JD. Emerging concepts for immune checkpoint blockade-based combination therapies. Cancer Cell. 2018;**33**(4):581–598. DOI: 10.1016/j.ccell.2018.03.005

[200] Bando H, Kotani D, Tsushima T, Hara H, Kadowaki S, Kato K, et al. TENERGY: Multicenter phase II study of Atezolizumab monotherapy following definitive Chemoradiotherapy with 5-FU plus Cisplatin in patients with unresectable locally advanced esophageal squamous cell carcinoma. BMC Cancer. 2020;**20**(1):336. DOI: 10.1186/s12885-020-06716-5

[201] Sha Y, Yang L, Jiang J, Cao J, Sun M, Yin L, et al. Pre-silencing of TNF-α by targeted siRNA delivery mitigates glucocorticoid resistance of dexamethasone in rheumatoid arthritis. Journal of Controlled Release. 2025;**386**:114122

[202] Hu C, Ma J, Chen X, Chen Y, Song Y, Tang Q, et al. Microenvironment-driven transformable self-assembly nanoplatform enables spatiotemporal remodeling for rheumatoid arthritis therapy. Science Advances. 2025;**11**(36):eadu5245. DOI: 10.1126/sciadv.adu5245

[203] Zhang X, Zhang Y, Liu Y. Fibroblast activation and heterogeneity in fibrotic disease. Nature Reviews Nephrology. 2025;**21**(9):613–632. DOI: 10.1038/s41581-025-00969-8

[204] Diao W, Jiao Y, Deng T, Gu J, Wang B, Zhang Q, et al. Synovium-On-A-Chip: Simulating the microenvironment of the rheumatoid arthritis synovium via multicell interactions to Target Fibroblast-Like Synoviocytes. Advanced Science (Weinheim). 2025:e11945. DOI: 10.1002/advs.202511945

[205] Wang X, Liang Q, Luo Y, Ye J, Yu Y, Chen F. Engineering the next generation of theranostic biomaterials with synthetic biology. Bioactive Materials. 2023;**32**:514–529. DOI: 10.1016/j.bioactmat.2023.10.018

[206] Liu L, Zhong Q, Tian T, Dubin K, Athale SK, Kupper TS. Epidermal injury and infection during poxvirus immunization is crucial for the generation of highly protective T cell-mediated immunity. Nature Medicine. 2010;**16**(2):224–227. DOI: 10.1038/nm.2078

[207] Zens KD, Chen JK, Farber DL. Vaccine-generated lung tissue-resident memory T cells provide heterosubtypic protection to influenza infection. JCI Insight. 2016;**1**(10):e85832. DOI: 10.1172/jci.insight.85832

[208] Lapuente D, Storcksdieck Genannt Bonsmann M, Maaske A, Stab V, Heinecke V, Watzstedt K, et al. IL-1beta as mucosal vaccine adjuvant: The specific induction of tissue-resident memory T cells improves the heterosubtypic immunity against

influenza A viruses. Mucosal Immunology. 2018;**11**(4):1265–1278. DOI: 10.1038/s41385-018-0017-4

[209] Wakim LM, Smith J, Caminschi I, Lahoud MH, Villadangos JA. Antibody-targeted vaccination to lung dendritic cells generates tissue-resident memory CD8 T cells that are highly protective against influenza virus infection. Mucosal Immunology. 2015;**8**(5):1060–1071. DOI: 10.1038/mi.2014.133

[210] Belongia EA, Naleway AL. Smallpox vaccine: The good, the bad, and the ugly. Clinical Medicine Research. 2003;**1**(2):87–92. DOI: 10.312 1/cmr.1.2.87

[211] Pan Y, Liu L, Tian T, Zhao J, Park CO, Lofftus SY, et al. Epicutaneous immunization with modified vaccinia Ankara viral vectors generates superior T cell immunity against a respiratory viral challenge. NPJ Vaccines. 2021;**6**(1):1. DOI: 10.1038/s41541-020-00265-5

[212] Kingstad-Bakke B, Lee W, Chandrasekar SS, Gasper DJ, Salas-Quinchucua C, Cleven T, et al. Vaccine-induced systemic and mucosal T cell immunity to SARS-CoV-2 viral variants. Proceedings of the National Academy of Sciences of the United States of America. 2022;**119**(20):e2118312119. DOI: 10.1073/pnas.2118312119

[213] Lai JCY, Cheng WK, Hopkins PD, Komba M, Carlow DA, Dutz JP. Topical adjuvant application during subcutaneous vaccination promotes resident memory T Cell generation. Journal of Immunology. 2019;**203**(9):2443–2450. DOI: 10.4049/jimmunol.1900199

[214] Chen H, Li Z, Qiu L, Dong X, Chen G, Shi Y, et al. Personalized neoantigen vaccine combined with PD-1 blockade increases $CD8^+$ tissue-resident memory T-cell infiltration in preclinical hepatocellular carcinoma models. Journal for Immunotherapy of Cancer. 2022;**10**(9):e004389. DOI: 10.1136/jitc-2021-004389

[215] Li ZY, Zhang Z, Cao XZ, Feng Y, Ren SS. Platinum-based neoadjuvant chemotherapy for triple-negative breast cancer: A systematic review and meta-analysis. Journal of International Medical Research. 2020;**48**(10):300060520964340. DOI: 10.1177/0300060520964340

[216] Zhang L, Chen Y, Cheng MY, Zhuang X, Zou J, Wei D, et al. Homologous recombination deficiency predicts the response to platinum-based neoadjuvant chemotherapy in early-stage triple-negative breast cancer patients: A systematic review and meta-analysis. Therapeutic Advances in Medical Oncology. 2022;**14**:17588359221096253

[217] Colton M, Cheadle EJ, Honeychurch J, Illidge TM. Reprogramming the tumour microenvironment by radiotherapy: Implications for radiotherapy and immunotherapy combinations. Radiation Oncology. 2020;**15**(1):254. DOI: 10.1186/s13014-020-01678-1

[218] Mami-Chouaib F, Blanc C, Corgnac S, Hans S, Malenica I, Granier C, et al. Resident memory T cells, critical components in tumor immunology. Journal for Immunotherapy of Cancer. 2018;**6**(1):87. DOI: 10.1186/s40425-018-0399-6

[219] Chen HHW, Kuo MT. Improving radiotherapy in cancer treatment: Promises and challenges. Oncotarget.

2017;**8**(37):62742–62758. DOI: 10.18632/oncotarget.18409

[220] Zhang X, Zhu L, Zhang H, Chen S, Xiao Y. CAR-T Cell Therapy in Hematological Malignancies: Current Opportunities and Challenges. Frontiers in Immunology. 2022;**13**:927153. DOI: 10.3389/fimmu.2022.927153

[221] Mackay LK, Wynne-Jones E, Freestone D, Pellicci DG, Mielke LA, Newman DM, et al. T-box transcription factors combine with the Cytokines TGF-beta and IL-15 to control tissue-resident memory T Cell fate. Immunity. 2015;**43**(6):1101–1111. DOI: 10.1016/j.immuni.2015.11.008

[222] Richmond JM, Strassner JP, Zapata Jr L, Garg M, Riding RL, Refat MA, et al. Antibody blockade of IL-15 signaling has the potential to durably reverse vitiligo. Science Translational Medicine. 2018;**10**(450): eaam7710. DOI: 10.1126/scitranslmed.aam7710

[223] Lin R, Zhang H, Yuan Y, He Q, Zhou J, Li S, et al. Fatty acid oxidation controls CD8+ tissue-resident memory T-cell survival in gastric adenocarcinoma. Cancer Immunology Research. 2020;**8**(4):479–492. DOI: 10.1158/2326-6066.CIR-19-0702

Section 3

T Cell Development, Repertoire and Autoimmune Targeted Therapy

Chapter 8

T- and B-Cell–Targeted Depletion Strategies: Emerging Therapeutics in Autoimmune Disease

Parv Barot and Sanjay Rathod

Abstract

T and B-cell–targeted depletion has become a cornerstone of advanced immunotherapeutic strategies aimed at recalibrating dysregulated adaptive immunity in autoimmune disease. By selectively removing autoreactive lymphocyte subsets, T-cell depletion disrupts pathogenic T-cell activation, cytokine amplification loops, and aberrant T–B cell interactions that drive autoimmune pathogenesis. Complementarily, B-cell depletion attenuates antigen presentation, germinal center reactions, and autoantibody generation, thereby mitigating downstream inflammatory cascades. Contemporary depletion modalities, spanning monoclonal antibodies, Fc-engineered biologics, bispecific platforms, and cellular immunotherapies, enable refined immunomodulation with improved specificity and reduced off-target immunosuppression. Mechanistic insights into lymphocyte reconstitution, tolerance reestablishment, and compensatory immune pathways further inform the optimization of these interventions. This chapter synthesizes current evidence and emerging therapeutic innovations to elucidate how dual T- and B-cell depletion strategies reshape autoimmune trajectories and offer a precision framework for targeted, durable disease control.

Keywords: autoimmune disease, B-cell depletion, T-cell depletion, chimeric antigen receptor T-cells, bispecific T-cell engagers, immune tolerance, pharmacological modeling

1. Introduction

Autoimmune diseases comprise a diverse and complex group of chronic, debilitating conditions that arise from a steady breakdown of both central and peripheral immune tolerance. Autoimmune diseases affect ~ 10% of the global population and result from a complex interaction of genetic, environmental, and sex-related factors. Their impact is rising globally, with reported increases of ~ 12.5% per year in prevalence and ~ 19.1% per year in incidence, emerging as a growing public health challenge [1]. They are driven by autoreactive lymphocytes that mistakenly attack self-antigens, leading to chronic inflammation and progressive tissue damage. Conditions such as systemic lupus erythematosus (SLE), rheumatoid arthritis (RA), multiple sclerosis (MS), and systemic sclerosis are mainly managed with broad immunosuppressants and glucocorticoids (used in ~70–80% of cases), but long-term use increases infection risk (~30–50%) along with systemic toxicity. While these therapies control symptoms, they do not address the underlying immune memory [1, 2].

The current approach of targeted biologic therapies has transformed clinical immunology, shifting the treatment regimen from broad immunosuppression to precise immune modulation-based therapeutics. Mechanistic insights have redefined disease biology, showing that B-cells function not only as autoantibody-producing effectors but also as key antigen-presenting and cytokine-secreting regulators of adaptive immunity. In parallel, pathogenic T cells contribute directly to tissue injury through cytotoxic effector functions and proinflammatory signaling, while also sustaining B-cell activation, together reinforcing disease persistence. Despite these advances, clinical outcomes with isolated B- or T-cell depletion remain inconsistent, with many patients experiencing partial or transient responses due to tissue-resident memory cells and the rapid reemergence of autoreactive clones. To overcome these limitations, therapeutic development has progressed from conventional monoclonal antibodies to engineered immune-modulating platforms, including Fc-enhanced monoclonal antibodies, bispecific T-cell engagers (TCEs), and chimeric antigen receptor (CAR)-T cell therapies. Collectively, these strategies aim to achieve deeper immune reset and sustained, treatment-free remission in refractory autoimmune disease [1, 3].

2. Immunopathogenesis of B and T lymphocytes in autoimmune disease

Systemic autoimmune disease is driven by ongoing, bidirectional interactions between dysregulated T and B lymphocytes. Understanding how these immune compartments play their roles at the cellular and molecular levels is central to the rationale behind modern lymphocyte depletion strategies.

2.1 The multifaceted roles of B lymphocytes

B-cells are now recognized as primary, hierarchical drivers of autoimmune pathology. They function not merely as terminal precursors of plasma cells but as active immune regulators that sustain chronic adaptive dysregulation. In diseases such as SLE and RA, autoreactive B cells exhibit highly efficient antigen-presenting capacity via B-cell receptor (BCR)-mediated antigen capture. This mechanism enables the selective uptake of low-abundance self-antigens [4]. Once processed, these peptides are presented on major histocompatibility complex (MHC) class II molecules alongside potent costimulatory signals. This presentation amplifies CD4 + T-cell activation and stabilizes the pathogenic T–B cell feedback loops that ensure disease chronicity [5].

Sustained germinal center activity and extranodal B-cell maturation niches give rise to long-lived plasma cells. These specialized cells reside deep within the bone marrow and inflamed tissues, evading most conventional immunosuppressive regimens. They maintain the durable production of high-affinity pathogenic autoantibodies, including antidouble-stranded DNA (anti-dsDNA) antibodies in SLE and anticitrullinated protein antibodies (ACPA) in RA. The immune complexes formed by these autoantibodies aggressively engage complement cascades and Fc receptor-bearing effector pathways. This engagement triggers sustained vascular injury, pathological tissue remodeling, and ultimate end-organ dysfunction. Due to their central role, targeting B cells is critical. However, simple depletion often triggers powerful compensatory survival mechanisms, which are detailed in Section 7 [6].

2.2 T-cell dysregulation, metabolic stress, and exhaustion

T lymphocytes act as the central systemic drivers of autoimmunity. They serve both as direct effectors of tissue injury and as critical amplifiers of B-cell–mediated humoral pathology. Within affected organs, clonally expanded CD4 + subsets – specifically T helper 1 (Th1) and T helper 17 (Th17) cells – are maintained by persistent antigenic stimulation within the inflamed tissue site. Their effector secretions are dominated by interferon-gamma (IFN-γ) and IL-17. These cytokines converge on stromal, endothelial, and myeloid compartments to induce massive chemokine amplification. This induces vascular activation and the continuous recruitment of inflammatory leukocytes, effectively stabilizing chronic, nonresolving inflammation [7, 8].

At the intracellular signaling level, autoreactive T cells exhibit a fundamentally altered activation landscape. This dysregulation is characterized by reduced T-cell receptor (TCR) signaling thresholds. Furthermore, epigenetically imprinted effector programs strictly favor persistent cytokine production. The dysregulation is compounded by the functional erosion of critical immune checkpoint pathways. Failures in cytotoxic T-lymphocyte-associated Protein 4 (CTLA-4) and programmed cell death protein 1 (PD-1) signaling impair the termination of activation sequences and disrupt the enforcement of peripheral tolerance. The inflamed tissue microenvironment further reinforces T-cell persistence through localized hypoxia, severe nutrient limitation, and intense metabolic competition. These hostile conditions artificially select for metabolically adaptable T-cell clones. These selected clones are uniquely capable of sustaining effector function under severe stress while actively resisting apoptosis. In parallel, the progressive collapse and phenotypic instability of FoxP3 + regulatory T-cell (Treg) populations remove a key suppressive axis. This regulatory collapse shifts the immunologic balance decisively toward unchecked effector dominance. Together, these processes establish a self-amplifying T-cell circuit that sustains chronic tissue destruction [9, 10].

2.3 Immunological synapse and T- and B-cell collaboration

The critical intersection of T- and B-cell pathology physically manifests within ectopic lymphoid structures and tertiary germinal centers, where intense, bidirectional costimulation drives continuous disease amplification. This cellular collaboration relies upon the formation of physical immunological synapses, stabilized by a dense network of molecular pairings. Crucial molecular interactions driving this process include the binding of the CD40 receptor on the surface of B cells with CD40 Ligand (CD40L) expressed on activated T-cells, alongside the high-affinity engagement of B-cell-expressed CD80 and CD86 with the T-cell-expressed CD28 receptor. Additionally, the Inducible T-cell costimulator (ICOS) heavily interacts with its corresponding ligand (ICOSL) to sustain cytokine cross-talk [11]. These integrated costimulatory signals are absolutely indispensable for the downstream mechanisms of B-cell class switching, affinity maturation, and successful terminal differentiation into both long-lived memory B cells and autoantibody-secreting plasma cells. Disrupting this intimate T–B collaboration is the primary, overarching objective of selective lymphocyte depletion therapies. By systematically eliminating the B-cell compartment, pathogenic T-cells are rapidly deprived of their most critical source of autoantigen presentation and vital costimulation, leading to subsequent T-cell anergy or activation-induced cell death. Conversely, effective T-cell depletion starves developing B-cells of the essential helper cytokine signals required for ectopic germinal center formation and continuous autoantibody generation [12, 13].

3. Monoclonal antibodies and Fc-engineered biologics

The initial translation of lymphocyte depletion concepts into routine clinical practice relied almost exclusively on monoclonal antibodies directed against lineage-specific surface antigens. Over recent decades, the pharmacological design of these agents has evolved dramatically, progressing from partially immunogenic chimeric constructs to fully humanized, precision Fc-engineered biologics specifically designed to overcome historical resistance mechanisms and achieve unprecedented depth of depletion.

3.1 The evolution of anti-CD20 cytotoxic monoclonal antibodies

Rituximab, a pioneering chimeric murine–human IgG1 monoclonal antibody targeting the CD20 surface antigen, established the clinical foundation of modern B-cell depletion therapy in autoimmune disease. Classified as a Type I anti-CD20 antibody, its cytotoxic activity is primarily mediated through complement-dependent cytotoxicity (CDC) and Fcγ receptor-driven antibody-dependent cellular cytotoxicity (ADCC). Rituximab efficiently engages natural killer (NK) cells and macrophages to eliminate circulating $CD20^+$ B cells via antibody-dependent cellular phagocytosis (ADCP) [14].

Despite proving clinically transformative across multiple indications, rituximab frequently induces incomplete and transient B-cell depletion within tissue-resident compartments. This limitation is attributable to several intrinsic biological factors. First, CD20 is not expressed on early B-cell precursors or terminally differentiated plasma cells, leaving these specific compartments entirely untouched and capable of sustaining disease. Second, antibody penetration and effector cell access are physically restricted within dense, fibrotic, inflamed tissue microenvironments. Finally, target antigen modulation occurs through Fc-mediated mechanisms such as trogocytosis. In this process, macrophages strip the rituximab-CD20 complex from the B-cell surface, allowing the B cell to survive and evade further detection [15].

To overcome these limitations, next-generation anti-CD20 strategies were meticulously developed. Obinutuzumab is a glycoengineered, humanized Type II anti-CD20 monoclonal antibody designed with dramatically enhanced affinity for the activating FcγRIIIa (CD16A) receptor. This structural modification results in improved engagement of innate effector cells and increased ADCC potential. Furthermore, obinutuzumab binds a distinct CD20 epitope, inducing a different pattern of lipid raft membrane organization. This reduces antigen internalization and promotes direct, actin-dependent, nonapoptotic cell death. Together, these mechanistic upgrades enable deeper and more durable depletion of both circulating and tissue-resident B-cell populations [16].

Together, these mechanistic advances enable deeper and more durable depletion of both circulating and tissue-resident B-cell populations, expanding the therapeutic effectiveness of CD20-directed therapy in refractory autoimmune diseases.

3.2 Inhibitory bifunctional antibodies: The paradigm of obexelimab

A key advancement in B-cell modulation is the shift from cytotoxic depletion to a precision functional inhibition approach, aimed at suppressing autoreactive signaling while preserving naive and memory B-cell compartments. Obexelimab is a first-in-class bifunctional humanized monoclonal antibody engineered to coengage CD19 and the inhibitory FcγRIIb (CD32B) receptor across the B-cell lineage. Its Fc domain is engineered for enhanced Fc γ RIIb affinity (~230-fold relative to native IgG1). This design functionally recapitulates endogenous immune complex–mediated negative feedback, reinforcing FcγRIIb-driven suppression of B-cell activation without inducing cellular depletion. By coengaging CD19 and FcγRIIb (CD32B), obexelimab enforces receptor coligation that drives phosphorylation of FcγRIIb immunoreceptor tyrosine-based inhibitory motifs (ITIMs), initiating recruitment of SH2 domain–containing inositol phosphatase-1 (SHIP-1) [17]. SHIP-1 attenuates PI3K signaling through PIP3 hydrolysis, thereby suppressing downstream AKT and NF-κB activation and rapidly dampening BCR-driven calcium flux, proliferation, cytokine release, and antigen presentation. This inhibitory signaling program operates independently of complement activation and Fc-mediated cytotoxicity, preserving B-cell viability while inducing a reversible hyporesponsive state rather than cellular depletion. As a result, immune homeostasis can be reestablished rapidly upon treatment cessation, in contrast to the prolonged immune reconstitution observed with B-cell ablative strategies [18].

Rigorous clinical evaluations of obexelimab have demonstrated profound systemic efficacy across multiple challenging indications. In the pivotal Phase 3 INDIGO trial investigating the agent in Immunoglobulin G4-related disease (IgG4-RD), obexelimab successfully met all primary and key secondary endpoints, cementing its regulatory submission trajectory projected for 2026. Similarly, the robust Phase 2 MoonStone trial in relapsing multiple sclerosis (RMS) reported a highly statistically significant 95% relative reduction in cumulative new gadolinium-enhancing T1 hyperintense brain lesions compared to a placebo cohort. Concurrently, the global Phase 2 SunStone trial continues to evaluate the capacity of obexelimab to drastically reduce systemic disease activity in complex SLE patients, pointing to its broad pan-autoimmune applicability [19]. **Table 1** provides an overview of the pharmacological characteristics and clinical applications of monoclonal and Fc-engineered biologics currently used or under investigation for autoimmune diseases.

3.3 T-cell directed monoclonal antibodies

While B-cell–directed therapies have dominated the treatment spectrum, T-cell–targeted approaches have reemerged with substantially refined mechanistic precision. Early anti-CD3 antibodies, exemplified by muromonab-CD3 (OKT3), mediated profound T-cell depletion but were limited by Fc receptor–dependent cross-linking, leading to widespread T-cell activation, severe cytokine release syndrome, and rapid antidrug antibody formation driven by their murine origin. In contrast, next-generation Fc receptor–nonbinding (FcRNB) anti-CD3 antibodies

Therapeutic agent	Primary molecular target(s)	Mechanism of action	Clinical stage	Indication
Rituximab	CD20 (Type I)	ADCC, CDC, macrophage phagocytosis	Standard of care (off-label)	SLE, RA, MS, and Vasculitis
Obinutuzumab	CD20 (Type II)	Direct actin-dependent apoptosis, enhanced ADCC	Phase II/III	Refractory SLE, LN, and Vasculitis
Obexelimab	CD19 and Fc γ RIIb	Bifunctional inhibition via ITIM/SHIP-1 phosphorylation	Phase III and Phase II	Immunoglobulin G4-related disease and relapsing multiple sclerosis, systemic lupus erythematosus
Alemtuzumab	CD52	Panlymphocyte depletion via CDC and ADCC.	Approved	Relapsing-remitting multiple sclerosis

Table 1.
Pharmacological profiles of monoclonal and Fc-engineered biologics in autoimmunity.

are engineered to eliminate Fc-mediated engagement with innate immune effector cells, thereby preventing systemic immune activation. This structural modification shifts signaling outcomes from global activation toward selective induction of activation-induced cell death in highly stimulated effector T-cells. At the same time, these agents preferentially spare and, in some contexts, support the expansion of Tregs, thereby rebalancing effector and regulatory arms of immunity. Collectively, this refined signaling control enables restoration of peripheral tolerance while minimizing cytokine-mediated toxicity [20, 21].

Alemtuzumab is a humanized monoclonal antibody targeting CD52, a surface glycoprotein broadly expressed on mature T and B lymphocytes and subsets of innate immune cells, resulting in rapid, profound lymphodepletion. In relapsing–remitting MS, this depletion is used as an immune reconstitution strategy that effectively resets adaptive immune activity. Reconstitution occurs primarily through peripheral homeostatic expansion rather than thymic output, yielding a repopulated T-cell compartment that is numerically restored but compositionally altered. Early recovery is characterized by the expansion of memory-derived clones and a relative increase in regulatory immune signals, along with reduced IL-17–associated effector activity. However, this nonphysiological repopulation trajectory can constrain TCR diversity and transiently disrupt immune equilibrium, which is associated with secondary autoimmune manifestations, including thyroid autoimmunity such as Graves' disease [22, 23]. This reflects a key limitation of broad lymphocyte ablation: disease control is achieved at the expense of the full restoration of physiological immune repertoire diversity.

4. Bispecific antibodies and TCEs

With the limited bandwidth of conventional monoclonal antibodies to effectively penetrate hypoxic, structurally complex inflamed lesions/sites and to overcome local immunoregulatory networks, the development of more functionally dynamic immunotherapeutic platforms has been driven. Among these, bispecific TCEs, originally established in the context of hematologic malignancies, have been increasingly adapted for autoimmune diseases. These engineered molecules are designed to simultaneously bind CD3 on T cells and defined surface antigens on pathogenic immune cells, thereby bypassing conventional antigen presentation and directly redirecting endogenous T-cell cytotoxic activity toward disease-driving cell populations within otherwise inaccessible tissue microenvironments.

4.1 Structural configurations and synaptic stabilization

TCEs are engineered fusion proteins, macromolecules containing at least two distinct and independent antigen-binding arms: one designed to target a pathogenic autoimmune-associated antigen (such as CD19, CD20, or B-cell maturation antigen [BCMA] on the B-cell lineage), and the other designed with high affinity for the CD3ε subunit of the TCR complex. By physically bridging endogenous T cells with pathogenic B cells, bispecific TCEs enforce the formation of a synthetic cytolytic synapse independent of conventional antigen presentation. This engineered interaction bypasses MHC-restricted peptide recognition and classical costimulatory requirements by directly juxtaposing CD3-mediated T-cell activation with a defined target-cell surface antigen. Synapse formation triggers potent localized T-cell activation, resulting in the release of perforin and granzymes toward the engaged target cell, culminating in caspase-dependent apoptosis and selective elimination of pathogenic immune cells [24, 25].

The structural configuration of TCEs is a key determinant of their pharmacodynamic activity and safety profile. Asymmetric 2:1 formats, with bivalent engagement of target antigens such as CD20 and monovalent CD3 binding, increase avidity and prolong binding time at the target cell interface, stabilizing the cytolytic synapse. This promotes efficient T-cell activation, polarization, and granule exocytosis even in the setting of low antigen density, enabling clearance of tissue-resident or antigen-dim B-cell populations that are less responsive to conventional monoclonal antibodies. Additional engineering features, including optimized linker flexibility and spatial orientation, further influence synapse geometry and signaling strength[26]. Trispecific constructs incorporating costimulatory interactions, such as CD2 engagement, enhance LFA-1–mediated adhesion and lower the activation threshold for T-cells, supporting sustained cytotoxic function without excessive CD3 hyperstimulation. Together, these design elements improve target selectivity, deepen cellular depletion within protected niches, and provide tighter control over systemic cytokine release [27].

4.2 T clinical application of TCEs in autoimmune syndromes

The clinical application of bispecific TCEs beyond hematologic malignancies into autoimmune diseases has enabled levels of B-cell depletion that exceed the pharmacodynamic limits of conventional monoclonal antibodies, particularly within tissue-resident compartments. Blinatumomab, a CD19 × CD3 construct originally developed for acute lymphoblastic leukemia, has demonstrated the capacity to induce deep, systemic B-cell aplasia accompanied by sustained clinical improvement in refractory RA and systemic sclerosis, without a corresponding increase in severe opportunistic infections [28]. This suggests that targeted cytolytic redirection can achieve profound immune modulation while preserving critical host defense functions. Parallel efforts with CD20 × CD3 bispecific antibodies, including Glofitamab, Epcoritamab, and Mosunetuzumab, are under active clinical evaluation in SLE and MS. Early-phase data with Mosunetuzumab indicate rapid and substantial reductions in circulating autoantibody titers and disease activity, with a safety profile characterized by controlled cytokine release and the absence of dose-limiting toxicity. More advanced multispecific designs aim to overcome lineage heterogeneity and antigen escape. Trispecific constructs such as LBL-051 simultaneously target CD19 and BCMA, thereby spanning the B-cell differentiation continuum from early memory populations to long-lived plasma cells. This dual-lineage targeting enables broader eradication of autoreactive clones and more complete suppression of autoantibody production, addressing a central limitation of single-antigen strategies and supporting more durable disease control [29, 30].

4.3 Expanding multispecificity beyond CD19 and CD20

Beyond cellular depletion, bispecific antibody therapeutics are now being deployed to modulate cytokine networks that sustain autoimmune inflammation. A central advantage of these agents lies in their ability to simultaneously intercept parallel and partially redundant signaling pathways that limit the efficacy of single-cytokine blockade. ABT-122, designed to coneutralize TNF-α and IL-17A, has demonstrated coordinated suppression of inflammatory signaling, with downstream reductions in chemokines such as CXCL9, CXCL10, CCL23, and E-selectin – key mediators of leukocyte recruitment and retention within inflamed tissues [31].

More refined approaches extend this principle to structurally and functionally related cytokine families. Sonelokimab, a trispecific nanobody, targets both IL-17A and IL-17 F, thereby inhibiting the full spectrum of IL-17 homo and heterodimer signaling and attenuating Th17-driven inflammation at its source. Similarly, Lutikizumab simultaneously neutralizes IL-1α and IL-1β, achieving comprehensive blockade of IL-1–dependent inflammatory cascades. By converging on multiple cytokine nodes within the same inflammatory axis, these multispecific biologics enable more complete and sustained suppression of pathogenic signaling networks, particularly in settings where compensatory pathway activation undermines conventional monotherapies [32, 33].

5. Cellular immunotherapies: Redefining depletion with living drugs

The revolutionary application of CAR T-cell therapy to the field of autoimmune disease represents a historical watershed moment in precision medicine. By meticulously engineering a patient's own autologous T cells ex vivo to express synthetic, customized receptors that recognize specific B-cell antigens, CAR-T therapy achieves an unparalleled depth of tissue clearance. Acting as a dynamic "living drug," CAR-T cells are uniquely capable of active in vivo migration, serial cytotoxicity, and localized proliferation at the site of pathology.

5.1 CD19-targeted CAR-T cells

CD19 is a hot target currently for systemic immune reset strategies due to its broad expression across B-cell ontogeny, spanning from early pro-B cells through mature naïve and memory B cells, and extending into early plasmablast stages prior to terminal plasma cell differentiation. This continuous expression window enables efficient clearance of the autoreactive B-cell compartment while minimizing the need to directly target long-lived plasma cells. Autologous CD19-directed CAR T cells are engineered by introducing a synthetic chimeric receptor composed of an extracellular single-chain variable fragment (scFv) for antigen recognition, linked via a transmembrane domain to intracellular signaling modules. These typically include the CD3ζ activation domain in combination with a costimulatory domain such as 4-1BB or CD28, which collectively regulate activation, proliferative capacity, metabolic fitness, and in vivo persistence [34].

In autoimmune disease, the clinical translation of CD19 CAR T-cell therapy has produced striking evidence of a deep immune reset. In early clinical cohorts of patients with treatment-refractory SLE, idiopathic inflammatory myopathies, and systemic sclerosis, a single infusion following lymphodepleting conditioning with fludarabine and cyclophosphamide resulted in the rapid ablation of circulating B cells, normalization of autoantibody profiles (including anti-dsDNA), restoration of complement levels, and marked clinical improvement across multiorgan disease manifestations, including nephritis and interstitial lung disease [35, 36]. Notably, these responses were sustained without maintenance immunosuppression, even after endogenous B-cell reconstitution, indicating durable reprogramming of the autoimmune network rather than transient suppression.

Subsequent larger clinical evaluations of autologous CD19 CAR T-cell platforms, including rapid-manufacturing next-generation products such as BMS-986353 (CC-97540), have further supported these findings. Across heavily pretreated systemic autoimmune cohorts, high rates of deep clinical responses have been observed, accompanied by substantial reductions in disease activity indices and clinically meaningful improvements in organ function metrics. Importantly, toxicity has remained largely manageable, with cytokine release syndrome predominantly low-grade and rare severe neurotoxicity, reflecting improved control of activation kinetics and dosing strategies in modern CAR T-cell constructs [37].

5.2 Dual-targeted CAR architectures: Synergizing CD19 and BCMA

Although CD19 is widely expressed across most stages of B-cell development, terminally differentiated, long-lived plasma cells within bone marrow niches lack CD19 expression and can persist following CD19-directed depletion. These cells constitute a durable source of autoantibody production and represent a potential substrate for disease recurrence. To address this limitation, dual-target CAR T-cell approaches have been developed to extend targeting across the full B-cell lineage. These constructs incorporate recognition domains for both CD19 and BCMA, the latter being selectively expressed on mature plasma cells [38]. Targeting of these compartments enables more complete depletion of autoreactive clones and more sustained suppression of pathogenic antibody production.

The clinical rationale for dual CD19/BCMA targeting is reinforced by allogeneic CAR T-cell platforms designed to achieve lineage-spanning B-cell eradication. CTA313 is an off-the-shelf dual CAR construct targeting CD19 and BCMA, thereby encompassing both precursor B cells and terminal plasma cell compartments. To enable allogeneic application, endogenous TCR and HLA class I loci are disrupted via CRISPR-Cas9 editing to mitigate graft-versus-host reactivity and host immune rejection. In addition, engineered modulation of host–immune recognition pathways

CAR-T product	Target antigen(s)	Construct features	Clinical indications investigated
BMS-986,353 (CC-97,540)	CD19	Autologous; 5-day NEX-T manufacturing	SLE, systemic sclerosis-associated interstitial lung disease, idiopathic inflammatory myopathies
CTA313	CD19/ BCMA	Allogeneic; TCR/HLA-I knockout, ANSWER™ molecule	Refractory SLE, lupus nephritis
GC012F	CD19/ BCMA	Autologous; FasTCAR-T manufacturing	SLE
C-CAR168	CD20/ BCMA	Autologous bispecific	SLE, neuromyelitis optica spectrum disorder, secondary progressive multiple sclerosis

Table 2.
Clinical efficacy and specifications of emerging cellular therapies in autoimmune diseases.

is incorporated to support in vivo persistence and functional activity. In early clinical evaluation of refractory SLE, CTA313 has been associated with rapid and deep serological responses, including marked suppression of autoantibody titers and normalization of disease activity indices. Clinically, this has translated into early achievement of low disease activity states and discontinuation of background immunosuppression in a substantial proportion of patients, consistent with durable ablation of autoreactive B-cell and plasma cell networks [39].

GC012F, a BCMA/CD19 dual FasT CAR-T construct, simultaneously targets CD19 + B-cell precursors and CD19-BCMA + long-lived plasma cells, thereby disrupting both upstream clonal expansion and downstream autoantibody production. In SLE, this lineage-spanning depletion has been associated with DORIS criteria, along with durable resolution of renal involvement, including normalization of proteinuria, reflecting effective suppression of the autoreactive humoral axis. Extending this strategy, C-CAR168 targets both CD20 + B cells and BCMA + plasma cells, enabling coordinated depletion of B-lineage compartments [40]. **Table 2** summarizes the key characteristics of emerging CAR-T cell therapies for autoimmune diseases, including their target antigens, construct features, and clinical indications currently under investigation.

5.3 Precision antigen targeting: CAAR-T and tissue-specific car-tregs

To tackle hypogammaglobulinemia and the risks associated with infections linked to total, pan-B-cell depletion, a targeted iteration of CAR technology was engineered: the chimeric autoantibody receptor (CAAR) T-cell. Rather than utilizing a broad scFv directed against a universal lineage marker like CD19, CAAR-T cells substitute the targeting domain with the exact structural autoantigen implicated in the specific indication. Consequently, the engineered CAAR-T cell acts as a specific biological "bait," selectively engaging, forming a synapse, and destroying pathogenic B-cell clones that express a BCR specific to that particular autoantigen. At the same time, the B-cell repertoire of healthy cells is preserved from depletion [41].

In clinical translation, MuSK-CAAR T cells have completed their Phase 1 trials (NCT05451212) for the treatment of Muscle-Specific Kinase (MuSK)-positive myasthenia gravis. CABA-201 met its primary endpoint, with both patients achieving rapid and sustained clinical responses alongside deep B-cell modulation after a four-day inpatient dosing protocol. Treatment was well-tolerated, with no Cytokine Release Syndrome (CRS), ICANS, serious adverse events, or infections observed, and all chronic immunosuppressive therapies were discontinued during follow-up, except for a planned prednisone taper in the SLE case. Similarly, DSG3-CAAR-T therapies are advancing through clinical stages (NCT04422912) by recruiting for the treatment of Pemphigus Vulgaris, directly and lethally targeting the rare desmoglein-3-reactive B-cells that are responsible for the severe, life-threatening mucosal blistering characteristic of the disease [41, 42].

CAR-engineered regulatory T-cells (CAR-Tregs) represent a targeted strategy for restoring tissue-localized immune tolerance without systemic immunosuppression. Autologous CD4 + FoxP3 + Tregs are modified to express CARs directed against disease-relevant tissue antigens (e.g., HLA-A2 in transplant settings or myelin-associated epitopes in neuroinflammation), enabling selective homing and retention at sites of ongoing immune injury. Following antigen engagement within inflamed tissue microenvironments, CAR-Tregs undergo local activation and expansion, reinforcing suppressive programs through the secretion of IL-10 and TGF-β, together with enhanced expression of inhibitory receptors such as CTLA-4. This coordinated activity attenuates effector T- and B-cell activation, dampens antigen presentation, and reestablishes local immune quiescence while preserving systemic immune competence. A representative clinical application is the ongoing first-in-human pilot study of AutoCD6-CAR Treg cells (NCT0,7395,050) in patients with stage 3 Type 1 diabetes. This autologous CAR-Treg platform is engineered to recognize CD6, a marker enriched on activated effector T-cells, with the rationale of selectively suppressing pathogenic T-cell activity while sparing regulatory T-cell populations. The study is designed to evaluate safety, tolerability, and feasibility in a disease context characterized by progressive autoimmune destruction of pancreatic β-cells and lifelong dependence on exogenous insulin therapy [43, 44].

5.4 In vivo engineering and next-generation delivery platforms

Despite its unparalleled efficacy, the clinical scalability of autologous CAR-T therapy is severely constrained by complex, incredibly costly, four to six-week "vein-to-vein" manufacturing processes. During this prolonged ex vivo expansion period, a patient's severe autoimmune disease may rapidly progress unmitigated. To entirely circumvent this massive logistical bottleneck, a revolutionary new approach is currently in development that bypasses ex vivo cell manipulation entirely. Utilizing the advanced lipid nanoparticle (LNP) technologies perfected during the rapid deployment of global viral vaccines, researchers are developing complex LNP vectors loaded with optimized messenger RNA (mRNA) that specifically encodes the CAR construct. Upon simple intravenous infusion, these highly targeted nanoparticles specifically bind to and transfect host T-cells circulating in vivo, directly delivering the genetic instructions required for temporary, robust CAR expression right within the patient's bloodstream. This pioneering in vivo engineering approach holds the explosive potential to utterly transform cellular therapy from a highly specialized, multistage hospital procedure into a routine, scalable pharmaceutical injection, drastically democratizing access for millions of patients suffering from severe autoimmunity. The primary pharmacological advantage of this modality lies in its immediate "off-the-shelf" kinetics, which bypasses the requirement for leukapheresis and high-dose lymphodepletive conditioning, thereby mitigating the risk of neutropenic sepsis and opportunistic infections. Furthermore, the transient, nonintegrating nature of mRNA-mediated transcription provides a critical safety buffer, facilitating a "hit-and-run" immune reset that avoids the protracted B-cell aplasia or insertional mutagenesis inherent to permanent lentiviral or retroviral integration. Conversely, these benefits are countered by significant bioengineering hurdles, most notably the requirement for high-affinity targeting ligands – such as anti-CD5 or anti-CD8 monoclonal antibodies – to ensure cell-type specificity and the potential for dose-limiting toxicities arising from the innate immunogenicity of ionizable lipids. Variable in vivo transfection efficiency also remains a hurdle, as the resulting CAR-T dosage is subject to individual physiological clearance rates and hepatic sequestration of the LNP vehicle [45].

Recent preclinical data from 2025 and early 2026 have significantly validated the therapeutic utility of these platforms in resolving complex autoimmune phenotypes. In humanized lupus mouse models, CD19-targeted "panCAR" LNPs have demonstrated robust B-cell depletion in both peripheral blood and lymphoid tissues at doses as low as 0.03 mg/kg, resulting in a statistically significant reduction in anti-dsDNA titers compared to traditional monoclonal antibody therapies like rituximab [46]. Furthermore, advances in extrahepatic delivery have achieved over 60% transfection efficiency in splenic T-cells in nonhuman primates (NHPs) without requiring complex targeting ligands, suggesting high translational potential for systemic immune resetting. Beyond B-cell aplasia, fibroblast activation protein (FAP)-targeted mRNA-LNPs have shown high efficacy in normalizing the microenvironment; recent studies in 2026 reported that a single intravenous dose achieved transient CAR expression in approximately 69% of circulating T cells, effectively degrading excess extracellular matrix and restoring organ compliance in models of cardiac and pulmonary fibrosis [47]. These findings suggest that for conditions including systemic lupus erythematosus, systemic sclerosis-associated interstitial lung disease (SSc-ILD), and idiopathic inflammatory myopathies (IIM), in vivo LNP-mediated intervention can disrupt the feed-forward loop of chronic inflammation and fibrosis, reestablishing homeostasis without the risks associated with long-term genomic modification [48, 49].

6. Mechanistic insights into lymphocyte reconstitution and the "immune reset"

The ultimate long-term objective of deep, aggressive lymphocyte depletion is not merely the temporary suppression of active clinical symptoms but the permanent achievement of an authentic "immune reset." This foundational concept posits that systematically wiping the immunological slate completely clean of pathogenic memory physically allows for the de novo repopulation of a naive, fundamentally self-tolerant lymphocyte repertoire, permanently altering the patient's disease trajectory.

6.1 Kinetics and phenotype of B-cell reconstitution

Following complete depletion of the peripheral B-cell compartment, immune reconstitution proceeds through a regulated, stepwise regenerative process originating within the bone marrow. Longitudinal multiparametric flow cytometry, coupled with single-cell RNA sequencing analyses in patients treated for systemic autoimmunity, has delineated a highly ordered and reproducible architecture of

B-cell recovery with marked divergence from the pretreatment immunologic state. In the early phase of reconstitution, the peripheral B-cell pool is predominantly composed of transitional (CD24hiCD38hi, IgM +) and immature B-cell subsets emerging directly from bone marrow output. This phase is followed by the gradual expansion of naive B cells (IgD + CD27-), which collectively constitute the dominant and most stable compartment during immune reconstitution. In contrast, class-switched memory B cells (IgD-CD27 +) and antibody-secreting plasmablast populations, previously expanded and transcriptionally primed in the setting of chronic autoimmune activation, remain depleted for extended periods, with some studies suggesting sustained or near-complete absence even during long-term follow-up [50].

At the transcriptional level, newly emerging B cells display a developmental gene signature consistent with early ontogeny and peripheral maturation. This includes elevated expression of genes associated with transitional programming and B-cell development (e.g., PLD4 and related maturation-associated transcripts), alongside a coordinated downregulation of pathways previously implicated in autoreactive activation, including chronic BCR signaling, NF-κB-driven inflammatory cascades, and plasmablast differentiation programs [51]. The resulting repertoire is not merely numerically restored but qualitatively reshaped, reflecting a fundamentally reset immunologic landscape. A critical feature of this reconstitution phase is the altered immunologic context in which lymphopoiesis occurs. In the absence of established autoreactive memory clones and their associated inflammatory crosstalk with T follicular helper cells, newly generated B cells undergo maturation under conditions of reduced antigenic pressure and diminished proinflammatory cytokine signaling. This environment appears to favor the restoration of central and peripheral tolerance mechanisms, allowing negative selection and anergy induction to operate with greater fidelity. Collectively, these processes contribute to the reemergence of a B-cell compartment that is developmentally naive, transcriptionally quiescent, and functionally distinct from the predepletion autoimmune state [52, 53].

6.2 Thymopoiesis, T-cell repertoire, and the Type I interferon signature

Although CD19-directed CAR-T cell therapy is mechanistically restricted to B-lineage depletion, its immunologic impact extends far beyond the B-cell compartment, producing profound secondary remodeling of T-cell homeostasis and innate immune signaling networks. Integrated transcriptomic and pathway-level analyses of peripheral blood mononuclear cells from patients with SLE treated with CD19 CAR-T consistently demonstrate a global attenuation of Type I interferon (IFN-I)-driven inflammatory programs. Following B-cell aplasia, there is a marked and sustained reduction in canonical IFN-stimulated gene (ISG) expression across both T cells and myeloid populations. Key interferon-regulated transcripts, including IRF7, ISG15, MX1, and related downstream effectors, show significant transcriptional downregulation, reflecting a collapse of the previously sustained IFN-I amplification loop. This is accompanied by broad suppression of interferon-response signatures at the pathway level, as demonstrated by gene set enrichment and single-cell differential expression analyses. The loss of antigen-presenting B-cell activity, together with reduced immune-complex–mediated Toll-like receptor engagement, is thought to be a principal upstream driver of this systemic recalibration [54, 55].

Importantly, this immunologic reprogramming occurs without measurable erosion of intrinsic TCR diversity. High-resolution repertoire profiling using probabilistic generative models of V(D)J recombination (including OLGA-based likelihood frameworks) demonstrates that the underlying probability landscape governing TCR-α and TCR-β chain generation remains largely invariant pre- and posttreatment. These findings indicate that CAR-T-mediated immune reset preserves the stochastic architecture of T-cell repertoire formation while decoupling it from pathological inflammatory signaling circuits [56]. In contrast, in settings of more profound lymphoablative interventions, such as autologous hematopoietic stem cell transplantation (AHSCT) combined with intensive conditioning regimens, long-term immune reconstitution becomes critically dependent on thymic regenerative capacity. Sustained clinical remission in such contexts correlates strongly with evidence of active thymopoiesis, including increased frequencies of CD31 + CD45RA + recent thymic emigrants within the CD4 + compartment, as well as the reemergence of thymus-derived FoxP3 + regulatory T cells. These populations collectively reflect de novo T-cell generation rather than peripheral expansion of preexisting clones. When thymic function is compromised due to age-related involution or prior cytotoxic injury, immune reconstitution shifts toward homeostatic peripheral proliferation of residual memory T-cell pools. This compensatory expansion occurs in a lymphopenic cytokine environment enriched for IL-7 and IL-15, promoting oligoclonal skewing of the TCR repertoire. Such contraction in diversity is associated with impaired regulatory buffering and an increased propensity for immune dysregulation, creating conditions that may favor secondary autoimmunity or inflammatory relapse in susceptible individuals [57].

6.3 High-dimensional profiling of TCR and BCR repertoires

High-throughput TCR and BCR repertoire sequencing enables quantitative reconstruction of adaptive immune clonality through CDR3 profiling derived from bulk and single-cell RNA-seq or targeted V(D)J amplification. In active SLE and RA, repertoires exhibit marked clonal contraction with oligoclonal expansions of antigen-experienced CD8 + T cells and class-switched B-cell clones, accompanied by restricted V/J gene usage and reduced Shannon diversity, consistent with chronic antigen-driven selection. Postlymphocyte-depleting therapy, longitudinal immune profiling demonstrates eradication of dominant preexisting clonotypes with reconstitution of a highly polyclonal repertoire. This is characterized by increased clonotype richness, restoration of near-normal V(D)J distribution, and recovery of diversity metrics (e.g., Shannon and Simpson indices). Newly emergent sequences predominantly originate from naïve lymphocyte pools, indicating de novo hematopoietic output and effective reset of antigen-experienced immune memory [58, 59].

7. Compensatory immune pathways and therapeutic resistance

The rapid and extensive depletion of established lymphocyte populations triggers strong homeostatic feedback responses driven by cytokine-mediated survival and proliferation signals. In the setting of lymphopenia, increased availability of cytokines such as IL-7 and IL-15, along with reduced cellular competition, promotes compensatory expansion of residual immune cells. If even small pools of pathogenic clones remain, these conditions can preferentially support their survival and proliferation, leading to the reemergence of autoreactive responses and eventual clinical relapse despite initial successful depletion.

7.1 The postdepletion B-cell activating factor and a proliferation-inducing ligand surge

The B-cell activating factor (BAFF) and a proliferation-inducing ligand (APRIL) cytokine system are absolutely critical for B-cell survival, maturation, and differentiation. B-cell depletion dramatically and immediately perturbs this delicate cytokine axis. The mass eradication of B cells from the periphery rapidly removes the primary cellular "sinks" that normally absorb circulating BAFF. Consequently, the immediate postdepletion phase is characterized by an acute, massively pronounced elevation in circulating serum BAFF concentrations. This post-depletion "BAFF surge" is highly pathogenic. The wildly elevated BAFF levels hyper-stimulate any surviving tissue-resident B-cells that escaped the initial mAb clearance or newly emerging transitional B cells exiting the bone marrow. This massive cytokine signal rescues them from programmed apoptosis and actively, forcefully promotes their rapid differentiation into mature, autoantibody-secreting plasma cells. Elegant mechanistic studies in murine models reveal that the primary source of this excess BAFF is heavily localized to splenic and lymphoid neutrophils. In states of high inflammation or specific genetic deficiencies (such as the downregulation of the BCMA receptor), these hyperactive neutrophils physically migrate directly into T-cell zones and secrete massive quantities of BAFF, acting as an emergency, localized survival niche for autoreactive lymphocytes. Clinically, the measured magnitude of the BAFF surge inversely correlates with the duration of patient remission, serving as a highly accurate biomarker predicting imminent disease flares and rapidly rising anti-dsDNA titers [60, 61].

To actively short-circuit this dangerous compensatory loop, sophisticated sequential and combinatorial therapeutic regimens have been instituted. The sequential administration of rituximab (utilized to violently deplete the primary B-cell bulk), followed immediately by maintenance dosing of belimumab (a human monoclonal antibody that physically binds and neutralizes soluble BAFF), directly counteracts the BAFF surge. By actively starving the residual, rituximab-resistant B-cells of their absolute requisite survival factor, this synergistic dual approach induces a far deeper and substantially more enduring total depletion. This strategy results in significantly lower rates of severe clinical flares in highly refractory SLE and complex autoimmune blistering diseases like bullous pemphigoid [62]. Clinically, the magnitude and duration of postdepletion BAFF elevation have been associated with the risk of disease reactivation, with higher levels correlating with earlier relapse and resurgence of autoantibody titers such as anti-dsDNA. Therapeutically, this compensatory axis can be attenuated through sequential or combinatorial targeting strategies. Initial B-cell depletion with anti-CD20–based approaches, followed by BAFF neutralization (e.g., belimumab-mediated blockade), reduces survival signaling available to residual and nascent B cells, thereby enhancing the depth and durability of depletion and contributing to improved disease control in refractory systemic autoimmunity [63, 64].

7.2 Tissue microenvironmental resistance and epigenetic bottlenecks

Resistance to lymphocyte-targeted therapies extends beyond antigen loss and is increasingly recognized at the level of tissue microenvironmental adaptation and epigenetic remodeling. In the context of CAR-T cells and bispecific TCEs, disease-intrinsic escape mechanisms include transcriptional downregulation, alternative splicing, or complete loss of target antigen expression at the cell surface (e.g., CD19-negative relapse), effectively abrogating immune recognition despite the persistence of effector cells. In parallel, the tissue microenvironment imposes potent extrinsic constraints that limit sustained cytotoxic function. Inflamed lymphoid and peripheral tissue niches in autoimmune disease exhibit features analogous to solid tumor microenvironments, including elevated TGF-β signaling, chronic antigen stimulation, hypoxia, and nutrient deprivation. These conditions collectively impair effector T-cell metabolism, restrict glycolytic and oxidative capacity, and promote progressive functional decline [65].

At the transcriptional and epigenetic level, chronic stimulation drives T-cell exhaustion programs characterized by stable chromatin remodeling and fixation of dysfunctional states. This is orchestrated, in part, by transcriptional regulators such as T-cell exhaustion factor (TOX) and the Nuclear receptor subfamily 4, group A (NR4A) family, which reinforce epigenetic accessibility patterns associated with reduced cytokine production, impaired proliferative capacity, and loss of cytolytic function. Once established, these epigenetic programs can become partially irreversible, limiting the durability of engineered T-cell responses [66, 67].

To overcome these constraints, next-generation cellular therapies are being designed with intrinsic resistance to suppressive signaling pathways. "Armored" CAR-T platforms, incorporating dominant-negative TGF-β receptors or cytokine-enhancing genetic circuits, have been developed to preserve effector function within suppressive tissue environments. In parallel, metabolic reprogramming strategies aim to sustain mitochondrial fitness and glycolytic flux under hypoxic and nutrient-limited conditions. Complementary pharmacologic approaches targeting exhaustion-associated transcriptional networks, including TOX and NR4A-linked pathways, are under investigation to restore functional plasticity in exhausted T cells and reinforce sustained clearance of pathogenic clones [68].

8. Biomarker-driven stratification and quantitative pharmacology

As the mechanistic understanding of immune resetting deepens and the available therapeutic arsenal expands, the next major clinical frontier focuses on overcoming logistical barriers and perfectly matching the highly aggressive depletion modality to the specific biological state of the individual patient.

8.1 Systems pharmacology and quantitative systems pharmacology modeling

The extreme biological heterogeneity of autoimmune diseases mandates stringent, highly accurate patient selection to maximize therapeutic efficacy and mitigate the inherent, potentially lethal risks of severe immunosuppression. To this end, quantitative systems pharmacology (QSP) modeling is being aggressively deployed to mathematically predict individual patient responses to CAR-T therapies. These complex QSP models integrate vast amounts of temporal patient data, encompassing the exact kinetics of lymphodepletion chemotherapy, the predicted in vivo expansion rates of the infused CAR-T cells, the logarithmic clearance of CD19 + B-cells, and the wildly fluctuating concentrations of surrogate biomarkers (such as complement C3 and IFN-alpha levels). By correlating these dynamic physiological parameters via advanced linear regression algorithms directly with clinical severity indices like the Systemic Lupus Erythematosus Disease Activity Index (SLEDAI) score, researchers and clinicians can highly accurately forecast the long-term trajectory of disease progression. This mathematical modeling allows for the pinpoint identification of the optimal therapeutic dosing window and helps determine exactly which patients require dual-targeted CARs versus those who will achieve remission with a simpler monoclonal antibody intervention [69].

8.2 Noninvasive biomarker panels

Concurrently, highly invasive and painful diagnostic procedures are being rapidly supplanted by high-resolution molecular biomarkers. In the management of severe lupus nephritis, novel, highly specific urinary biomarker panels, which evaluate local intrarenal inflammatory proteins and specific molecular markers like the E3 ligase/GILZ regulatory axis, are currently demonstrating exceptional predictive validity. These advanced noninvasive assays are remarkably capable of accurately reflecting the underlying destructive renal histology and precisely forecasting longitudinal patient responses to targeted depletion therapies. This breakthrough technology enables real-time, precision-guided adjustments to intensive treatment protocols, allowing clinicians to escalate or taper immunosuppression based on molecular realities without subjecting highly vulnerable patients to the risks of repeated kidney biopsies [69].

9. Conclusion

The definitive clinical transition from reliance on conventional, broad-spectrum immunosuppression to highly targeted, mechanistically precise T- and B-cell depletion strategies marks a profound, irreversible inflection point in the modern management of severe, treatment-refractory autoimmune diseases. Early-generation monoclonal antibodies successfully laid the conceptual groundwork by explicitly demonstrating the immense clinical validity of lineage-specific cellular ablation. Yet, their long-term efficacy is frequently and severely curtailed by incomplete deep-tissue penetration, receptor internalization, and the rapid emergence of compensatory biological survival pathways, most notably the highly pathogenic BAFF cytokine surge [70]. The brilliant structural innovation inherent in modern Fc-engineered biologics, such as the bifunctional inhibitor obexelimab, offers a highly refined alternative, achieving extraordinarily potent functional inhibition and remarkably rapid cellular recovery while meticulously preserving the underlying healthy, naive immune repertoire [71].

The subsequent introduction of bispecific TCEs and adoptively transferred CAR-T cells has successfully translated the formidable, unmatched cytotoxic power of the endogenous T-cell compartment directly into the autoimmune niche. Through advanced dual-targeting architectures – particularly the simultaneous, aggressive targeting of both CD19 and BCMA – these revolutionary cellular therapies execute an unparalleled depth of total clearance. They successfully eradicate both the actively proliferating B-cell precursors and the deeply entrenched, historically untouchable long-lived plasma cells residing in the bone marrow. The resulting clinical outcomes, explicitly defined by durable, totally drug-free remissions and the profound, permanent downregulation of systemic inflammatory transcriptomic signatures, unequivocally substantiate the biological reality of a true "immune reset" [25, 72].

As the field of precision immunology continues its rapid advance, the seamless integration of these extraordinarily potent depleting agents with mathematically predictive systems pharmacology models, highly accurate noninvasive biomarker surveillance, and infinitely scalable in vivo LNP mRNA engineering platforms will be absolutely essential [69]. By surgically and permanently excising the autoreactive memory compartments while deliberately and carefully fostering the healthy repopulation of a tolerant, perfectly balanced immune repertoire, dual T and B-cell targeted depletion strategies offer a highly mechanistically grounded, precision-driven therapeutic framework. This framework is not merely capable of suppressing symptoms but of permanently and fundamentally altering the long-term trajectory of autoimmune disease, finally bringing the concept of a definitive cure into clinical reality [71, 73].

Acknowledgments

The author gratefully acknowledges Nrupa Dinesh Patel for assistance with Zotero reference management and citation organization. Zotero was used for referencing throughout this manuscript. The author also acknowledges the Hillman Library, University of Pittsburgh, for providing comprehensive access to scientific journals and literature resources. Grammarly was utilized for grammatical corrections and language refinement during the writing process. Finally, sincere thanks are extended to the author's family for their continuous support and encouragement throughout the preparation of this manuscript.

Conflict of Interest

The authors declare no conflicts of interest

Abbreviations

AHSCT	Autologous hematopoietic stem cell transplantation
AKT	Protein kinase B
APRIL	A Proliferation-inducing ligand
BAFF	B-cell activating factor
BCMA	B-cell MATURATION ANTIGEN
BCR	B-cell receptor
CAR	Chimeric antigen receptor
CAR-T	Chimeric antigen receptor T cell
CAAR-T	Chimeric autoantibody receptor T cell
CD	Cluster of differentiation
CDC	Complement-dependent cytotoxicity
CDR3	Complementarity-determining region 3
CRISPR-Cas9	Genome editing system
CXCL13	Chemokine ligand 13
CXCL9	Chemokine ligand 9
CXCL10	Chemokine ligand 10

DORIS	Definition of remission in SLE
Fc	Fragment crystallizable
FcγRIIb (CD32B)	Inhibitory Fc receptor
FcγRIIIa (CD16A)	Activating Fc receptor
FoxP3	Regulatory T-cell transcription factor
HLA	Human leukocyte antigen
IFN-α/β	Type I interferon
IFN-γ	Interferon gamma
Ig	Immunoglobulin
IgG4-RD	IgG4-related disease
IL	Interleukin
IRF7	Interferon regulatory factor 7
ISG15	Interferon-stimulated gene 15
MX1	Myxovirus resistance protein 1
LNP	Lipid nanoparticle
MHC II	Major histocompatibility complex II
MS	Multiple sclerosis
NF-κB	Nuclear factor kappa B
NR4A	Nuclear receptor subfamily 4 group A
OLGA	Repertoire modeling framework
PD-1	Programmed cell death protein 1
PI3K	Phosphoinositide 3-kinase
PIP3	Phosphatidylinositol (3,4,5)-trisphosphate
PLD4	Phospholipase D4
RA	Rheumatoid arthritis
RMS	Relapsing multiple sclerosis
RTE	Recent thymic emigrant
scRNA-seq	Single-cell RNA sequencing
SHIP-1	SH2-domain inositol phosphatase-1
SLE	Systemic lupus erythematosus
SRI-4	SLE responder index-4
TACI	Transmembrane activator and CAML interactor
TCE	T-cell engager
TCR	T-cell receptor
Tfh	T follicular helper cell
TGF-β	Transforming growth factor beta
Th1	T helper 1 cell
Th17	T helper 17 cell
TLR	Toll-like receptor
TNF-α	Tumor necrosis factor alpha
TOX	T-cell exhaustion factor
Treg	Regulatory T cell
V(D)J	Variable-diversity-joining recombination

Author details

Parv Barot* and Sanjay Rathod
Novasenta Inc., Pittsburgh, Pennsylvania, USA

*Address all correspondence to: parv.barot@novasenta.com

References

[1] Kumar M, Yip L, Wang F, Marty SE, Fathman CG. Autoimmune disease: Genetic susceptibility, environmental triggers, and immune dysregulation. Where can we develop therapies? Frontiers in Immunology. 2025;**16**:1626082. DOI: 10.3389/fimmu.2025.1626082

[2] Vukovic J, Abazovic D, Vucetic D, Medenica S. CAR-engineered T cell therapy as an emerging strategy for treating autoimmune diseases. Frontiers in Medicine. 2024;**11**:1447147. DOI: 10.3389/fmed.2024.1447147

[3] Blüml S, McKeever K, Ettinger R, Smolen J, Herbst R. B-cell targeted therapeutics in clinical development. Arthritis Research & Therapy. 2013;**15**(S1):S4. DOI: 10.1186/ar3906

[4] Sarrand J, Soyfoo M. B-Cells and plasmablasts as architects of autoimmune disease: From molecular footprints to precision therapeutics. Cells. 2026;**15**(2):119. DOI: 10.3390/cells15020119

[5] Merino-Vico A, Frazzei G, Van Hamburg JP, Tas SW. Targeting B cells and plasma cells in autoimmune diseases: From established treatments to novel therapeutic approaches. European Journal of Immunology. 2023;**53**(1):2149675. DOI: 10.1002/eji.202149675

[6] Żurawek M, Ziółkowska-Suchanek I, Iżykowska K. Fibrosis in immune-mediated and autoimmune disorders. Journal of Clinical Medicine. 2025;**14**(18):6636. DOI: 10.3390/jcm14186636

[7] Song X, Liang H, Nan F, Chen W, Li J, He L, et al. Autoimmune diseases: Molecular pathogenesis and therapeutic targets. MedComm. 2025;**6**(7):e70262. DOI: 10.1002/mco2.70262

[8] Heintzman DR, Fisher EL, Rathmell JC. Microenvironmental influences on T cell immunity in cancer and inflammation. Cellular & Molecular Immunology. 2022;**19**(3):316–326. DOI: 10.1038/s41423-021-00833-2

[9] Yamaguchi T, Wing JB, Sakaguchi S. Two modes of immune suppression by Foxp3+ regulatory T cells under inflammatory or non-inflammatory conditions. Seminars in Immunology. 2011;**23**(6):424–430. DOI: 10.1016/j.smim.2011.10.002

[10] Wang R, Lan C, Benlagha K, Camara NOS, Miller H, Kubo M, et al. The interaction of innate immune and adaptive immune system. MedComm. 2024;**5**(10):e714. DOI: 10.1002/mco2.714

[11] Zhao L, Jin S, Wang S, Zhang Z, Wang X, Chen Z, et al. Tertiary lymphoid structures in diseases: Immune mechanisms and therapeutic advances. Signal Transduction and Targeted Therapy. 2024;**9**(1):225. DOI: 10.1038/s41392-024-01947-5

[12] Deenick EK, Ma CS. The regulation and role of T follicular helper cells in immunity: T follicular helper cells in immunity. Immunology. 2011;**134**(4):361–367. DOI: 10.1111/j.1365-2567.2011.03487.x

[13] Mintz MA, Cyster JG. T follicular helper cells in germinal center B cell selection and lymphomagenesis. Immunological Reviews. 2020;**296**(1):48–61. DOI: 10.1111/imr.12860

[14] Kessel A, Rosner I, Rituximab TE. Beyond simple B cell depletion. Clinical Reviews in Allergy & Immunology. 2008;**34**(1):74–79. DOI: 10.1007/s12016-008-8074-1

[15] Uzzan M, Ko HM, Rosenstein AK, Pourmand K, Colombel J, Mehandru S. Efficient long-term depletion of CD20+ B cells by rituximab does not affect gut-resident plasma cells. Annals of the New York Academy of Sciences. 2018;**1415**(1):5–10. DOI: 10.1111/nyas.13577

[16] Tobinai K, Klein C, Oya N, Fingerle-Rowson G. A Review of Obinutuzumab (GA101), a Novel Type II Anti-CD20 Monoclonal Antibody, for the Treatment of Patients with B-Cell Malignancies. Advances in Therapy. 2017;**34**(2):324–356. DOI: 10.1007/s12325-016-0451-1

[17] Morelli DM, Craig HC, Feng X, Youd M, Matijevic MI, Kerfoot SM. CD19 and Fc γ RIIb co-engagement inhibits processes essential to T cell–dependent B-cell responses. The Journal of Immunology. 2026;**215**(1):vkaf247. DOI: 10.1093/jimmun/vkaf247

[18] Chu SY, Pong E, Bonzon C, Yu N, Jacob CO, Chalmers SA, et al. Inhibition of B cell activation following in vivo co-engagement of B cell antigen receptor and Fc γ receptor IIb in non-autoimmune-prone and SLE-prone mice. Journal of Translational Autoimmunity. 2021;**4**:100075. DOI: 10.1016/j.jtauto.2020.100075

[19] Culver EL, Baker MC, Della-Torre E, Zhang W, Perugino CA, Wells A, et al. Efficacy and Safety of Obexelimab to Treat IgG4-Related Disease: Protocol for a Global, Randomized, Placebo-Controlled Trial. Rheumatology and Therapy. 2026. DOI: 10.1007/s40744-026-00835-4

[20] Han X, et al. Stimulating T Cells Against Cancer With Agonist Immunostimulatory Monoclonal Antibodies. In International Review of Cell and Molecular Biology Department of Immunobiology, Yale School of Medicine, New Haven, CT 06510: Elsevier; 2019. p. 1–25. DOI: 10.1016/bs.ircmb.2018.07.003

[21] Herold KC, Burton JB, Francois F, Poumian-Ruiz E, Glandt M, Bluestone JA. Activation of human T cells by FcR nonbinding anti-CD3 mAb, hOKT3γ1(Ala-Ala). Journal of Clinical Investigation. 2003;**111**(3):409–418. DOI: 10.1172/JCI16090

[22] Von Essen MR, Chow HH, Holm Hansen R, Buhelt S, Sellebjerg F. Immune reconstitution following alcmtuzumab therapy is characterized by exhausted T cells, increased regulatory control of proinflammatory T cells and reduced B cell control. Frontiers in Immunology. 2023;**14**:1249201. DOI: 10.3389/fimmu.2023.1249201

[23] Ruck T, Bittner S, Wiendl H, Meuth S. Alemtuzumab in multiple sclerosis: Mechanism of action and beyond. International Journal of Molecular Sciences. 2015;**16**(7):16414–16439. DOI: 10.3390/ijms160716414

[24] Michaelson JS, Baeuerle PA. CD19-directed T cell–engaging antibodies for the treatment of autoimmune disease. Journal of Experimental Medicine. 2024;**221**(5):e20240499. DOI: 10.1084/jem.20240499

[25] Kang X, Zhao Y, Ling H, Huang X. Bispecific and multispecific T-cell engagers: Advancing the future of immunotherapy. Antibody Therapeutics. 2026;**9**(1):58–69. DOI: 10.1093/abt/tbaf026

[26] Cech P, Skórka K, Dziki L, Giannopoulos K. T-Cell Engagers—The Structure and Functional Principle and Application in Hematological Malignancies. Cancers. 2024;**16**(8):1580. DOI: 10.3390/cancers16081580

[27] Lei T, Wang Y, Zhang Y, Yang Y, Cao J, Huang J, et al. Leveraging CRISPR gene editing technology to optimize the efficacy, safety and accessibility of CAR T-cell therapy. Leukemia. 2024;**38**(12):2517–2543. DOI: 10.1038/s41375-024-02444-y

[28] Subklewe M, Magno G, Gebhardt C, Bücklein V, Szelinski F, Arévalo HJR, et al. Application of blinatumomab, a bispecific anti-CD3/CD19 T-cell engager, in treating severe systemic sclerosis: A case study. European Journal of Cancer. 2024;**204**:114071. DOI: 10.1016/j.ejca.2024.114071

[29] Liu X, Zhao J, Guo X, Song Y. CD20 × CD3 bispecific antibodies for lymphoma therapy: Latest updates from ASCO 2023 annual meeting. Journal of Hematology & Oncology. 2023;**16**(1):90. DOI: 10.1186/s13045-023-01488-4

[30] Zhang Z, Markmann C, Yu M, Agarwal D, Rostami S, Wang W, et al. Immunotherapy targeting B cells and long-lived plasma cells effectively eliminates pre-existing donor-specific allo-antibodies. Cell Reports Medicine. 2023;**4**(12):101336. DOI: 10.1016/j.xcrm.2023.101336

[31] Genovese MC, Weinblatt ME, Aelion JA, Mansikka HT, Peloso PM, Chen K, et al. ABT-122, a Bispecific Dual Variable Domain Immunoglobulin Targeting Tumor Necrosis Factor and Interleukin-17A, in Patients With Rheumatoid Arthritis With an Inadequate Response to Methotrexate. Arthritis & Rheumatology. 2018;**70**(11):1710–1720. DOI: 10.1002/art.40580

[32] Iznardo H, Puig L. Dual inhibition of IL-17A and IL-17F in psoriatic disease. Therapeutic Advances in Chronic Disease. 2021;**12**:20406223211037846. DOI: 10.1177/20406223211037846

[33] Cao Z, Li Y, Wang W, Jie S, Hu X, Zhou J, et al. Is Lutikizumab, an Anti–Interleukin-1α/β Dual Variable Domain Immunoglobulin, efficacious for Osteoarthritis? Results from a Bayesian network meta-analysis. BioMed Research International. 2020;**2020**(1):9013283. DOI: 10.1155/2020/9013283

[34] Forsthuber TG, Cimbora DM, Ratchford JN, Katz E, Stüve O. B cell-based therapies in CNS autoimmunity: Differentiating CD19 and CD20 as therapeutic targets. Therapeutic Advances in Neurological Disorders. 2018;**11**:1756286418761697. DOI: 10.1177/1756286418761697

[35] McCue AC, Yao Z, Kuhlman B. Advances in modular control of CAR-T therapy with adapter-mediated CARs. Advanced Drug Delivery Reviews. 2022;**187**:114358. DOI: 10.1016/j.addr.2022.114358

[36] Lee BW, Kwon EJ, Ju JH. Chimeric Antigen Receptor T-cell therapy in systemic autoimmune rheumatic diseases: Current insights and future prospects. Journal of Rheumatic Diseases. 2025;**32**(3):154–165. DOI: 10.4078/jrd.2024.0122

[37] Reshef R, Azzi J, Ayala E, Cherry M, Nash R, Hütter-Krönke ML, et al. Clinical Outcomes from the Pooled

Safety Analysis of CD19 Nex-TTM (BMS-986353), a Chimeric Antigen Receptor (CAR) T cell Therapy Manufactured Using a Next-Generation Process, in Severe Refractory Autoimmune Diseases: Results from Phase 1 Breakfree Studies. Transplantation and Cellular Therapy. 2026;**32**(2):S1. DOI: 10.1016/j.jtct.2025.12.014

[38] Bachiller M, Barceló-Genestar N, Rodriguez-Garcia A, Alserawan L, Dobaño-López C, Giménez-Alejandre M, et al. ARI0003: Co-transduced CD19/BCMA dual-targeting CAR-T cells for the treatment of non-Hodgkin lymphoma. Molecular Therapy. 2025;**33**(1):317–335. DOI: 10.1016/j.ymthe.2024.11.028

[39] Bumma N, Devarakonda S, Khan A. Dual attack on multiple myeloma: Targeting BCMA and CD19. AME Clinical Trials Review. 2025;**3**:41–41. DOI: 10.21037/actr-24-275

[40] Qiang W, Lu J, Jia Y, Liu J, Liu J, He H, et al. B-Cell Maturation Antigen/CD19 Dual-Targeting Immunotherapy in Newly Diagnosed Multiple Myeloma. JAMA Oncology. 2024;**10**(9):1259. DOI: 10.1001/jamaoncol.2024.2172

[41] Doan A, Pulsipher MA. Hypogammaglobulinemia due to CAR T-cell therapy. Pediatric Blood & Cancer. 2018;**65**(4):e26914. DOI: 10.1002/pbc.26914

[42] Oh S, Mao X, Manfredo-Vieira S, Lee J, Patel D, Choi EJ, et al. Precision targeting of autoantigen-specific B cells in muscle-specific tyrosine kinase myasthenia gravis with chimeric autoantibody receptor T cells. Nature Biotechnology. 2023;**41**(9):1229–1238. DOI: 10.1038/s41587-022-01637-z

[43] Lee J, Lundgren DK, Mao X, Manfredo-Vieira S, Nunez-Cruz S, Williams EF, et al. Antigen-specific B cell depletion for precision therapy of mucosal pemphigus vulgaris. Journal of Clinical Investigation. 2020;**130**(12):6317–6324. DOI: 10.1172/JCI138416

[44] Arjomandnejad M, Kopec AL, Keeler AM. CAR-T Regulatory (CAR-Treg) Cells: Engineering and Applications. Biomedicines. 2022;**10**(2):287. DOI: 10.3390/biomedicines10020287

[45] Gao Y, Hu J, An N, Wen X, Li C. In vivo engineering of CAR-T cells: Delivery strategies and clinical translation. Biomarker Research. 2026;**14**(1):23. DOI: 10.1186/s40364-026-00899-y

[46] Hu K, Srivastava S, Ma B, Yang Y, Wang H, Mangolini M, et al. Engineering armoured in vivo CAR T cells through targeted delivery and transient mRNA gating. openRxiv. 2026. DOI: 10.64898/2026.03.10.710759

[47] Asadi G, Rajabinejad M. In vivo CAR-T engineering: Insights from the 2025 ASH annual meeting. Experimental Hematology & Oncology. 2026;**15**(1):30. DOI: 10.1186/s40164-026-00762-8

[48] Wei C, Shan X, Huang Y, Ma B, Zhao Z, Fang Y, et al. FAP-Synergistic Organ-Targeted mRNA-LNP for Overcoming Delivery Barriers in Hepatic and Pulmonary Fibrosis. Journal of the American Chemical Society. 2026;**148**(9):9309–9327. DOI: 10.1021/jacs.5c16886

[49] Schroeder A, Suissa N, Yeini E, Abu-Hariri H, Nudelman I, Rosin G,

et al. Machine Learning-Driven Discovery of a Lipid Nanoparticle for In-Vivo T-Cell Transfection in Non-Human Primates. Mana.bio & Sheba Medical Center Research Square. 2025. DOI: 10.21203/rs.3.rs-7848619/v1

[50] Allman D, Pillai S. Peripheral B cell subsets. Current Opinion in Immunology. 2008;**20**(2):149–157. DOI: 10.1016/j.coi.2008.03.014

[51] Gómez-Manríquez J, Hernández-Bello J, Muñoz-Valle JF, Sifuentes-Franco S, Graciano-Machuca O, Morales-Núñez JJ. B cell development: Transcriptional regulation and immunological mechanisms in homeostasis. Frontiers in Immunology. 2025;**16**:1593338. DOI: 10.3389/fimmu.2025.1593338

[52] Rothenberg EV. Transcriptional Control of Early T and B Cell Developmental Choices. Annual Review of Immunology. 2014;**32**(1):283–321. DOI: 10.1146/annurev-immunol-032712-100024

[53] Baliu-Piqué M, Tesselaar K, Borghans JAM. Are homeostatic mechanisms aiding the reconstitution of the T-cell pool during lymphopenia in humans? Frontiers in Immunology. 2022;**13**:1059481. DOI: 10.3389/fimmu.2022.1059481

[54] Wilhelm A, Chambers D, Müller F, Bozec A, Grieshaber-Bouyer R, Winkler T, et al. Selective CAR T cell–mediated B cell depletion suppresses IFN signature in SLE. JCI Insight. 2024;**9**(12):e179433. DOI: 10.1172/jci.insight.179433

[55] Mostafavi S, Yoshida H, Moodley D, LeBoité H, Rothamel K, Raj T, et al. Parsing the Interferon Transcriptional Network and Its Disease Associations. Cell. 2016;**164**(3):564–578. DOI: 10.1016/j.cell.2015.12.032

[56] Elhanati Y, Sethna Z, Callan CG, Mora T, Walczak AM. Predicting the spectrum of TCR repertoire sharing with a data-driven model of recombination. Immunological Reviews. 2018;**284**(1):167–179. DOI: 10.1111/imr.12665

[57] Atilla E, Ataca Atilla P, Demirer T. A Review of Myeloablative vs Reduced Intensity/Non-Myeloablative Regimens in Allogeneic Hematopoietic Stem Cell Transplantations. Balkan Medical Journal. 2017;**34**(1):1–9. DOI: 10.4274/balkanmedj.2017.0055

[58] Pai JA, Satpathy AT. High-throughput and single-cell T cell receptor sequencing technologies. Nature Methods. 2021;**18**(8):881–892. DOI: 10.1038/s41592-021-01201-8

[59] Enrich E, Antón-Iborra M, Hobeich C, Mora-Buch R, Lara-de-león AG, Parra-Martínez A, et al. A high-throughput sequencing strategy for clinical repertoire profiling of T cell receptor beta chain: Development and reference values across healthy adults, paediatrics, and cord blood units. International Journal of Molecular Sciences. 2025;**26**(19):9590. DOI: 10.3390/ijms26199590

[60] Gorbacheva V, Ayasoufi K, Fan R, Baldwin WM, Valujskikh A. B Cell Activating Factor (BAFF) and a Proliferation Inducing Ligand (April) Mediate CD40-Independent Help by Memory CD4 T Cells. American Journal of Transplantation. 2015;**15**(2):346–357. DOI: 10.1111/ajt.12984

[61] Mackay F, Silveira PA, Brink R. B cells and the BAFF/April axis:

Fast-forward on autoimmunity and signaling. Current Opinion in Immunology. 2007;**19**(3):327–336. DOI: 10.1016/j.coi.2007.04.008

[62] Batten M, Groom J, Cachero TG, Qian F, Schneider P, Tschopp J, et al. Baff Mediates Survival of Peripheral Immature B Lymphocytes. The Journal of Experimental Medicine. 2000;**192**(10):1453–1466. DOI: 10.1084/jem.192.10.1453

[63] Carter LM, Isenberg DA, Ehrenstein MR. Elevated serum BAFF levels are associated with rising anti–double-stranded dna antibody levels and disease flare following B Cell Depletion Therapy in systemic lupus erythematosus. Arthritis & Rheumatism. 2013;**65** (10):2672–2679. DOI: 10.1002/art.38074

[64] Smulski CR, Eibel H. BAFF and BAFF-Receptor in B Cell Selection and Survival. Frontiers in Immunology. 2018;**9**:2285. DOI: 10.3389/fimmu.2018.02285

[65] Legato L, Bisio M, Fasano F, Benevolo Savelli C, Secreto C, Dellacasa CM, et al. Mechanisms of Resistance to CAR T-Cells and How to Overcome Them. Methods and Protocols. 2025;**8**(5):108. DOI: 10.3390/mps8050108

[66] Battistello E, Hixon KA, Comstock DE, Collings CK, Chen X, Rodriguez Hernaez J, et al. Stepwise activities of mSWI/SNF family chromatin remodeling complexes direct T cell activation and exhaustion. Molecular Cell. 2023;**83**(8):1216–1236.e12. DOI: 10.1016/j.molcel.2023.02.026

[67] Tian Y, Li Y, Shao Y, Zhang Y. Gene modification strategies for next-generation CAR T cells against solid cancers. Journal of Hematology & Oncology. 2020;**13**(1):54. DOI: 10.1186/s13045-020-00890-6

[68] Wang Y, Shao W, Mao J, Ye Q. Overcoming Resistance and Relapse in CAR-T and CAR-NK Cell Therapies: From Bench to Bedside. Research. 2026;**9**:1068. DOI: 10.34133/research.1068

[69] Kiaie SH, Majidi Zolbanin N, Ahmadi A, Bagherifar R, Valizadeh H, Kashanchi F, et al. Recent advances in mRNA-LNP therapeutics: Immunological and pharmacological aspects. Journal of Nanobiotechnology. 2022;**20**(1):276. DOI: 10.1186/s12951-022-01478-7

[70] Schweighoffer E, Tybulewicz VL. BAFF signaling in health and disease. Current Opinion in Immunology. 2021;**71**:124–131. DOI: 10.1016/j.coi.2021.06.014

[71] Robinson WH, Fiorentino D, Chung L, Moreland LW, Deodhar M, Harler MB, et al. Cutting-edge approaches to B-cell depletion in autoimmune diseases. Frontiers in Immunology. 2024;**15**:1454747. DOI: 10.3389/fimmu.2024.1454747

[72] De Bousser E, Callewaert N, Festjens N. T cell engaging immunotherapies, highlighting chimeric antigen receptor (CAR) T cell therapy. Cancers. 2021;**13**(23):6067. DOI: 10.3390/cancers13236067

[73] Lu Y, Ruan Y, Hong P, Rui K, Liu Q, Wang S, et al. T-cell senescence: A crucial player in autoimmune diseases. Clinical Immunology. 2023;**248**:109202. DOI: 10.1016/j.clim.2022.109202

Chapter 9

T-Cell Ontogeny

Cynthia Guadalupe Pelayo Mena, Yanet Ventura Enríquez, Claudia Mondragón Albarrán, Adán Germán Gallardo Rodríguez, Gabriel Aceves Castillo, Aldo Mujica Martínez, Moises Leonardo Mendoza Torres, Monica Alethia Cureño Diaz, Estibeyesbo Said Plascencia Nieto, Erika Gómez Zamora, Christian Omar Ramos Peñafiel and Verónica Fernández Sánchez

Abstract

Hematopoiesis is a highly organized process that begins during embryonic life and is maintained throughout the lifespan. The transition from fetal hematopoietic sites to adult bone marrow establishes an efficient cellular production system. Differentiation of hematopoietic stem cells (HSCs) into the lymphoid lineage is essential for adaptive immunity and depends on a complex network of interactions among molecular signals, the hematopoietic niche, and subsequent maturation within the thymic niche. Understanding these mechanisms is not only of biological importance but also has diagnostic and therapeutic implications for multiple hematological and immunological diseases. This chapter describes the ontogeny of T lymphocytes, as well as their stages of commitment, selection, and immunological function.

Keywords: thymus, T-cell development, positive selection, negative selection, hematopoietic stem cells

1. Introduction

T lymphocytes originate from hematopoietic progenitors derived from the bone marrow (BM) that migrate to the thymus, where they undergo highly regulated processes of maturation, selection, and subsequent export to the peripheral immune system. Peripheral T lymphocytes comprise several functional subsets, including naïve T cells capable of responding to new antigens, memory T cells derived from prior antigenic activation that contribute to long-term immunity, and regulatory T cells (Tregs) that play a central role in maintaining immune tolerance and controlling excessive immune responses [1].

The homeostasis of the T-cell system is regulated by multiple factors. In addition to thymopoiesis, T-cell populations are maintained through mechanisms such as post-thymic homeostatic proliferation, antigen-driven expansion, apoptosis, and cellular turnover, all of which contribute to defining the size and composition of this cellular compartment. The total number of T lymphocytes in humans has been estimated at approximately 3×10^{11} cells. Moreover, the diversity of the T-cell receptor (TCR) repertoire is remarkably extensive. In young individuals, the diversity of the TCR-β chain is estimated to range from 2×10^6 to 2×10^7 variants, each of which can pair with multiple TCR-α chains, generating a potential repertoire of approximately 10^8 distinct TCRs. Naïve T-cell clones are estimated to contain roughly 1,000 cells per clonotype, reflecting the balance between thymic output and peripheral homeostatic expansion [2].

With aging, the thymic epithelial space progressively decreases, declining by approximately 3% per year during middle age. Nevertheless, islands of intact thymic cortex and medulla persist and continue to support ongoing TCR rearrangement and T-cell development. Despite this residual activity, the capacity of the thymus to sustain a highly diverse T-cell repertoire declines over time. Studies suggest that by the seventh decade of life, a critical period is reached in which T-cell homeostasis becomes increasingly compromised, and the diversity of the naïve T-cell repertoire begins to collapse. Thymic involution is therefore a hallmark of immunological aging. Importantly, this process is not merely a passive, age-dependent degeneration of an organ system but rather an active and regulated biological process whose underlying mechanisms remain incompletely understood. Furthermore, the minimal level of thymic activity required to maintain a large and diverse pool of peripheral T lymphocytes remains unclear [3].

In this context, understanding the cellular and molecular mechanisms that regulate T-cell development is essential for interpreting the organization and long-term maintenance of the adaptive immune system. This chapter, therefore, examines the key processes that govern T-cell ontogeny, from the origin of hematopoietic progenitors and their migration to the thymus, to the sequential events of lineage commitment, thymic selection, and the generation of mature, functional T-cell populations.

2. Hematopoiesis

Hematopoiesis is the dynamic process by which blood cells (erythrocytes, megakaryocytes [MKs], granulocytes, lymphocytes, and monocytes) are continuously generated, maintained, and renewed from a reservoir of hematopoietic stem cells (HSCs) [4]. This system is essential for immune homeostasis, oxygen transport, hemostasis, and infection response. Throughout life, hematopoiesis undergoes anatomical, functional, and molecular changes that begin during embryonic development and are established in the adult BM. The regulation of HSC differentiation into myeloid and lymphoid lineages is tightly controlled by intrinsic factors and signals from the microenvironment or hematopoietic niche [5].

2.1 Stages of hematopoiesis (embryonic, fetal, and adult)

Hematopoiesis arises from niches that change over time and space and follows two overlapping waves: the primitive, or extraembryonic, wave and the definitive, or intraembryonic, wave.

Extraembryonic hematopoiesis begins in the yolk sac during the first three weeks of development and gives rise to transient cell populations, primarily erythroid cells, macrophages, and MKs. The yolk sac is composed of the visceral endoderm and mesoderm. Mesodermal cells form blood islands that not only participate in hematopoiesis but also give rise to the vascular system. It is believed that a common precursor, the hemangioblast, gives rise to both lineages, as endothelial and hematopoietic cells share the expression of several molecular markers.

During the fourth and fifth weeks of development, definitive or intraembryonic waves of hematopoiesis occur in the aorta–gonad–mesonephros (AGM) region, which is composed of the surrounding mesenchyme and urogenital ridges. The AGM has the capacity to generate multipotent cells committed to both myeloid and lymphoid lineages [6]. Hematopoietic progenitor cells also arise in the umbilical and vitelline arteries, which are likely responsible for colonizing the developing fetal liver. The fetal liver serves as the main organ for hematopoietic expansion and differentiation until the end of fetal life, while hematopoiesis is simultaneously established in the BM [7].

Mesenchymal stem cells (MSCs) also originate during this phase in the AGM region of the embryo. These cells give rise to osteogenic, adipogenic, and chondrogenic lineages and are responsible for organizing and maintaining the microenvironment for HSCs, as they are associated with extracellular matrix (ECM) molecules, hematopoietic cytokines, and chemokines [8].

From the sixth week of development until birth, the fetal liver becomes the primary hematopoietic organ of the body. At this site, HSCs retain the capacity to differentiate into all hematopoietic lineages. During this stage, definitive erythropoiesis and megakaryopoiesis occur, along with the initiation of primary lymphopoiesis. The spleen and lymph nodes also partially contribute to hematopoiesis. During this period, the foundation of the immune system is established, with the migration of precursors to the thymus for T-lymphocyte differentiation.

From the third trimester onward, the BM progressively replaces the liver as the primary hematopoietic site. After birth, the BM becomes the dominant organ, maintaining continuous blood cell production throughout the lifetime. In adults, hematopoiesis occurs primarily in the red bone marrow, which is mainly located in the sternum, ribs, vertebrae, pelvis, and proximal epiphyses of long bones. HSCs reside in specialized niches composed of stromal cells, osteoblasts, endothelial cells, fibroblasts, adipocytes, and ECM components. Within these niches, self-renewal, quiescence, proliferation, differentiation, and migration are tightly regulated by signals such as CXCL12, SCF, TPO, IL-7, and the Notch signaling pathway. With aging, a bias toward myelopoiesis is observed, accompanied by a relative decline in lymphopoiesis, a phenomenon that is associated with immunosenescence [7–9].

2.2 HSCs and the hierarchy of differentiation

Hematopoietic stem cells are defined by two fundamental properties: self-renewal capacity and multipotency. Phenotypically, human HSCs are characterized as $CD34^{+}CD38^{-}CD90^{+}CD45RA^{-}$. HSCs give rise to multipotent progenitors (MPPs), which lose their self-renewal capacity and progressively commit to the common myeloid progenitor (CMP) and common lymphoid progenitor (CLP). This process is regulated by transcription factors such as RUNX1, GATA2, IKZF1, PU.1, and

NOTCH1. Lymphoid progeny arise from CLP and are responsible for adaptive immunity and specialized innate immune responses [9, 10].

3. Migration and maturation of T lymphocytes

T cells develop within the thymic microenvironment; however, they originate from HSCs in the BM. Currently, there is no consensus regarding the precise characteristics of the cells that exit the BM and colonize the thymus. Under physiological homeostatic conditions, the thymus does not contain self-renewing precursors capable of sustaining thymopoiesis. Therefore, a continuous influx of progenitors into the thymus is required for T-cell development. These cells are known as thymic seeding progenitors (TSPs) and are derived from HSCs that originate in the fetal liver and, later, in the BM [11, 12].

The HSC-derived hematopoietic progenitor cells can be divided into two groups: bone marrow–resident hematopoietic progenitor cells (BM-HPCs) and circulating hematopoietic progenitor cells (cHPCs), which differ in their immunohistochemical profiles. The cHPCs display a "pre-activated" state that is associated with greater differentiation efficiency in vitro compared with BM-HPCs [13]. This designation reflects transcriptional and functional characteristics that distinguish circulating progenitors from their bone marrow–resident counterparts. Transcriptomic analyses have demonstrated enrichment of genes associated with migratory capacity, cytokine responsiveness, and early lymphoid priming, suggesting a heightened readiness for differentiation upon thymic entry. Functionally, cHPCs exhibit increased efficiency in generating T-lineage cells in Notch-dependent coculture systems, supporting the concept that these progenitors are molecularly poised for thymic homing and lineage commitment. Continuous thymic seeding contributes to the maintenance of normal thymopoiesis and prevents clonal dominance of thymic progenitors [11].

Thymic seeding progenitors enter the corticomedullary junction of the thymus, where they differentiate into early T-cell progenitors (ETPs) within the thymic cortex. These cells comprise a heterogeneous group of progenitors with the potential to differentiate into granulocytic cells, monocytes/macrophages, dendritic cells, natural killer (NK) cells, and B lymphocytes, review **Figure 1** [12–16].

Cells with a $CD34^{+}CD7^{+}$ phenotype, also present in fetal BM and umbilical cord blood, have the potential to differentiate into T cells. $CD7^{+}$ cells have been described in the embryonic thymus, suggesting that they may represent T-cell precursors. However, Lavaert et al. [11, 17] defined these cells as TSP2 and described a novel population of TSP1. TSP1 cells ($CD34^{+}CD44^{+}CD10^{+}CD7^{-}CD123^{-}CD127^{-}$) were identified as T-cell precursors, whereas TSP2 cells ($CD34^{+}CD44^{+}CD10^{-}CD7^{+}$CD123^lo^CD127^lo^) give rise to both T cells and dendritic cells (DCs).

Stromal compartments within the thymus support the entry and differentiation of ETPs and express Notch ligands, including JAG1, JAG2, DLL1, and DLL4, which activate distinct signaling pathways that promote T-cell differentiation. Studies in mice have demonstrated that several chemokines (CCL21 and CCL25 acting through CCR7 and CCR9, respectively) are involved in the recruitment and entry of circulating TSPs into the thymus. Additionally, interactions between the integrins $\alpha L\beta 2$ and $\alpha 4\beta 1$ and their ligands ICAM1 and VCAM1 on endothelial cells mediate the adhesion and extravasation of circulating progenitors. Likewise, signaling through

DOI: http://dx.doi.org/10.5772/intechopen.1015349

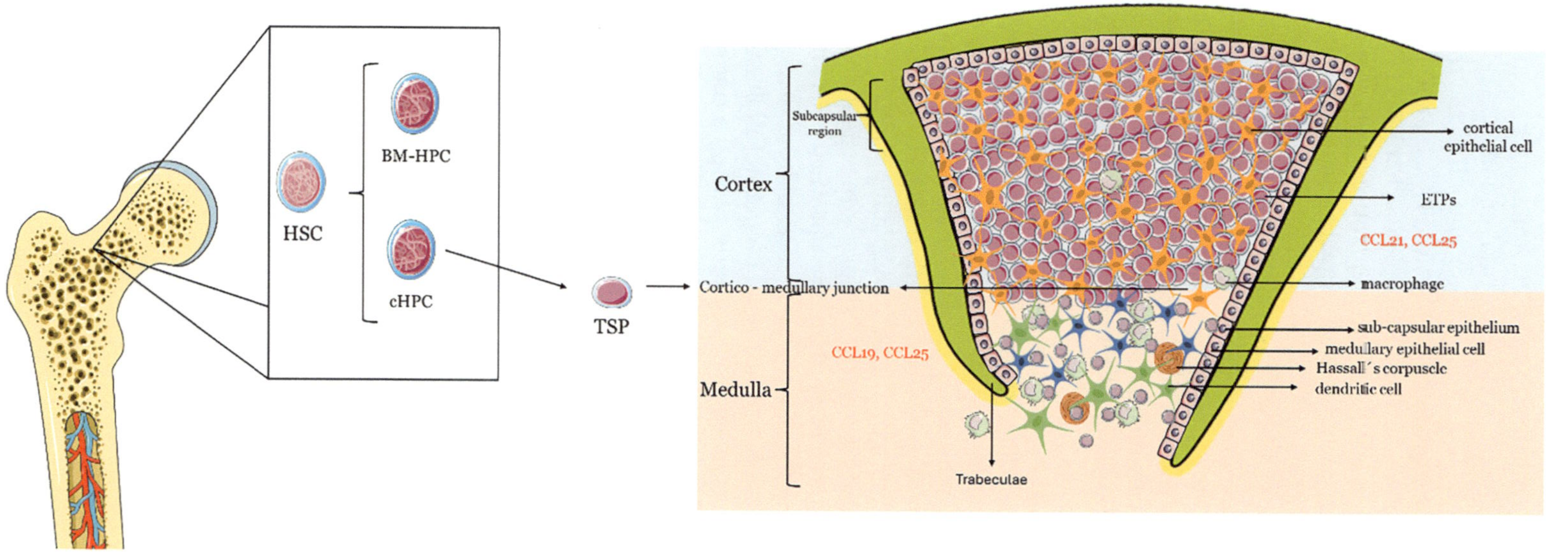

Figure 1.
Bone marrow origin and thymic migration of T-cell progenitors. HSC-derived hematopoietic progenitor cells can be divided into two groups: bone marrow-resident hematopoietic progenitor cells (BM-HPC) and circulating hematopoietic progenitor cells (CHCP).

the lymphotoxin-β receptor (LTβR), in addition to its roles in T-cell development and thymic organization, contributes to HSPC homing by promoting the differentiation of several classes of thymic portal endothelial cells located in the perivascular space, which facilitates progenitor entry into the thymus. LTβR signaling also regulates the expression of VCAM1, CCL19, and CCL21, thereby controlling progenitor homing through multiple mechanisms [11, 12, 14].

Early T-cell specification is critically dependent on signals provided by the thymic microenvironment, with the Notch signaling pathway playing a central role. Engagement of Notch receptors on incoming progenitor cells by ligands expressed on thymic stromal cells initiates and sustains the T-lineage transcriptional program while actively repressing gene expression associated with alternative lineages. This signaling axis establishes the foundational identity of developing thymocytes and represents the earliest step toward T-lineage commitment. Consequently, progenitor multipotency is progressively restricted following Notch engagement, leading to the upregulation of T-lineage–associated genes, such as *GATA3* and the interleukin-7 receptor (*IL7R*) [18].

Additionally, in addition to Notch-mediated instruction, other microenvironmental cues act in a coordinated manner to reinforce and refine early T-cell specification. Cytokines, such as interleukin-7 (IL-7), promote cell survival and controlled expansion, whereas chemokine-driven migration ensures that developing progenitors traverse distinct thymic regions in a spatially and temporally regulated sequence. Together with the Notch signaling pathway, these cues establish stage-specific gene regulatory networks that guide the transition from multipotent thymus-seeding progenitors to early T-lineage–specified cells [19].

At this stage, T-cell specification remains reversible. Although progenitor cells initiate a T-lineage–associated transcriptional program, full lineage commitment has not yet been achieved. Instead, early thymocytes occupy a transitional state characterized by a partial restriction of developmental potential and heightened sensitivity to environmental signals. The transition from specification to irreversible commitment occurs later during defined intrathymic developmental stages and is enforced by additional regulatory checkpoints.

Thus, thymic entry and early specification represent the foundational phase of T-cell ontogeny, during which MPPs are instructed toward a T-cell fate while retaining developmental flexibility. This early developmental window establishes the conditions necessary for subsequent commitment, selection, and maturation events that ultimately define the T-cell lineage.

T cells generated within the thymic microenvironment during fetal, perinatal, or adult stages differ in composition and function. For example, memory $CD8^+$ T cells and regulatory T cells (Tregs) produced in the perinatal thymus persist into adulthood, where they play a key role in early-life protection against pathogens [20].

4. Thymus: Structural formation, composition, and function

4.1 Structural formation

The thymus is an essential primary lymphoid organ composed of a three-dimensional epithelial network of thymic stroma that provides a specialized microenvironment for the phenotypic and functional maturation of lymphoid progenitors. It is located in the superior mediastinum and has a bilobed morphology, measuring approximately 30–40 mm in length and 25–35 mm in width. The thymus is surrounded by an external mesenchymal capsule that penetrates the organ at regular intervals to form trabecular structures. Histologically, the thymus contains two main compartments, the cortex and medulla, which are separated by the corticomedullary junction.

The thymus is composed primarily of epithelial, dendritic, mesenchymal, and endothelial cells and is considered the principal site for the production and selection of an immunocompetent and self-tolerant T-cell repertoire [20].

Human thymic development occurs during fetal life, and the organ is colonized by hematopoietic progenitors between the 7th and 8th weeks of gestation. These early migrating cells contribute to lymphopoiesis and the development and organization of the thymic microenvironment. Unlike most organs, which coordinate growth and size throughout postnatal life, the thymus reaches full maturation in utero and undergoes progressive involution beginning at puberty.

Thymic involution involves structural remodeling, characterized by the gradual replacement of functional thymic tissue with fibro-adipose tissue, a decline in naïve T-cell production, alterations in the thymic stromal microenvironment, a reduction in both cortical and medullary thymic epithelial cells (TECs), reduced stromal cellularity, and an increase in perivascular space. Collectively, these changes negatively impact immune function, resulting in reduced resistance to pathogens, increased susceptibility to autoimmunity, and diminished immunosurveillance of tumors [21, 22].

4.2 Thymic composition

The thymic microenvironment contains abundant lymphoid progenitor cells (LPCs) integrated into a three-dimensional epithelial stromal network. This network is primarily composed of TECs, dendritic cells, endothelial cells, macrophages, fibroblasts, and mesenchymal and vascular elements. The three-dimensional organization of the thymic stroma allows close spatial interactions between LPCs and developing TECs. Based on their anatomical location, molecular profiles, and functional properties, TECs are classified into two major lineages: cortical TECs (cTECs) and medullary TECs (mTECs) [20–25].

Thymic epithelial cells display diverse morphologies and gene expression patterns and provide migratory cues through the secretion of multiple cytokines that support LPC homing and the guided migration of developing thymoblasts through distinct thymic compartments [25]. In addition, TECs create specialized niches in which thymocytes receive essential signals for differentiation. Cortical TECs are required for thymocyte commitment, T-cell receptor expression, and positive selection, enabling the recognition of major histocompatibility complex (MHC) molecules. In contrast, medullary TECs support negative selection by eliminating strongly self-reactive T cells, thereby inducing central self-tolerance [20, 25–28].

Additionally, mesenchymal cells derived from the neural crest ectoderm contribute to the formation of the thymic capsule, septa, fibroblasts, and pericytes. In contrast, mesoderm-derived mesenchymal cells give rise to endothelial cells [20].

4.3 Function

The immunological function of the thymus was first demonstrated in 1961 by Jacques Miller, when mice thymectomized immediately after birth exhibited a severe deficiency in a specific lymphocyte population that was later identified as T lymphocytes [28]. Therefore, the thymus is regarded as the primary site for the production and maturation of T cells, which are subsequently supplied to peripheral lymphoid tissues.

In adulthood, thymic output declines progressively; however, longitudinal and repertoire-based analyses have demonstrated that, in humans, maintenance of the naïve T-cell compartment relies predominantly on peripheral homeostatic proliferation rather than sustained thymic export [29]. Furthermore, diversity studies of the human T-cell receptor repertoire indicate that naïve T cells can persist for approximately 5–10 years while preserving broad clonal representation [30]. As individuals age, T-cell function gradually declines, accompanied by increased susceptibility to infections, malignancy, and autoimmunity [31].

5. Stages of T-lymphocyte commitment

While thymic entry and early T-lineage specification establish the initial transcriptional program, irreversible lineage commitment is achieved only after thymocytes progress through defined intrathymic developmental stages. These stages mark the transition from a reversible, microenvironment-dependent state to a stabilized, permanently restricted T-cell identity. Within this framework, lineage commitment is best understood as a progressive restriction of developmental potential, enforced by sequential regulatory checkpoints [32].

In T lymphocytes, commitment occurs in two interconnected phases: the initial stabilization of T-lineage identity during intrathymic progression, followed later by functional specialization into $CD4^{+}$ or $CD8^{+}$ subsets through antigen receptor–dependent selection.

This critical intrathymic process involves extensive changes in genomic activity that culminate in the conversion of multipotent hematopoietic precursors into cells irreversibly committed to a T-cell fate. The signaling pathways and transcriptional regulatory programs guiding these transitions have been extensively characterized, in part due to the availability of experimental systems that allow causal interrogation of gene regulatory networks during T-cell specification and differentiation [33].

The thymus provides the structural and signaling context in which these later commitment transitions occur, offering a specialized three-dimensional stromal environment that delivers spatially and temporally coordinated signals required for cell survival, proliferation, differentiation, and selection. Importantly, the thymus does not generate lymphoid progenitors de novo; rather, it functions as an instructional organ that guides incoming progenitor cells through successive stages of lineage commitment, ensuring both functional competence and self-tolerance of the T cells.

From a conceptual standpoint, T-cell ontogeny exemplifies several fundamental principles of developmental biology, including the progressive restriction of cell fate, dependence on niche-derived signals, use of developmental checkpoints to enforce lineage fidelity, and coupling of differentiation with selective survival.

Consequently, the study of T-cell commitment has contributed not only to advances in immunology but also to a broader understanding of how complex cellular identities are established and stabilized during development. These principles have been experimentally supported by in vitro thymic surrogate systems, such as OP9–DLL stromal cocultures, which recapitulate key aspects of thymic signaling and allow for controlled analysis of early T-lineage specification from defined hematopoietic precursors [34].

Thus, the intrathymic stages of T-cell development illustrate how lineage identity becomes progressively stabilized through sustained signaling, transcriptional reinforcement, and checkpoint-dependent selection. These mechanisms ensure that commitment is not abrupt but rather consolidated through defined developmental transitions.

5.1 Progressive commitment during early intrathymic stages

After initial thymic specification, developing thymocytes enter a series of defined intrathymic stages characterized by progressive restriction of developmental potential. These early phases are collectively known as the double-negative (DN) stages, defined by the absence of the coreceptors CD4 and CD8. Rather than constituting arbitrary subdivisions, DN stages represent successive phases of proliferation, lineage restriction, and selection that ultimately culminate in irreversible commitment to the T-cell lineage. Conventionally, the DN compartment is subdivided into DN1–DN4 based on the differential expression of CD44 and CD25. Within this framework, DN1 and DN2 correspond to the early stages of expansion and progressive lineage restriction, whereas DN3 marks the emergence of progenitors that are fully restricted to the T-cell fate [35].

The earliest DN population, commonly referred to as DN1, consists of early intrathymic thymocytes that retain residual developmental plasticity during the initial phases of lineage restriction. At this stage, thymocytes remain capable of adopting alternative hematopoietic fates under permissive conditions, highlighting the distinction between lineage specification and irreversible commitment to a specific fate. As cells transition to the DN2 stage, there is a marked reduction in the non–T-lineage potential. DN2 represents a critical developmental window during which T-lineage–associated transcriptional programs are reinforced, whereas alternative lineage options are progressively silenced. This process reflects continued intrathymic signaling, including sustained Notch1 activity in cooperation with transcription factors such as Runx1 and GATA3, which collectively reinforce T-lineage restriction and repress alternative lineage programs [36].

A key developmental transition occurs within the DN2 compartment, commonly referred to as the commitment point, at which thymocytes lose their capacity to differentiate into non–T-cell lineages. Passage through this point reflects the integration of sustained thymic signals, including continuous Notch-mediated instruction, persistent stromal interactions, cytokine-mediated support, and spatial cues within the thymic cortex. Once this threshold is crossed, developing cells become irreversibly committed to the T-cell lineage, even if they are removed from the thymic environment.

Subsequent progression to the DN3 stage is marked by the initiation of TCR β-chain gene rearrangement and the engagement of a major developmental checkpoint, known as β-selection. At this stage, thymocytes are tested for their ability to generate functional pre-TCR complexes. Successful signaling through the pre-TCR promotes cell survival, clonal expansion, and further differentiation, whereas failure to generate productive signals results in developmental arrest and apoptosis. This checkpoint ensures that only thymocytes with functional antigen receptor rearrangements are permitted to advance to the next stage.

Thymocytes that successfully pass β-selection enter the DN4 stage, which is characterized by rapid proliferation and preparation for the transition into the double-positive (DP) stage, during which both CD4 and CD8 coreceptors are expressed. By the DN3–DN4 transition, T-lineage commitment is complete and irreversible. At this point, subsequent developmental decisions no longer determine whether a cell will become a T lymphocyte but instead define the functional subtype it will adopt within the T-cell lineage. This committed state is reinforced by the stable suppression of alternative lineage potentials, including dendritic, myeloid, NK, and other non–T-cell fates.

Taken together, the DN stages demonstrate that T-cell commitment is achieved through a progressive multistep process rather than a single binary event. This developmental logic exemplifies a fundamental principle of ontogeny: Lineage identity is stabilized through the sequential integration of extrinsic environmental signals and intrinsic regulatory programs, enforced by developmental checkpoints that tightly couple differentiation to selective survival. This framework establishes the basis for subsequent DP thymocyte maturation, during which antigen receptor–dependent signaling guides further differentiation and lineage bifurcation toward CD4 or CD8 single-positive fates. **Figure 2** illustrates the progressive commitment and maturation of T lymphocytes in the thymus [37].

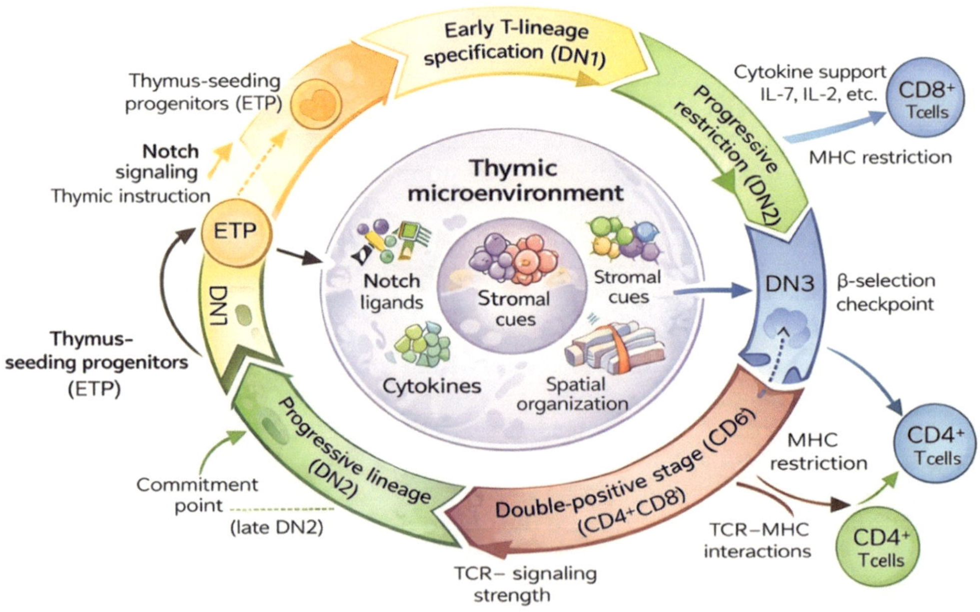

Figure 2.
Progressive commitment and maturation of T lymphocytes in the thymus.

6. Selection and lineage choice during the DP stage

Following the completion of irreversible T-lineage commitment, thymocytes enter the DP stage, which is defined by the simultaneous expression of CD4 and CD8 coreceptors. This stage represents a pivotal phase of T-cell ontogeny, in which developmental decisions no longer concern lineage identity but instead focus on functional specialization within the T-cell lineage.

The DP stage is characterized by extensive selection processes that ensure antigen receptor functionality and self-tolerance. During this phase, thymocytes undergo rearrangement of the TCRα locus, completing the assembly of a functional αβ T-cell receptor. Concurrently, positive selection is initiated, whereby cortical DP thymocytes that receive appropriate αβTCR-mediated signals from self-peptides presented by MHC molecules are rescued from apoptosis and allowed to progress toward single-positive differentiation [38]. The expression of a complete TCR enables productive interactions with TECs and initiates the central processes of thymic selection.

Positive selection ensures the survival of thymocytes whose TCRs recognize self-MHC molecules with sufficient, but not excessive, affinity. Thymocytes that fail to receive adequate TCR-mediated signals undergo apoptosis, a process commonly referred to as "death by neglect." Through this mechanism, the thymus establishes a T-cell repertoire that is both MHC-restricted and capable of mounting effective adaptive immune responses against foreign antigens. Importantly, MHC restriction also imparts functional directionality, guiding positively selected thymocytes toward differentiation into either the $CD4^+$ or $CD8^+$ single-positive lineage, depending on whether their TCRs engage MHC class II or MHC class I molecules, respectively [39].

In parallel, negative selection eliminates thymocytes bearing TCRs that bind to self-peptide–MHC complexes with excessively high affinity. This process is essential for establishing central tolerance and preventing autoimmunity. Together, positive and negative selection function as complementary checkpoints that sculpt the developing T-cell repertoire by coupling differentiation to selective survival. Positively selected DP thymocytes subsequently migrate to the thymic medulla, where they mature into $CD4^+$ or $CD8^+$ single-positive cells through coreceptor downregulation guided by the MHC specificity of their TCR interactions.

Within the DP compartment, thymocytes that successfully complete selection are directed toward one of two major functional lineages: $CD4^+$ helper T cells or $CD8^+$ cytotoxic T cells. This lineage choice is primarily determined by the nature, strength, and duration of TCR signaling elicited by interactions with MHC class II or class I molecules. Although multiple mechanistic models have been proposed to explain this process, a unifying concept is that qualitative and quantitative differences in TCR signaling are translated into distinct transcriptional programs that stabilize either the CD4 or CD8 lineage fate, respectively.

Two principal models have been proposed to explain how TCR–MHC interactions instruct lineage fate. The kinetic signaling model posits that sustained TCR signaling, typically associated with MHC class II engagement, promotes CD4 lineage differentiation, whereas interruption of TCR signaling following MHC class I interaction favors CD8 commitment. In contrast, the duration-of-signal model emphasizes the total length and persistence of TCR-mediated signaling as the critical determinant of lineage choice, with prolonged signaling biasing toward CD4 differentiation and shorter signaling intervals promoting CD8 fate. Although these models differ in mechanistic emphasis, both underscore the importance of temporally regulated TCR signaling thresholds in directing CD4/CD8 lineage specification [39].

In this context, the CD4/CD8 lineage decision represents a second intralineage commitment event that is fundamentally distinct from the earlier T-lineage commitment. Rather than extinguishing alternative hematopoietic fates, this decision refines functional specialization within an already-committed lineage. Once established, CD4 or CD8 identity is maintained through stable gene regulatory networks that preserve lineage-specific effector function.

Thus, the DP stage constitutes a critical developmental bottleneck in T cell ontogeny, integrating antigen receptor signaling with selection and lineage choice. Through these tightly coordinated processes, the thymus ensures that only T cells that are both self-tolerant and functionally competent proceed to full maturation as single-positive $CD4^+$ or $CD8^+$ T lymphocytes [39].

7. Positive and negative selection

The random nature of TCR gene rearrangements generates receptor specificities directed against foreign and self-antigens. Autoreactive T cells can be highly detrimental if they escape the thymic environment of the host. Therefore, the thymus has evolved mechanisms that selectively preserve useful lymphocytes, eliminate nonfunctional TCRs, and delete potentially harmful autoreactive clones [40].

Selection begins at the DP stage, when TCR is expressed at relatively low levels on the thymocyte surface. If a TCR recognizes a self-peptide presented by MHC molecules, the developmental outcome of each DP thymocyte is determined by the strength and quality of the TCR–peptide–MHC interactions. Thymocytes whose TCRs bind to self-peptide–MHC complexes with low affinity undergo positive selection, whereas those expressing high-affinity TCRs are eliminated through negative selection. Thymocytes whose TCRs fail to bind to self-peptide–MHC complexes with sufficient avidity undergo apoptosis and are removed from the repertoire.

In positively selected thymocytes, the expression of recombination-activating genes (*RAG1* and *RAG2*), which encode proteins required for V(D)J recombination in B lymphocyte and T lymphocyte, as well as *PTCRA*, is downregulated. Concurrently, the expression of the CD4 and CD8 coreceptors is partially reduced. These cells subsequently migrate from the thymic cortex to the medulla, where reexpression of one coreceptor occurs and lineage commitment to either the $CD4^+$ or $CD8^+$ fate is finalized [41].

Signaling through the Src family kinases (SFKs) Lck plays a central role in regulating both positive and negative selection. Thymic selection mechanisms are severely compromised in the absence of Lck. Lck interacts with the CD4 and CD8 coreceptors through cysteine residues located within the cytoplasmic domains of each coreceptor and the corresponding cysteines within Lck, enabling efficient coupling of TCR engagement to downstream signaling cascades.

Cortical thymic epithelial cells are primarily responsible for mediating positive selection, whereas hematopoietic stromal cells, particularly antigen-presenting cells (APCs), are key inducers of negative selection. Interactions between the TCR and peptide–MHC (pMHC) complexes shape the developing T-cell repertoire, a process that is further influenced by the presence of specialized cellular populations, such as dendritic cells [42, 43].

7.1 Molecular and cellular mechanisms of regulation

T-lymphocyte function is governed by tightly coordinated molecular and cellular regulatory mechanisms that ensure effective immune responses while preserving tolerance to self-antigens. These mechanisms operate at multiple levels, integrating signals derived from antigen recognition, costimulatory pathways, cytokine networks, and the cellular microenvironment to precisely regulate T-cell activation, differentiation, and effector function [44]. Central to this regulation is the integration of signals initiated by TCR engagement and modulated by activating and inhibitory inputs, which together determine the functional outcome of effector and regulatory T cells [45].

At the molecular level, T-cell activation is initiated by the engagement of the TCR with antigenic peptides presented by MHC molecules on APCs. However, TCR signaling alone is insufficient to induce full T-cell activation. Productive immune responses require additional costimulatory signals, most notably through CD28 engagement, which amplifies intracellular signaling cascades and promotes T-cell survival, proliferation, and cytokine production. These activating signals are further shaped by cytokine-mediated pathways, particularly those involving JAK–STAT signaling, which supports the clonal expansion and differentiation of antigen-specific T cells [46].

In contrast, inhibitory receptors, such as CTLA-4 and PD-1, attenuate TCR-mediated signaling and function as critical negative regulators that restrain immune activation and maintain immune homeostasis. The cellular context in which T cells encounter APCs, whether within secondary lymphoid organs or peripheral tissues, further influences the strength, quality, and duration of these signaling events. Together, the activating and inhibitory pathways regulate key aspects of T-cell biology, including metabolic reprogramming, lineage differentiation, and effector function [47].

Importantly, inhibitory receptors such as CTLA-4 and PD-1 are not confined to peripheral immune regulation but intersect directly with developmental signaling pathways during thymic ontogeny. CTLA-4 competes with CD28 for binding to CD80/CD86, thereby modulating the strength of costimulatory signaling that influences thymocyte survival and differentiation. Similarly, PD-1 engagement attenuates proximal TCR signaling by recruiting phosphatases that dampen downstream activation cascades, effectively recalibrating selection thresholds during positive and negative selection. Through these mechanisms, inhibitory receptor signaling contributes to the fine-tuning of central tolerance, influencing both clonal deletion and the development of regulatory T cells. These observations underscore that pathways now therapeutically targeted in immune checkpoint blockade are embedded within physiological mechanisms that shape T-cell repertoire formation, lineage stability, and immune homeostasis from early developmental stages.

Downstream of receptor engagement, intracellular signaling pathways coordinate the transcriptional and epigenetic programs that define T-cell fate. Transcription factors, such as NF-κB, NFAT, and AP-1, are activated following TCR stimulation and regulate gene expression programs involved in cytokine production, metabolic adaptation, and lineage specification. These molecular programs are reinforced by cytokine cues that guide the polarization of naïve T cells into distinct functional subsets, thereby integrating environmental signals with antigen recognition [48].

At the cellular level, T-cell regulation is shaped by interactions with other immune cell populations and the tissue microenvironment. Antigen-presenting cells modulate TCR signal strength through antigen density, costimulatory molecule expression, and cytokine secretion, whereas regulatory T cells suppress excessive immune activation by limiting antigen presentation and delivering inhibitory signals. These mechanisms are reinforced by the induction of coinhibitory receptors, establishing feedback loops that prevent sustained inflammation after antigen clearance [49].

In addition to signal integration at the receptor level, emerging evidence highlights the importance of metabolic regulation in shaping T-cell responses. Activation-induced metabolic reprogramming toward glycolysis supports rapid proliferation and effector differentiation, whereas alternative metabolic states favor memory formation and regulatory phenotypes. These metabolic programs are tightly linked to signaling cascades downstream of the TCR and costimulatory receptors, reinforcing the concept that lineage decisions and functional specialization are coordinated at multiple regulatory layers.

Collectively, these molecular and cellular regulatory mechanisms ensure that T lymphocytes respond efficiently to immunological challenges while avoiding pathological immune activation. Disruption of these regulatory processes contributes to immune dysregulation, autoimmunity, chronic inflammation, and cancer, underscoring the clinical relevance of understanding T-cell regulation in both physiological and pathological contexts [50].

7.2 Function of T lymphocytes and their clinical relevance

T lymphocytes are central components of the adaptive immune system and play a fundamental role in immune surveillance, host defense, and the maintenance of immunological homeostasis. Their functional relevance derives from their capacity to recognize specific antigens, coordinate immune responses, and eliminate infected or abnormal cells while preserving tolerance to self. These functions are mediated by the expression of a unique TCR, which enables antigen recognition in the context of MHC molecules on APCs and represents the functional outcome of tightly regulated developmental processes occurring within the thymus [51].

Importantly, the functional competence of mature T lymphocytes is intrinsically linked to the developmental checkpoints established during thymic ontogeny. Processes such as positive and negative selection not only ensure MHC restriction and central tolerance but also shape the breadth and specificity of the peripheral T-cell repertoire. Thus, the qualitative characteristics of immune responses in adulthood are directly influenced by the efficiency and stringency of intrathymic selection mechanisms.

From a functional perspective, mature T lymphocytes are broadly classified into two principal subsets: $CD4^+$ helper T cells and $CD8^+$ cytotoxic T cells. $CD4^+$ T cells primarily function as regulators and coordinators of immune responses. Upon antigen recognition, they differentiate into specialized effector populations that provide essential help to B lymphocytes, activate macrophages, and shape the magnitude and quality of immune responses through the secretion of cytokines. In this manner, CD4⁺ T cells orchestrate both humoral and cellular immunity [52].

In contrast, $CD8^+$ T cells constitute the principal effectors of cell-mediated cytotoxicity. These cells directly eliminate virus-infected cells, intracellular pathogen–harboring cells, and malignant cells through antigen-specific recognition. Cytotoxic activity is mediated by the formation of an immunological synapse with the target cell, followed by the directed release of cytotoxic granules containing effector molecules such as granzyme B, which induce apoptosis in the target cell [53].

In addition to immediate effector functions, a subset of activated T cells differentiates into long-lived memory T cells, which provide rapid and robust responses upon antigen reencounter. The establishment of immunological memory reflects coordinated transcriptional and metabolic adaptations that preserve antigen specificity while enhancing responsiveness. This capacity for durable immune protection represents a defining feature of adaptive immunity and underlies the effectiveness of vaccination strategies.

Beyond their effector roles, T lymphocytes are essential for maintaining immune equilibrium. Regulatory T cells, a specialized subset predominantly derived from the $CD4^+$ lineage, play a critical role in suppressing excessive or inappropriate immune activation and are indispensable for the maintenance of peripheral tolerance. Through the coordinated activity of effector and regulatory T-cell populations, immune responses are rendered effective yet tightly controlled, thereby limiting collateral tissue damage and preventing autoimmunity.

The clinical significance of T lymphocytes is underscored by their involvement in a wide spectrum of pathological conditions, including immunodeficiencies, autoimmune diseases, malignancies, and transplant rejection [54]. Defects in T-cell development or function lead to increased susceptibility to infections and impaired immune competence, whereas failures in tolerance mechanisms permit self-reactive T cells to drive chronic inflammation and tissue injury. Furthermore, aberrant T-cell proliferation and differentiation are central to the pathogenesis of T-cell leukemia and lymphomas, in which normal developmental checkpoints are bypassed or deregulated [55].

Finally, T lymphocytes have emerged as central targets of therapeutic intervention in modern clinical practice. Immune checkpoint inhibitors, by modulating PD-1 and CTLA-4 signaling pathways, restore T-cell effector function in cancer and chronic infections. Adoptive cellular therapies, including chimeric antigen receptor (CAR)-T cells, rely on *ex vivo* manipulation of T-cell activation and differentiation states to enhance persistence, cytotoxic capacity, and resistance to exhaustion. Moreover, strategies aimed at improving thymic function or accelerating T-cell reconstitution following HSC transplantation are directly informed by an understanding of intrathymic developmental checkpoints. Collectively, these therapeutic advances illustrate how insights into T-cell ontogeny have translated into transformative clinical applications.

8. Concluding remarks and biological relevance

T-cell development represents a paradigmatic model of lineage commitment, achieved through the cumulative integration of sequential instructional signals and tightly regulated developmental checkpoints. Throughout this process, the thymus functions as a central instructional organ, integrating microenvironmental cues with intrinsic gene regulatory programs to ensure lineage fidelity, functional competence, and self-tolerance.

A fundamental principle highlighted by this model is that cellular identity is stabilized through sustained signal integration rather than abrupt fate decisions. Early developmental stages preserve a degree of plasticity, allowing responsiveness to environmental inputs, whereas later transitions progressively enforce irreversible commitment. This gradual restriction of developmental potential underscores the importance of temporal and spatial coordination in cell fate determination.

Beyond its developmental significance, precise regulation of T-cell ontogeny is essential for maintaining immune homeostasis. Disruption of these tightly controlled processes can result in profound pathological consequences, including immunodeficiency, autoimmunity, and malignant transformation. Thus, understanding the molecular and cellular mechanisms governing T-cell development provides a critical framework for interpreting the ontogenetic basis of immune-related diseases and for designing therapeutic strategies that target immune dysfunction at its developmental root.

In contemporary clinical practice, insights into T-cell ontogeny have directly informed innovative therapeutic strategies. The manufacturing of CAR-T cells relies on the controlled manipulation of T-cell activation and differentiation states to optimize persistence and effector function. Likewise, approaches aimed at enhancing thymic regeneration or accelerating immune reconstitution following HSC transplantation are grounded in an understanding of intrathymic developmental checkpoints. These translational applications illustrate how fundamental principles of T-cell development continue to shape modern immunotherapy and regenerative medicine.

Acknowledgment

The authors acknowledge the use of artificial intelligence (ChatGPT) for language editing and refinement of the chapter. SmartArt and BioArt (NCBI) were used for the preparation of **Figure 1**, and BioRender was used for the preparation of **Figure 2**.

Author details

Cynthia Guadalupe Pelayo Mena[1], Yanet Ventura Enríquez[1], Claudia Mondragón Albarrán[1], Adán Germán Gallardo Rodríguez[2], Gabriel Aceves Castillo[1], Aldo Mujica Martínez[1], Moises Leonardo Mendoza Torres[1], Monica Alethia Cureño Diaz[3], Estibeyesbo Said Plascencia Nieto[4], Erika Gómez Zamora[5], Christian Omar Ramos Peñafiel[6] and Verónica Fernández Sánchez[7]*

1 Naval Medical Center, Mexico City, Mexico

2 School of Sport Sciences, Universidad Anáhuac México, Huixquilucan, México

3 Institutional Intelligence in Oncological Health/National Cancer Institute, Mexico City, Mexico

4 Postgraduate Studies and Research Section, Higher School of Medicine, National Polytechnic Institute, Mexico City, Mexico

5 Juarez Hospital of Mexico, Mexico City, Mexico

6 Hematology Department, Hospital General de México "Dr. Eduardo Liceaga," Mexico City, Mexico

7 Faculty of Higher Studies Iztacala, National Autonomous University of Mexico (UNAM), Mexico City, Mexico

*Address all correspondence to: alf2228@yahoo.com.mx

References

[1] Saule P, Trauet J, Dutriez V, Lekeux V, Dessaint JP, Labalette M. Accumulation of memory T cells from childhood to old age: Central and effector memory cells in CD4(+) versus effector memory and terminally differentiated memory cells in CD8(+) compartment. Mechanisms of Ageing and Development. 2006;**127**(3):274–281. DOI: 10.1016/j.mad.2005.11.001

[2] Goldrath AW, Bevan MJ. Selecting and maintaining a diverse T-cell repertoire. Nature. 1999;**402**(6759):255–262. DOI: 10.1038/46218

[3] Goronzy JJ, Weyand CM. T cell development and receptor diversity during aging. Current Opinion in Immunology. 2005;**17**(5):468–475. DOI: 10.1016/j.coi.2005.07.020

[4] Chapman J, Zhang Y. Histology, Hematopoiesis. 2023 May 1. In: StatPearls [Internet]. Treasure Island (FL): StatPearls Publishing; 2026

[5] Skulimowska I, Sosniak J, Gonka M, Szade A, Jozkowicz A, Szade K. The biology of hematopoietic stem cells and its clinical implications. FEBS Journal. 2022;**289**(24):7740–7759. DOI: 10.1111/febs.16192

[6] Julien E, El Omar R, Tavian M. Origin of the hematopoietic system in the human embryo. FEBS Letters. 2016;**590**(22):3987–4001. DOI: 10.1002/1873-3468.12389

[7] Mikkola HK, Orkin SH. The journey of developing hematopoietic stem cells. Development. 2006;**133**(19):3733–3744. DOI: 10.1242/dev.02568

[8] Belyavsky A, Petinati N, Drize N. Hematopoiesis during ontogenesis, adult life, and aging. International Journal of Molecular Sciences. 2021;**22**(17):9231. DOI: 10.3390/ijms22179231

[9] Hoffman CM, Calvi LM. Minireview: Complexity of hematopoietic stem cell regulation in the bone marrow microenvironment. Molecular Endocrinology. 2014;**28**(10):1592–1601. DOI: 10.1210/me.2014-1079

[10] Calvi LM, Link DC. Cellular complexity of the hematopoietic stem cell niche in the bone marrow. Calcified Tissue International. 2014;**94**(1):112–124. DOI: 10.1007/s00223-013-9805-8

[11] Liang KL, Boehme L, Paepens S, Hassan M, Taghon T. Thymic pioneers: Charting the origin, identity, and fate of human thymus seeding progenitors. Journal of Allergy and Clinical Immunology. 2025;**156**(4):854–866. DOI: 10.1016/j.jaci.2025.06.014

[12] Srinivasan J, Vasudev A, Shasha C, Selden HJ, Perez Jr E, LaFleur B, Sinari SA, Krueger A, Richie ER, Ehrlich LIR. The initial age-associated decline in early T-cell progenitors reflects fewer pre-thymic progenitors and altered signals in the bone marrow and thymus microenvironments. Aging Cell. 2023;**22**(8):e13870. DOI: 10.1111/acel.13870

[13] Quaranta P, Basso-Ricci L, Hernandez RJ, Pacini G, Naldini MM, Barcella M, et al. Circulating hematopoietic stem/progenitor cell subsets contribute to human hematopoietic homeostasis. Blood.

2024;**143**(19):1937–1952. DOI: 10.1182/blood.2023022666

[14] Shah DK, Zúñiga-Pflücker JC. An overview of the intrathymic intricacies of T cell development. Journal of Immunology. 2014;**192**(9):4017–4023. DOI: 10.4049/jimmunol.1302259

[15] Francelin C, Veneziani LP, Farias AS, Mendes-da-cruz DA, Savino W. Neurotransmitters modulate intrathymic T-cell development. Frontiers in Cell and Developmental Biology. 2021;**9**:668067. DOI: 10.3389/fcell.2021.668067

[16] Ruíz-Pérez M, Vandenabeele P, Tougaard P. The thymus road to a T cell: Migration, selection, and atrophy. Frontiers in Immunology. 2024;**15**:1443910. DOI: 10.3389/fimmu.2024.1443910

[17] Lavaert M, Liang KL, Vandamme N, Park JE, Roels J, Kowalczyk MS, et al. Integrated scRNA-seq identifies human postnatal thymus seeding progenitors and regulatory dynamics of differentiating immature thymocytes. Immunity. 2020;**52**(6):1088–1104.e6. DOI: 10.1016/j.immuni.2020.03.019

[18] Boehme L, Roels J, Taghon T. Development of γδ T cells in the thymus - A human perspective. Seminars in Immunology. 2022;**61-64**:101662. DOI: 10.1016/j.smim.2022.101662

[19] Hosokawa H, Rothenberg EV. Cytokines, transcription factors, and the initiation of T-cell development. Cold Spring Harbor Perspectives in Biology. 2018;**10**(5):a028621. DOI: 10.1101/cshperspect.a028621

[20] Nowell CS, Farley AM, Blackburn CC. Thymus organogenesis and development of the thymic stroma. Methods in Molecular Biology. 2007;**380**:125–162. DOI: 10.1007/978-1-59745-395-0_8

[21] Barthlott T, Keller MP, Krenger W, Holländer GA. A short primer on early molecular and cellular events in thymus organogenesis and replacement. Swiss Medical Weekly. 2006;**136**(23-24):365–369. DOI: 10.4414/smw.2006.11401

[22] Liang Z, Dong X, Zhang Z, Zhang Q, Zhao Y. Age-related thymic involution: Mechanisms and functional impact. Aging Cell. 2022;**21**(8):e13671. DOI: 10.1111/acel.13671

[23] Srinivasan J, Lancaster JN, Singarapu N, Hale LP, Ehrlich LIR, Richie ER. Age-related changes in thymic central tolerance. Frontiers in Immunology. 2021;**12**:676236. DOI: 10.3389/fimmu.2021.676236

[24] Tabilas C, Smith NL, Rudd BD. Shaping immunity for life: Layered development of $CD8^+$ T cells. Immunological Reviews. 2023;**315**(1):108–125. DOI: 10.1111/imr.13185

[25] Figueiredo M, Zilhão R, Neves H. Thymus inception: Molecular network in the early stages of thymus organogenesis. International Journal of Molecular Sciences. 2020;**21**(16):5765. DOI: 10.3390/ijms21165765

[26] Cosgrove D, Chan SH, Waltzinger C, Benoist C, Mathis D. The thymic compartment responsible for positive selection of CD4+ T cells. International Immunology. 1992;**4**(6):707–710. DOI: 10.1093/intimm/4.6.707

[27] Gotter J, Brors B, Hergenhahn M, Kyewski B. Medullary epithelial cells of the human thymus express a highly diverse selection of tissue-specific genes colocalized in chromosomal clusters. Journal of Experimental Medicine. 2004;**199**(2):155–166. DOI: 10.1084/jem.20031677

[28] Klein L, Kyewski B, Allen PM, Hogquist KA. Positive and negative selection of the T cell repertoire: What thymocytes see (and don't see). Nature Reviews Immunology. 2014;**14**(6):377–391. DOI: 10.1038/nri3667

[29] den Braber I, Mugwagwa T, Vrisekoop N, Westera L, Mogling R, de Boer AB, Willems N, Schrijver EH, Spierenburg G, Gaiser K, et al. Maintenance of peripheral naive T cells is sustained by thymus output in mice but not humans. Immunity. 2012;**36**:288–297

[30] Qi Q, Liu Y, Cheng Y, Glanville J, Zhang D, Lee JY, Olshen RA, Weyand CM, Boyd SD, Goronzy JJ. Diversity and clonal selection in the human T-cell repertoire. Proceedings of the National Academy of Sciences of the United States of America. 2014;**111**:13139–13144. DOI: 10.1073/pnas.1409155111

[31] Kumar BV, Connors TJ, Farber DL. Human T-cell development, localization, and function throughout life. Immunity. 2018;**48**(2):202–213. DOI: 10.1016/j.immuni.2018.01.007

[32] Issuree PD, Ng CP, Littman DR. Heritable gene regulation in the CD4:CD8 T cell lineage choice. Frontiers in Immunology. 2017;**8**:291. DOI: 10.3389/fimmu.2017.00291

[33] Rothenberg EV. Programming for T-lymphocyte fates: Modularity and mechanisms. Genes and Development. 2019;**33**(17-18):1117–1135. DOI: 10.1101/gad.327163.119

[34] Golzari-Sorkheh M, Yoganathan K, Chen ELY, Singh J, Zúñiga-Pflücker JC. T cell development: From T-lineage specification to intrathymic maturation. Advances in Experimental Medicine and Biology. 2025;**1471**:81–137. DOI: 10.1007/978-3-031-77921-3_4

[35] Yui MA, Rothenberg EV. Developmental gene networks: A triathlon on the course to T cell identity. Nature Reviews Immunology. 2014;**14**(8):529–545. DOI: 10.1038/nri3702

[36] Carpenter AC, Bosselut R. Decision checkpoints in the thymus. Nature Immunology. 2010;**11**(8):666–673. DOI: 10.1038/ni.1887

[37] Gottimukkala KP, Jangid R, Patta I, Sultana DA, Sharma A, Misra-Sen J, Galande S. Regulation of SATB1 during thymocyte development by TCR signaling. Molecular Immunology. 2016;**77**:34–43. DOI: 10.1016/j.molimm.2016.07.005

[38] Alpdogan O, van den Brink MR. Immune tolerance and transplantation. Seminars in Oncology. 2012;**39**(6):629–642. DOI: 10.1053/j.seminoncol.2012.10.001

[39] Kurd N, Robey EA. T-cell selection in the thymus: A spatial and temporal perspective. Immunological Reviews. 2016;**271**(1):114–126. DOI: 10.1111/imr.12398

[40] Jameson SC, Hogquist KA, Bevan MJ. Positive selection of thymocytes. Annual Review of Immunology. 1995;**13**:93–126. DOI: 10.1146/annurev.iy.13.040195.000521

[41] Sprent J, Webb SR. Function and specificity of T cell subsets in the mouse. Advances in Immunology. 1987;**41**:39–133. DOI: 10.1016/s0065-2776(08)60030-9

[42] Bommhardt U, Basson MA, Krummrei U, Zamoyska R. Activation of the extracellular signal-related kinase/mitogen-activated protein kinase pathway discriminates CD4 versus CD8 lineage commitment in the thymus. Journal of Immunology. 1999;**163**(2):715–722

[43] Trobridge PA, Forbush KA, Levin SD. Positive and negative selection of thymocytes depends on LCK interaction with the CD4 and CD8 coreceptors. Journal of Immunology. 2001;**166**(2):809–818. DOI: 10.4049/jimmunol.166.2.809

[44] Hwang JR, Byeon Y, Kim D, Park SG. Recent insights of T cell receptor-mediated signaling pathways for T cell activation and development. Experimental and Molecular Medicine. 2020;**52**(5):750–761. DOI: 10.1038/s12276-020-0435-8

[45] Pascutti MF, Martinez GJ, Quiroga MF. Editorial: Strategies for modulating T cell responses in autoimmunity and infection. Frontiers in Immunology. 2020;**11**:208. DOI: 10.3389/fimmu.2020.00208

[46] Campos JS, Henrickson SE. Defining and targeting patterns of T cell dysfunction in inborn errors of immunity. Frontiers in Immunology. 2022;**13**:932715. DOI: 10.3389/fimmu.2022.932715

[47] Thaventhiran T, Sethu S. T cell co-inhibitory receptors-functions and signalling mechanisms. Journal of Clinical and Cellular Immunology. 2012;**1**. DOI: 10.4172/2155-9899.S12-004

[48] Pollizzi KN, Powell JD. Integrating canonical and metabolic signalling programmes in the regulation of T cell responses. Nature Reviews Immunology. 2014;**14**(7):435–446. DOI: 10.1038/nri3701

[49] Seliger B, Massa C. Modulation of lymphocyte functions in the microenvironment by tumor oncogenic pathways. Frontiers in Immunology. 2022;**13**:883639. DOI: 10.3389/fimmu.2022.883639

[50] van Panhuys N. TCR signal strength alters T-DC activation and interaction times and directs the outcome of differentiation. Frontiers in Immunology. 2016;**7**:6. DOI: 10.3389/fimmu.2016.00006

[51] Fuller JL, Samuel RE, Abraham JJ, Gad D, Padilla DM, Cottrell J. The role of T-lymphocytes in bone remodeling. Open Journal of Orthopedics. 2023;**13**(4):131. DOI: 10.4236/ojo.2023.134014

[52] Luckheeram RV, Zhou R, Verma AD, Xia B. $CD4^{+}$T cells: Differentiation and functions. Clinical and Developmental Immunology. 2012;**2012**:925135. DOI: 10.1155/2012/925135

[53] Kurihara S, Ishikawa A, Kaneko S. Genome editing iPSC to purposing enhancement of induce CD8 killer T cell function for regenerative immunotherapy. Inflammation and Regeneration. 2024;**44**(1):20. DOI: 10.1186/s41232-024-00328-3

[54] Sun L, Su Y, Jiao A, Wang X, Zhang B. T cells in health and disease. Signal Transduction and Targeted Therapy. 2023;**8**(1):235. DOI: 10.1038/s41392-023-01471-y

[55] Adu-Berchie K, Obuseh FO, Mooney DJ. T cell development and function. Rejuvenation Research. 2023;**26**(4):126–138. DOI: 10.1089/rej.2023.0015

Chapter 10

TCR Repertoire: Metrics, Structure and Clinical Implementation

Ksenia Zornikova

Abstract

The T-cell receptor (TCR) repertoire is continuously molded by immunological challenges, including pathogen exposure, tumor recognition, and hematological diseases: each influencing its diversity and clonality. Characterizing the structure and evolutionary dynamics of TCR repertoires provides critical insight into immune system function, persistence of antigen-specific clonotypes, and disease progression. This chapter will present foundational principles of repertoire analysis, focusing on measures of diversity (e.g., Shannon and Simpson indices), clonality (Gini index), and inter-sample overlap metrics, and their relevance for predicting disease outcomes and therapeutic responses. In addition, we will examine how antigen-specific TCR affinity shapes T-cell persistence, functionality, and promiscuity, with particular emphasis on their implications for TCR-based cell therapies. This chapter aims to bridge repertoire analytics with translational immunology, informing both fundamental understanding and clinical applications.

Keywords: TCR repertoire, TCR-based therapy, TCR analysis, T-cell receptors, TCR affinity

1. Introduction

T cells are central mediators of adaptive immunity. They recognize peptide fragments derived from pathogenic or abnormal antigens that are presented by major histocompatibility complex (MHC) molecules through T cell receptors (TCRs).

Advances in next-generation sequencing (NGS) technologies have enabled high-throughput profiling of TCR repertoires. These approaches provide detailed insight into T-cell diversity, clonality, antigen specificity, and clonal evolution during disease and treatment. They have also led to the development of quantitative metrics that characterize repertoire architecture and enable comparisons across individuals, tissues, and clinical conditions. Such analyses demonstrate that TCR repertoire composition and dynamics reflect both physiological immune development and pathological immune responses. TCR repertoire characteristics are influenced by age, infection, autoimmunity, and malignancy, and may serve as valuable biomarkers for immune competence, disease severity, and therapeutic response.

In oncology, the TCR repertoire has emerged as a critical component of antitumor immunity. Tumor development, progression, and response to therapy are closely linked to the presence, diversity, and functional state of tumor-reactive T cells. Furthermore, modern immunotherapeutic strategies, including immune checkpoint inhibitors (ICIs), cancer vaccines, and adoptive T-cell therapies, rely on the activation, expansion, or engineering of tumor-specific TCRs. Understanding TCR repertoire organization and antigen recognition mechanisms is therefore essential for optimizing these therapeutic approaches and improving patient outcomes.

2. TCR structure

TCRs are highly diverse heterodimers composed of either α and β chains or γ and δ chains, encoded by the *TRA*, *TRB*, *TRG*, and *TRD* genes, respectively. αβ TCRs account for approximately 95% of all TCRs and are primarily responsible for MHC-restricted antigen recognition. In contrast, γδ TCRs are less abundant, with only 1%–5% of T cells expressing them, and they mainly participate in innate-like immune responses to exogenous and endogenous antigens in an MHC-independent manner [1].

TCR chains are generated through somatic recombination of variable (V), diversity (D), and joining (J) gene segments, accompanied by random nucleotide insertions and deletions [2]. TCR diversity is concentrated within six hypervariable loops located in the variable domains of the α and β chains, known as complementarity-determining regions (CDRs), with three CDRs per chain (CDR1α, CDR2α, CDR3α, and CDR1β, CDR2β, CDR3β). During V(D)J recombination, CDR1 and CDR2 are encoded entirely by germline gene segments, whereas CDR3α and CDR3β arise from junctional diversity and are, therefore, the most variable regions of the TCR [3, 4]. The combined effects of V(D)J recombination, nucleotide insertion and deletion, and αβ chain pairing result in the potential generation of approximately 10^{15}–10^{20} unique TCR sequences [5].

During antigen recognition, CDR1α, CDR1β, CDR2α, and CDR2β primarily interact with the MHC molecule [6, 7], whereas CDR3α and CDR3β predominantly engage the peptide antigen [8, 9]. Interactions between peptide antigens and CDR1 and/or CDR2 regions have also been reported [10]; however, most of the studies analyzed only CDR3 regions and mainly focus on the β chain.

3. Sequencing approaches to capture the TCR repertoire

NGS has transformed TCR analysis and enabled the development of high-throughput TCR sequencing (TCR-seq) assays for profiling T-cell repertoires. Both DNA and RNA can serve as input material. DNA is present at a stable copy number per cell, allowing direct quantification of clonotype frequencies. However, DNA-based approaches are less sensitive and do not account for allelic exclusion, which can lead to overestimation of repertoire diversity. In contrast, RNA expression levels vary between cells and may affect quantitative accuracy, but RNA-based methods are more sensitive and avoid biases related to allelic exclusion. The incorporation of unique molecular identifiers (UMIs) further improves accuracy by correcting for amplification and sequencing errors [11, 12]

For bulk TCR repertoire analysis, three main approaches are commonly used: (1) TCR amplification by multiplex PCR [13], (2) 5′ rapid amplification of cDNA ends

(5′ RACE) PCR, which involves the addition of common adapters prior to PCR amplification [14], and (3) TCR amplification following gene capture [15, 16]. Multiplex PCR is the most widely used method; however, variability in primer efficiency can lead to inaccurate estimation of clonotype frequencies [17]. The 5′ RACE approach is limited by adapter ligation efficiency [18] and has been reported to be less reproducible than multiplex PCR [19, 20]. Consequently, bulk TCR-seq methods introduce biases in repertoire characterization and complicate accurate pairing of α and β chains.

To address these limitations, alternative sequencing and analytical approaches, such as pairSEQ [21] and TIRTL-seq [22], have been developed to improve αβ chain pairing. However, both methods require larger sample sizes and/or repeated sequencing of the same samples. A major advance in αβ chain pairing was achieved with the advent of single-cell TCR sequencing [23, 24], which also enables simultaneous analysis of the transcriptome and functional state of individual T cells [25]. Nevertheless, single-cell approaches are currently limited to profiling only several thousand cells, whereas the estimated TCR repertoire size in a healthy adult is approximately 3.8×10^8 clonotypes [26]. Therefore, bulk TCR-seq methods remain the most widely used approach for comprehensive assessment of TCR repertoires.

4. Characteristics of the TCR repertoire

The immune repertoire consists of a highly diverse set of unique clonotypes – T cells with certain TCRs. During infection or other immunological challenges, clonotypes specific to pathogen- or tumor-derived antigens undergo clonal expansion. These expanded clones differentiate into effector cells that mediate pathogen clearance or tumor control. Following the resolution of the immune response, a subset of antigen-specific T cells persists as long-lived memory cells, thereby establishing durable immunological memory [5, 27].

There is no gold standard for TCR-specific metrics, and most indices used to describe repertoire diversity, evenness, clonality, and uniqueness originate from ecology, where a species corresponds to a unique TCR, and the repertoire represents a population.

The repertoire is typically characterized by two parameters: richness (the number of clonotypes, denoted as N in the equations below) and evenness (or how (un) equally each clonotype is presented).

4.1 Repertoire richness

Richness can be defined simply as the number of unique clonotypes. However, some studies use indices that account for the contribution of rare clonotypes, such as the Chao1 [28] index and the abundance-based coverage estimator (ACE) [29].

The Chao1 index explicitly incorporates rare clonotypes, particularly singletons (n_1, clonotypes observed once) and doubletons (n_2, clonotypes observed twice), and is especially useful when many unique clonotypes are present, for example, in naïve T-cell compartments:

$$Chao1 = N + \left(\frac{n_1(n_1 - 1)}{2(n_2 + 1)}\right)$$

The ACE is a nonparametric estimator of species richness in a population. It estimates the impact of rare TCR sequences, where the threshold for rare sequences is by default set to 10. The threshold makes the ACE more reliable in cases of clonal expansion (e.g., in tumors or infections).

$$ACE = N_{abund} + \frac{N_{rare}}{C_{ace}} + \frac{n_1}{C_{ace}}\gamma_{ace}^2$$

where N_{abund} and N_{rare} are number of unique clonotypes with >10 copies and ≤10 copies, respectively; γ_{ace}^2 is the coefficient of variation for the rare clones; C_{ace} is the sample coverage estimator, calculated as:

$$C_{ace} = 1 - \frac{n_1}{N_{rare}}$$

For all of those indices, a higher value indicates a more diverse repertoire.

4.2 Repertoire clonality

Repertoire evenness, often referred to as clonality, reflects the extent of expansion of specific clonotypes. High clonality indicates the dominance of a few clones, whereas low clonality reflects a more evenly distributed repertoire.

The simplest, although not fully representative, way to describe repertoire composition is to calculate the proportion of highly expanded clones (HECs) [30]. This metric is calculated as the sum of all clonotypes with abundance exceeding a defined threshold. Common thresholds are 0.01% or 0.1%, although these can be adjusted according to specific research needs.

$$HEC = \sum_{i=1}^{N} p_i$$

where p_i is the proportion of the ith clonotype relative to the total number N of clones, this method excludes rare clonotypes and complicates comparisons between studies due to variability in threshold selection.

To overcome this bias, the diversity evenness score DE50 may be used [31]. DE50 describes the number of unique clonotypes (summed in rank order from highest to lowest frequency) required to account for 50% of the total TCR repertoire. However, DE50 considers only a fraction of the repertoire and is not suitable for comparing highly diverse repertoires with rare clonotypes.

A more sophisticated approach to quantifying clonality is the Pielou index, which is derived from Shannon entropy and is also known as the normalized Shannon index [32]:

$$Pielou\ index = -\frac{\sum_{i=1}^{N} p_i log_b p_i}{log_b(N)}$$

where p_i is the frequency of clonotype i in the repertoire with N unique sequences. Values close to 0 indicate dominance of specific clonotypes, whereas values close to 1 indicate even distribution. The Pielou index measures evenness and is well-suited for describing the overall structure of the repertoire; however, it is less sensitive to highly expanded clonotypes. Because the Pielou index is normalized by the number of clones, it is more appropriate for comparing multiple samples.

Another commonly used metric is the Gini coefficient [33]:

$$Gini\ coefficient = \frac{\sum_{i=1}^{N}\sum_{j=1}^{N}|p_i - p_j|}{2N^2\underline{p}}$$

where p_i and p_j are the frequencies of the ith and j^{th} clonotypes, and $\underline{p}$ is the average of clone frequency. The Gini coefficient ranges from 0 (maximal diversity with equal clone abundances) to 1 (extreme inequality, indicating high clonality). The Gini coefficient measures inequality in clonal size and is superior for detecting HECs. However, its values are more difficult to compare across samples with different sequencing depths, as it is not normalized by the number of unique clonotypes.

4.3 Repertoire diversity

Repertoire diversity is a combination of richness and evenness and is commonly quantified using Shannon entropy, the Simpson index, or the Gini–Simpson index.

The Shannon entropy (also known as the Shannon-Wiener index) [34] is defined as:

$$Shannon\ entropy = -\sum_{i=1}^{N} p_i log_b p_i$$

where p_i is the frequency of clonotype i in the repertoire with N unique sequences, Shannon entropy is close to 0 in the case of monoclonal (i.e., 1 TCR) or oligoclonal (i.e., the presence of a few dominant clones) repertoires and reaches its maximum when clones are evenly distributed. However, Shannon entropy can be higher in repertoires with one dominant clonotype and many evenly distributed minor clones than in strongly oligoclonal repertoires. Thus, Shannon entropy is sensitive to rare clonotypes and is particularly useful in contexts such as naïve T cells. However, changes in the number of rare clonotypes can influence the result: if one sample is sequenced deeper than another, the Shannon index may appear higher simply because more rare clones are detected.

The Simpson index [35] measures the probability that two randomly selected clones belong to the same clonotype:

$$Simpson\ index = \sum_{i=1}^{N} p_i^2$$

However, this parameter is not intuitive because higher values correspond to lower diversity; therefore, modified versions are often used, including the inverse Simpson index and the Gini–Simpson index.

The inverse Simpson index ranges from 1 (monoclonal repertoire) to ∞ (high diversity) and describes the effective number of equally abundant clonotypes.

$$Inverse\ Simpson\ index = \frac{1}{\sum_{i=1}^{N} p_i^2}$$

The Gini–Simpson index describes the probability that two randomly selected clones belong to different clonotypes:

$$Gini - Simpson\ index = 1 - \sum_{i=1}^{N} p_i^2$$

The Gini–Simpson index is close to 0 when the repertoire is highly oligoclonal and close to 1 in the case of a polyclonal repertoire with even clone distribution. Along with the Shannon index, the Gini–Simpson index decreases with the appearance of dominant clonotypes. However, in contrast to Shannon entropy, the Gini-Simpson index is more sensitive to the presence of dominant clonotypes and is more suitable for studying skewed repertoires and samples with unequal sequencing depths or cell counts. Moreover, normalization makes the Gini–Simpson index more suitable for statistical analysis.

Thus, in both cases, a repertoire with high richness and evenness is more diverse than a low-richness and low-evenness one. However, Shannon entropy, in contrast to the Gini–Simpson index, is generally higher in more abundant repertoires, even when frequency distributions are similar.

Aside from the indices described above, many others exist. They differ in robustness, and their results may be skewed by the size of the analyzed sample, the number of hyper-expanded clonotypes, the presence of rare clonotypes, and differences in their relative abundances [33, 36]. The choice of a particular metric typically depends on research objectives, methodological preference, variability in sample quality, sequencing depth, etc. (**Figure 1**).

4.4 Repertoires overlap

Monitoring changes in repertoire diversity provides insight into immune response dynamics, but a complete understanding also requires tracking specific clonotypes. Repertoire similarity analysis allows comparison of overlap in clonotypes across different time points and/or different sources.

A first similarity index is the Jaccard index, which measures the number of overlapping clonotypes (c_{ij}) divided by the number of clonotypes in both compared samples (N_i and N_j, respectively) [37]:

$$Jaccard\ index = \frac{c_{ij}}{N_i + N_j - c_{ij}}$$

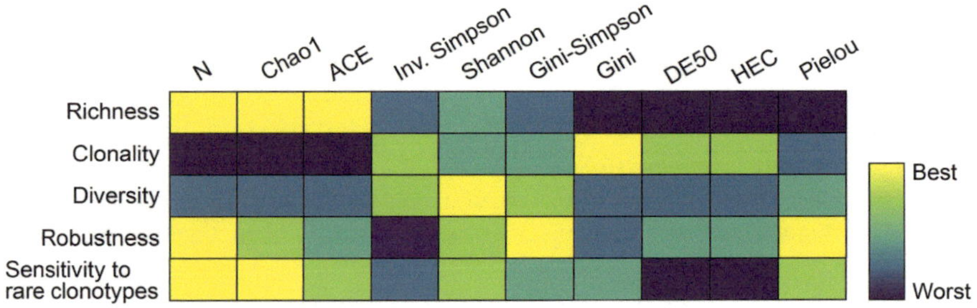

Figure 1.
Suitability of diversity indices for characterizing distinct parameters of the TCR repertoire. Robustness refers to the stability and reliability of a diversity index when sequencing depth changes.

The index ranges from 0 (no overlap) to 1 (complete overlap); however, it considers only the presence or absence of specific sequences and ignores the relative abundance of the overlapping clonotypes.

The Morisita-Horn overlap index is more informative and addresses this limitation, as it incorporates the relative frequency of clonotypes [38]:

$$Morisita - Horn\,index = \frac{2\sum_{i=1}^{N} x_i y_i}{\left(\sum_{i=1}^{N} f_i^2 + \sum_{i=1}^{N} g_i^2\right) XY}$$

where $f_i = x_i/X$ and $g_i = y_i/Y$, with x_i and y_i being the clone sizes of the ith sequence in sample 1 and sample 2, respectively; X and Y are the total number of clones in each sample; N is the total number of unique clonotypes found in both samples. This index also ranges from 0 (no overlap between repertoires) to 1 (identical repertoires in terms of richness and evenness). The Morisita–Horn index is highly effective for analyzing similarities between samples in which the expansion of specific clonotypes is important, such as during infection, cancer, or vaccination.

4.5 Clustering and sequence similarity

The Jaccard and Morisita–Horn indices measure the proportion of identical clonotypes shared between two samples. However, it has been shown that similar CDR3 patterns can be shared among TCRs specific to the same epitope [8, 39, 40].

Such TCRs may be found by constructing clusters. These clusters can be built based on a simple difference in amino acid sequences that takes into account only substitutions (e.g., Hamming distance) and/or insertions and deletions (e.g., Levenshtein distance). Such neighborhood enrichment algorithms may additionally incorporate a generative V(D)J recombination model and correct for intrinsic rearrangement biases (e.g., ALICE [41]) or rely on user-provided reference repertoires to additionally control for thymic selection and shared pathogen-driven T-cell expansions (e.g., TCRNET [39]). These clustering approaches are relatively simple and enable assessment of similarity within epitope-specific repertoires [42, 43]. However, they may be limited in predicting the specificity of novel TCRs, as some epitope-specific repertoires exhibit low sequence similarity. Moreover, certain methods, such as ALICE, are more appropriately applied to the identification of expanded clones within individual patient repertoires.

A more sophisticated clustering framework is implemented in TCRdist [40, 44], which computes a weighted mismatch distance across CDR1, CDR2, CDR2.5 (an MHC-facing loop), and CDR3 regions using the BLOSUM62 substitution matrix, together with gap penalties to account for CDR length variation. Pairwise distances are calculated for all TCRs and assembled into a distance matrix for downstream clustering.

A related approach is used in iSMART [45], which incorporates CDR3 sequences and, optionally, V-gene usage. iSMART computes alignment scores for subsets of CDR3 sequences using the BLOSUM62 matrix, with sequences pre-sorted by length, and gap penalties applied to CDR3s differing by a single insertion or deletion.

Another widely used method for predicting shared specificity is Grouping of Lymphocyte Interactions (GLIPH) by Paratope Hotspots [8]. GLIPH identifies epitope-specific clusters based on the enrichment of shared V-gene usage, CDR3 length distributions, clonal expansion, shared HLA alleles among donors, motif significance, and cluster size. Such an approach could be used to predict the specificity of a new TCR by verifying its affiliation to a specificity group determined by GLIPH. Updated and more robust versions of the algorithm, GLIPH2, as well as GLIPH3, which supports paired αβ TCR sequences, have been released recently (Wang et al., 2022).

A conceptually distinct clustering strategy was introduced by *Ostmeyer et al.* [46], who applied machine-learning methods to Atchley factors – biophysiochemical properties of CDR3β residues, including codon diversity, secondary structure propensity, molecular size, polarity, and electrostatic charge – rather than primary sequence similarity. However, this approach has not been extensively validated.

A broader integrative strategy is implemented in TCRDivER, which combines diversity and similarity metrics derived from either BLOSUM62-based distances or Atchley factors [47].

Despite broadly comparable performance and the ability to identify similar CDR3 motifs among TCRs recognizing common viral epitopes, these models may behave differently depending on the condition under investigation, the dataset in question, and the experimental methodology [48]. At present, clustering is used primarily as a research tool for investigating fundamental patterns of immune responses and has limited application in clinical practice.

5. TCR repertoire characteristics as predictors of immune status

5.1 Diversity and clonality

Age, prior medical history, and ongoing disease states strongly influence TCR repertoire characteristics. The fetal repertoire is more diverse than that of adults, although it demonstrates higher overlap between individuals [49]. From birth through adolescence, overall diversity and the number of unique clonotypes decline, with marked reductions in clonotype publicity and sequence similarity during the first year of life [50]. Rapid immune adaptation in early childhood primarily shapes memory T-cell populations generated during initial antigen exposures; these early-formed memory populations often become more abundant than those generated later in life. Aside from transient expansions and contractions during acute immune responses, the T-cell repertoire remains relatively stable throughout adulthood [51]. With aging, however, a two- to four-fold contraction in TCR diversity has been reported [51–53], accompanied by increased clonality [54–56], most likely driven by age-related thymic involution [57].

In theory, higher TCR diversity increases the probability that virus- or tumor-specific T cells will recognize cognate antigens and effectively control infection or malignant growth, thereby limiting immune escape. In line with this concept, age-associated contraction of the naïve T-cell repertoire results in impaired immune responses in a murine influenza virus model [58]. Human studies demonstrate that reduced repertoire diversity with aging is associated with increased disease severity during infection [54, 59].

Repertoire contraction is also observed in viral infections such as SARS-CoV-2 [42, 60], cytomegalovirus [61], and HIV [62], with severe disease associated with lower TCR diversity compared to mild disease. Patients with autoimmune diseases, including rheumatoid arthritis, type 1 diabetes mellitus, inflammatory bowel disease, and others, also demonstrate a decrease in the diversity of the T-cell repertoire [63].

A significant decrease in TCR repertoire diversity, accompanied by increased clonality, has been reported in peripheral blood from patients with different solid tumors, including glioblastoma, colorectal cancer, lung cancer, melanoma, cervical cancer, and pancreatic ductal adenocarcinoma [64–66]. These changes are particularly pronounced in older patients [64]. Similarly, patients with hematological malignancies, including acute myeloid leukemia, diffuse large B-cell lymphoma, and T-cell lymphoid malignancies, exhibit significantly higher clonality and lower TCR repertoire diversity in blood and lymph nodes, even after adjustment for age-related effects [64].

Most likely, reduced diversity arises from chronic antigen stimulation, leading to clonal expansion and T-cell exhaustion [67]. Thus, a skewed repertoire in cancer patients is associated with an increased risk of severe viral infections [42, 68–70], prolonged infection duration [71, 72], and reduced overall survival [73]. Although vaccination significantly reduces the risk of severe infection and mortality [74, 75], their T-cell responses remain weaker than those observed in healthy individuals [76, 77].

Reduced TCR diversity may influence not only susceptibility to infection in cancer patients but also the course of malignancy itself. Decreased repertoire diversity in peripheral blood, metastasis-positive lymph nodes, and tumor tissue has been associated with advanced disease stage [78–80] and poor prognosis [67, 80, 81] for different solid tumors. However, in lung cancer, higher TCR diversity within tumor tissue has been linked to worse outcomes, whereas greater diversity in peripheral blood correlates with longer progression-free survival [67, 82].

Despite broadly observed associations between higher repertoire diversity and prolonged survival, numerous studies report substantial differences between intratumoral and peripheral blood TCR repertoires, as well as between distinct regions of the same tumor or between primary and metastatic lesions [67, 83]. In some studies, TCR diversity in tumor tissue is lower than in adjacent normal tissue, whereas in others, the opposite has been observed [82]. These discrepancies may reflect differences in tumor stage and the complexity of the tumor microenvironment, which can vary substantially in the degree of T-cell infiltration [84, 85]. However, in some cases, limited but highly focused T-cell infiltration can lead to outcomes comparable to those of highly infiltrated tumors, underscoring the importance of TCR quality rather than quantity [86]. Although tumor-infiltrating TCRs may reflect responses to tumor-associated antigens [87], only a small fraction of intratumoral T cells are truly tumor-reactive [88]. As neoantigens emerge during tumor evolution, their spatial heterogeneity contributes to regional variation in TCR repertoires. This heterogeneity reflects selective clonal expansion within tumors and correlates with somatic mutation burden and tumor heterogeneity [89, 90], and in some cases, is associated with poor prognosis [91].

Overall, the relationship between TCR diversity and tumorigenesis remains complex, context-dependent, and influenced by the analyzed tissue compartment [92]. While low diversity is generally associated with severe infections or poorer survival, TCR repertoire characteristics cannot be reliably used as a sole predictor of disease outcome in clinical practice.

5.2 Repertoire publicity

Repertoire analysis may not only describe the dynamic patterns of immune response but also reveal public TCRs – clonotypes shared among multiple individuals. Although the expectation is that the TCR repertoire is mostly unique in each individual due to its high diversity, overlap of TCRβ in unrelated individuals has been reported at 5% of naive CD4 + and 3.5% of naive CD8 + T cells, and 2.3% of memory CD4 + and 0.4% of memory CD8 + T cells [39]. The presence of public clonotypes may be attributed to convergent recombination (numerous V(D)J recombination events converging to generate the same nucleotide sequence), recombinatorial biases (different gene segments having preferences in usage frequency and pairing), and precursor frequency (different naive T cell precursors being made across a wide range of frequencies) [40–42]. Enrichment of specific public TCRs in antigen-experienced populations indicates that antigen-driven selection plays a major role in shaping these shared clonotypes [43].

Such clonotypes are thought to play a crucial role in establishing an effective pathogen-specific response and in the infection control of pathogens like Cytomegalovirus, Epstein-Barr virus, SARS-CoV-2, HIV, and Adenovirus [43, 93–95]. HIV-associated public TCRs frequently exhibit high avidity and cross-reactivity, both critical determinants of antiviral efficacy. Similarly, patients with mild SARS-CoV-2 tend to have more public clonotypes than patients with severe disease [60, 96]. Public or similar clonotypes are generally more common in antiviral immune responses compared to anti-tumor immunity [42, 43, 97, 98]. It should also be noted, though, that not all viral antigens cause an immune response with a high level of CDR3 similarity or publicity [43]. Both highly homologous and highly diverse epitope-specific repertoires can recognize epitopes containing mutations [43]. However, long-term immunity is mediated by the clonal diversity of the antigen-specific T cell response [99, 100], whereas clonality does not appear to play a significant role [99].

Multiple common tumor and viral antigens were discovered. The presence of similar clonotypes among tumor-infiltrating lymphocytes [89, 101, 102] or the expansion of certain V/J genes [103, 104] suggested an extensive immune response to tumor-associated antigens (TAAs) within the tumor. Most tumor antigens are patient-specific neoantigens, which reduce the proportion of public TCRs. This effect is particularly pronounced in tumors with a high tumor mutation burden, which indicates a higher abundance of neoantigens [105]. Although public clonotypes can be detected in cancer patients [45, 106, 107], they are not necessarily tumor-specific and may reflect immune responses to unrelated antigens [108, 109].

Consequently, the presence of public clonotypes in cancer patients does not necessarily predict similar clinical outcomes. Instead, the activation state of T cells with specific clonotypes, rather than TCR specificity alone, appears to drive effective antitumor responses [110].

6. TCR repertoire and response to therapy

As crucial factors in the anticancer immune response, T cells affect and participate in the process of immunotherapy and traditional treatments [111, 112]. Thus, in-depth analysis of the TCR repertoire has the potential to provide necessary insights for understanding individual tumors and immunity and to guide treatment.

6.1 Traditional anti-cancer treatment

While traditional treatments, such as surgical tumor removal, do not impact lymphocytes on a molecular level, they also cause changes in the TCR repertoire. Patients with colorectal cancer demonstrated contraction of hyperexpanded clonotypes in peripheral blood after surgery [30]. On one hand, this may reflect the removal of tumor antigens, but it may also be related to the overall immune stress after surgery [113]. Although the reasons for these changes are complex, the TCR repertoire can characterize the overall immune state to some extent and has potential for predicting surgery prognosis. For example, higher intratumoral TCR clonality in patients with non-small cell lung cancer was associated with a reduced percentage of residual tumor at the time of surgery [114].

Radio and chemotherapy remain the primary treatments for hematological malignancies and are often combined with surgery to treat solid tumors.

Radiotherapy, although predominantly localized, can induce responses outside the radiation field. This effect is probably mediated by the release of TAAs that are captured by antigen-presenting cells and presented to naïve T cells in the lymph nodes, leading to the activation of tumor-reactive T-cells. Those T cells are then released into the blood stream and may target tumor cells both within and outside the radiation field [115, 116]. Radiotherapy also promotes immune activation through the release of pro-inflammatory cytokines and damage-associated molecular patterns [117]. Indeed, radiotherapy increased the clonality and abundance of tumor-specific clonotypes in patients with renal cell carcinoma [118] and non-small cell lung cancer [119]. However, these newly expanded clonotypes contracted over time, in contrast to the most expanded clonotypes present before therapy, which persisted after treatment. These findings suggest that T-cell responses to newly released TAAs are short-lived [120].

Chemotherapy generally does not prevent long-term reconstitution of blood TCR repertoire diversity to levels appropriate for patient age in either solid or hematological malignancies. However, it may result in near-complete renewal of the repertoire, with minimal overlap compared to the pre-treatment repertoire [64, 121]. Patients with breast and colorectal cancers have demonstrated reduced diversity and similarity compared with pre-treatment repertoires. Lower diversity in some patients has been associated with improved therapeutic response, possibly reflecting a more focused immune response [122, 123]. However, low diversity or high clonality prior to chemotherapy has been associated with poor treatment outcomes [123–126].

6.2 Immune checkpoint inhibitors

Immunotherapeutic strategies activate the immune system and enhance tumor-specific immune responses. The most effective current cancer immunotherapies include ICIs, tumor antigen-based vaccines, and adoptive cell transfer [127–129].

ICIs involve monoclonal antibodies that block inhibitory receptors such as cytotoxic T-lymphocyte–associated protein 4 (CTLA-4), programmed death receptor 1 (PD-1), or its ligand PD-L1. These therapies can produce durable complete responses in some patients, depending on the cancer type. CTLA-4 blockade has demonstrated substantial efficacy in metastatic melanoma [130], whereas anti-PD-1/PD-L1 therapies have shown greater effectiveness in other malignancies, including non-small cell lung cancer [131, 132], Hodgkin lymphoma [133], Merkel cell carcinoma [134], triple-negative breast cancer [135], renal cell carcinoma [136], urothelial carcinoma [137, 138], and head and neck squamous cell carcinoma [139].

CTLA-4 regulates the early stages of T-cell activation. Anti-CTLA-4 therapy has been associated with increased peripheral blood TCR diversity [140–142], largely through the generation of new clonotypes [143, 144], including tumor-specific clones [145]. However, the relationship between repertoire diversity and clinical outcomes remains inconsistent. Some studies report improved survival and clinical benefit in patients with high pre-treatment blood TCR diversity after anti-CTLA-4 monotherapy [143, 146], whereas others do not confirm this association [140, 147, 148]. Moreover, increased peripheral blood T-cell diversity has also been linked to treatment-associated toxicity, suggesting that CTLA-4 blockade may promote the expansion of autoreactive T-cell populations [140, 142, 148]. Nevertheless, it should be noted that most early clinical studies were performed with limited cohort sizes, and the effects of anti-CTLA-4 monotherapy are not clear because anti-CTLA-4 is mostly administered in combination with anti-PD-1/L1 or other adjuvant therapies in clinical studies.

Similarly to anti-CTLA-4, anti-PD-1 therapy increases peripheral TCR diversity [149]. However, more studies have shown that anti-PD-1 treatment mainly leads to TCR clonal expansion rather than the generation of new clonotypes. Increased clonality has been associated with clinical response in metastatic melanoma, non-small cell lung cancer, glioblastoma, and metastatic bladder cancer [147, 150–154]. This effect likely reflects the maintenance and expansion of pre-existing antitumor T-cell populations [152, 155].

6.3 Anti-cancer vaccines

Therapeutic cancer vaccines typically contain defined tumor antigens or antigen-loaded dendritic cells designed to enhance antitumor immunity, eliminate minimal residual disease, and establish durable immune memory [156]. Interestingly, while such vaccines increase the diversity of TCR in the tumor tissue [157, 158], high clonality and expansion of pre-existing clonotypes, rather than the generation of new clones, were observed [159, 160] and associated with better response and longer progression-free survival [160, 161]. The detection of identical TCR clonotypes in tumor tissue and peripheral blood has been linked to prolonged clinical response, likely reflecting sustained circulation of tumor-reactive T cells [161]. For example, in melanoma, longer progression-free survival correlates with higher cumulative frequency of persistent clones and the frequency of effector-memory/memory CD8 + and CD4 + T cells [160].

6.4 TCR-based cell therapies

The improved outcome that may be achieved by stimulation of tumor-infiltrating lymphocytes suggests that the immune system can generate receptors capable of recognizing tumor cells. Genetically engineered T-cells – CAR-T cells – have displayed remarkable clinical efficacy in hematological malignancies, with FDA-approved therapies targeting CD19 (Kymriah, Yescarta, Tecartus, Breyanzi) and BCMA (Abecma), while showing moderate success in solid tumors [162]. However,

CAR-T cells target only antigens on the cell surface, while T-cell receptor-engineered T-cells (TCR-T) have the advantage of targeting potentially any antigen. Moreover, TCRs bind their ligands with relatively low affinity, typically in the micromolar range (1–100 μM) [163, 164], and require substantially lower antigen density (approximately 1–50 complexes per cell) to initiate T-cell activation compared with CARs, which bind targets with nanomolar affinity [165] and require target densities exceeding 1000 molecules per cell [166–168]. This heightened sensitivity to low antigen concentration provides a major therapeutic advantage of TCR-T cells, especially for targeting intracellular tumor antigens presented through MHC molecules.

On the other hand, during thymic negative selection, highly self-reactive T cells are eliminated to prevent autoimmunity, resulting in a peripheral TCR repertoire that generally exhibits low to moderate affinity toward self-antigens. While this mechanism maintains immune tolerance, it also restricts the natural ability of T cells to recognize tumor-associated antigens, many of which are derived from self-proteins. Consequently, overcoming these affinity limitations has become a key objective in TCR-T therapeutic engineering.

TCR-T therapy involves the manufacturing and infusion of T cells genetically reengineered to express a certain TCR, specific to a tumor antigen. To improve anti-tumor efficacy, TCRs are usually engineered to increase affinity. High-affinity TCRs demonstrate superior effector function compared with lower-affinity receptors [169]. High-affinity TCRs may facilitate antigen recognition independently of the CD8 co-receptor, detect lower antigen levels, and enable broader recruitment of $CD4^+$ T cells, which provide cytokine-mediated immune support – all of which can improve tumor control following adoptive transfer [169–173]. However, excessively high-affinity TCRs may promote early exhaustion of T cells following target antigen recognition, limiting the durability of therapeutic responses.

For both CAR-T and TCR-T therapies, the main limitation is the same: the target antigen should be exclusively expressed on tumor cells. Common targets for TCR-T therapies include MART-1 and NY-ESO-1.

MART-1 is expressed in about 90% of melanoma cases [174]. Clinical trials demonstrate tumor regression in 30–69% of treated patients, although serious adverse events, including respiratory distress, ototoxicity, uveitis, and skin toxicity, have been reported [175–177]. NY-ESO-1–specific TCR-T therapies showed encouraging results, with a 45%–55% clinical response rate in metastatic melanoma patients [178, 179], 50%–61% in metastatic synovial sarcoma patients [178–180], and approximately 80% in multiple myeloma, including 70% complete responses [181], without significant side effects. Other antigens, including MAGE-A3 and CEA, have been evaluated, but clinical trials were discontinued due to severe toxicity [182, 183]. Therapies targeting other antigens, such as human endogenous retrovirus type E (HERV-E), demonstrated low toxicity but limited efficacy [184]. TCR-T therapy targeting MAGE-A4 or MAGE-A10 epitopes did not demonstrate clinical response in patients with esophageal cancer and non–small cell lung cancer, respectively [185, 186]; however, more promising results were demonstrated for MAGE-A4-specific TCRs with enhanced affinity [187, 188]. Other cancer antigens are being tested in the clinic, such as KK-LC-1 (NCT03778814 and NCT05035407) or PRAME (NCT03686124 and NCT02743611), with no clinical results yet published.

EBV- or CMV-specific T cells engineered to express a Wilms Tumor Antigen 1 (WT1)-specific T-cell receptor did not improve clinical outcomes in patients with relapsed or refractory acute myeloid leukemia (AML), despite prolonged persistence of transferred cells [189]. However, these engineered T cells were able to prevent AML recurrence in individuals at increased risk of post-hematopoietic cell transplantation relapse [190]. Notably, durable responses were predominantly driven by oligoclonal T-cell populations that were among the most abundant clonotypes in the infused products. This pattern suggests preferential expansion during both in vitro manufacturing and subsequent in vivo persistence [190].

Tumor neoantigens are another possible target for TCR-T therapy. These antigens are potentially expressed exclusively by tumor cells. High-avidity T cells specific to these neoantigens are not eliminated during negative thymic selection. Such T cells can be isolated from patient tumors or healthy donor peripheral blood [191]. Frequently mutated oncogenes, including TP53, KRAS, and PIK3CA, are being explored as targets [191]. In one case, a patient with breast cancer was treated with TCR-T cells targeting the $p53^{R175H}$ neoepitope and demonstrated a partial response with limited toxicity. However, disease progression occurred after six months due to the loss of MHC class I expression [192]. In another study, a patient with pancreatic cancer was treated with $KRAS^{G12D}$-specific TCR-T cells. After six months, tumor regression was still ongoing with no toxicity described, and functional TCR-engineered T cells were persisting in the circulation [193]. TCR-T cells targeting the $KRAS^{G12V}$ mutant are also being tested in the clinic (NCT03190941). However, the identification of epitopes containing recurrent ("public") mutations remains challenging because HLA restriction substantially limits the number of patients eligible for targeting a given neoantigen.

For TCR-T therapy, TCR cross-reactivity is an additional complicating factor. Cross-reactivity represents an intrinsic feature of TCR recognition. TCRs can recognize peptides differing by only one or two amino acids within typical 8–10 amino acid MHC class I-restricted epitopes. Thus, peptides not sharing a single residue may productively interact with the same TCR [194]. Considering that only approximately 1% of peptides are presented on MHC molecules, the estimated frequency of potential cross-reactive targets may be as high as one in 10^4 peptides [195, 196].

Physiologically, cross-reactivity is beneficial, particularly in antiviral immunity, where a single TCR may recognize multiple related or mutated epitopes. It helps to limit immune escape and provides protection against rapidly mutating viruses such as HIV, SARS-CoV-2, and dengue virus [43, 197–200]. Additionally, due to cross-reactivity, some memory T cells with low-affinity TCRs may be stimulated by mutated epitopes and recruited in the immune response during re-infection [201].

However, artificial TCR modification may bypass the negative selection that occurs in the thymus, increasing the risk of unintended recognition of self-peptides. Such off-target toxicity remains one of the major translational barriers for TCR-T therapy. In that context, cross-reactivity can result in severe and unpredictable toxicity.

MAGE-A3 was considered a genuinely tumor-specific target, and engineered anti-MAGE-$A3_{112-120}$ (KVAELVHFL) T cells were adoptively transferred to cancer patients. This caused severe neurological damage and even death due to unexpected cross-reactivity to MAGE-A12 (KMAELVHFL), which is expressed in the brain [202]. Another study reported cardiotoxicity in patients after infusion of affinity-enhanced TCRs against the MAGE-$A3_{168-176}$ peptide (EVDPIGHLY), caused by recognition of an unrelated peptide derived from the muscle protein titin

(ESDPIVAQY), which is presented by cardiomyocytes [203, 204]. However, some studies have described viral-specific and bacterial-derived epitopes that elicit cross-reactive responses to tumor antigens [205, 206], which sometimes may even lead to tumor reduction during infection [207].

On the other hand, cross-reactivity may be utilized to identify peptides that are not naturally processed and presented but can be used to elicit strong cross-reactive T cell responses against the original TAAs. However, this approach has not yet resulted in the development of an effective therapeutic cancer vaccine. While mutated peptides induce a rapid and persistent expansion of specific effector memory CD8 + T cells, those cells demonstrated limited cross-recognition of wild-type peptides, and such immunization was not associated with a significant increase in disease-free or overall survival [208, 209].

While traditional therapies do not directly target T-cell populations, ICIs and anticancer vaccines specifically engage these cells. In theory, all such therapies aim to reactivate the immune response and generate T cells specific to new antigens. However, evidence suggests that, in most cases, pre-existing rather than newly generated tumor-specific clonotypes are more effective. In this instance, TCR-T therapy appears to be a promising solution; however, to date, it has demonstrated only moderate efficacy and is frequently associated with significant toxicity. Another major limitation is the lack of universality of this approach. First, neoantigen diversity is high, and most of them are patient-specific. Second, both public tumor antigens and neoantigens must be presented by specific HLA molecules. This substantially restricts the number of eligible patients, as most studies focus on common alleles such as HLA-A*02. Moreover, TCR cross-reactivity appears to be more frequent and less predictable than that observed with CAR-T cells, raising additional safety concerns. Overall, balancing TCR affinity and cross-reactivity remains a fundamental challenge in TCR-T therapy development, requiring optimization strategies that maximize tumor specificity and functional potency while minimizing off-target toxicity. Therefore, modulation of the immunosuppressive tumor microenvironment and reduction of antigen-specific T-cell exhaustion may ultimately have a greater therapeutic impact. Nonetheless, the number of available studies is still too limited to draw definitive conclusions.

7. Conclusion

T-cell receptor repertoire analysis provides a comprehensive framework for understanding adaptive immune responses in cancer and pathogen-associated diseases. Advances in high-throughput sequencing and computational analysis have enabled detailed characterization of repertoire diversity, clonality, and antigen specificity, supporting their use as biomarkers for disease progression, immune competence, therapeutic response, and patient stratification. The increasing integration of bulk and single-cell sequencing approaches is further improving the resolution of T-cell functional states and tumor-specific immune dynamics.

TCR repertoire profiling is a powerful approach in the analysis of viral infections, cancer outcomes, and response to therapies (**Figure 2**). Despite these advances, challenges remain, including limitations in predicting antigen specificity, sampling-related biases in diversity estimation, and the lack of standardized analytical methodologies. Continued development of multimodal experimental strategies and

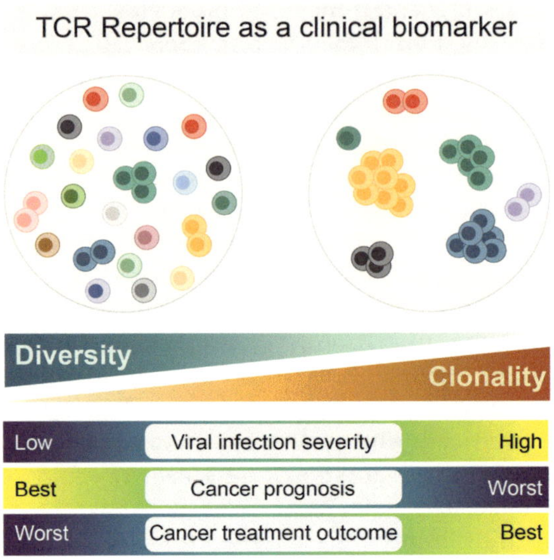

Figure 2.
TCR repertoire diversity and clonality can serve as biomarkers for prognosis in viral infections, malignancies, and responses to anticancer therapies.

machine-learning-based analytical tools is expected to improve the interpretation of repertoire data and enhance its clinical applicability.

Overall, TCR repertoire profiling represents a promising component of precision oncology. Its continued refinement is likely to improve understanding of host-tumor interactions, guide immunotherapeutic development, and support personalized treatment strategies in cancer care.

Conflict of Interest

The author declares no conflict of interest.

Author details

Ksenia Zornikova
University College London, London, United Kingdom

*Address all correspondence to: kvzornikova@gmail.com

References

[1] Morath A, Schamel WW. αβ and γδ T cell receptors: Similar but different. Journal of Leukocyte Biology. 2020;**107**:1045–1055. DOI: 10.1002/JLB.2MR1219-233R

[2] Bassing CH, Swat W, Alt FW. The Mechanism and Regulation of Chromosomal V(D)J Recombination. Cell. 2002;109:S45–55. DOI: 10.1016/S0092-8674(02)00675-X

[3] Mora T, Walczak AM. Quantifying Lymphocyte Receptor Diversity. BioRxiv. 2016. DOI: 10.1101/046870

[4] Davis MM, Bjorkman PJ. T-cell antigen receptor genes and T-cell recognition. Nature. 1988;**334**:395–402. DOI: 10.1038/334395a0

[5] Zarnitsyna VI, BD E, LN S, JN B, Antia R. Estimating the diversity, completeness, and cross-reactivity of the T cell repertoire. Frontiers in Immunology. 2013;**4**. DOI: 10.3389/fimmu.2013.00485

[6] Blevins SJ, Pierce BG, Singh NK, Riley TP, Wang Y, Spear TT, et al. How structural adaptability exists alongside HLA-A2 bias in the human αβ TCR repertoire. Proceedings of the National Academy of Sciences. 2016;**113**. DOI: 10.1073/pnas.1522069113

[7] Sharon E, Sibener LV, Battle A, Fraser HB, Garcia KC, Pritchard JK. Genetic variation in MHC proteins is associated with T cell receptor expression biases. Nature Genetics. 2016;**48**:995–1002. DOI: 10.1038/ng.3625

[8] Glanville J, Huang H, Nau A, Hatton O, Wagar LE, Rubelt F, et al. Identifying specificity groups in the T cell receptor repertoire. Nature. 2017;**547**:94–98

[9] Cole DK, Miles KM, Madura F, Holland CJ, Schauenburg AJA, Godkin AJ, et al. T-cell Receptor (TCR)-peptide specificity overrides affinity-enhancing TCR-major histocompatibility complex interactions. Journal of Biological Chemistry. 2014;**289**:628–638

[10] Wu D, Kolesnikov A, Yin R, Guest JD, Gowthaman R, Shmelev A, et al. Structural assessment of HLA-A2-restricted SARS-CoV-2 spike epitopes recognized by public and private T-cell receptors. Nature Communications. 2022;**13**:19

[11] Shugay M, Britanova OV, Merzlyak EM, Turchaninova MA, Mamedov IZ, Tuganbaev TR, et al. Towards error-free profiling of immune repertoires. Nature Methods. 2014;**11**:653–655

[12] Kivioja T, Vähärautio A, Karlsson K, Bonke M, Enge M, Linnarsson S, et al. Counting absolute numbers of molecules using unique molecular identifiers. Nature Methods. 2012;**9**:72–74

[13] Fernandes S, Chavan S, Chitnis V, Kohn N, Pahwa S. Simplified fluorescent multiplex PCR method for evaluation of the T-cell receptor Vβ-chain repertoire. Clinical and Vaccine Immunology. 2005;**12**:477–483. DOI: 10.1128/CDLI.12.4.477-483.2005

[14] Freeman JD, Warren RL, Webb JR, Nelson BH, Holt RA. Profiling the T-cell receptor beta-chain repertoire by

massively parallel sequencing. Genome Research. 2009;**19**:1817–1824. DOI: 10.1101/gr.092924.109

[15] Mulder DT, Mahé ER, Dowar M, Hanna Y, Li T, Nguyen LT, et al. CapTCR-seq: Hybrid capture for T-cell receptor repertoire profiling. Blood Advances. 2018;**2**:3506–3514

[16] Linnemann C, Heemskerk B, Kvistborg P, Kluin RJC, Bolotin DA, Chen X, et al. High-throughput identification of antigen-specific TCRs by TCR gene capture. Nature Medicine. 2013;**19**:1534–1541

[17] Polz MF, Cavanaugh CM. Bias in template-to-product ratios in multitemplate PCR. Applied and Environmental Microbiology. 1998;**64**:3724–3730. DOI: 10.1128/AEM.64.10.3724-3730.1998

[18] Wulf MG, Maguire S, Humbert P, Dai N, Bei Y, Nichols NM, et al. Non-templated addition and template switching by Moloney murine leukemia virus (MMLV)-based reverse transcriptases co-occur and compete with each other. Journal of Biological Chemistry. 2019;**294**:18220–18231

[19] Liu X, Zhang W, Zeng X, Zhang R, Du Y, Hong X, et al. Systematic comparative evaluation of methods for investigating the TCRβ repertoire. PLoS One. 2016:11e0152464. DOI: 10.1371/journal.pone.0152464

[20] Rosati E, Dowds CM, Liaskou E, Henriksen EKK, Karlsen TH, Franke A. Overview of methodologies for T-cell receptor repertoire analysis. BMC Biotechnology. 2017;**17**:61. DOI: 10.1186/s12896-017-0379-9

[21] Howie B, Sherwood AM, Berkebile AD, Berka J, Emerson RO, Williamson DW, et al. High-throughput pairing of T cell receptor α and β sequences. Science Translational Medicine. 2015;7. DOI: 10.1126/scitranslmed.aac5624

[22] Pogorelyy MV, Kirk AM, Adhikari S, Minervina AA, Sundararaman B, Vegesana K, et al. TIRTL-seq: Deep, quantitative and affordable paired TCR repertoire sequencing. Nature Methods. 2026;**23**:56–64

[23] Pai JA, Satpathy AT. High-throughput and single-cell T cell receptor sequencing technologies. Nature Methods. 2021;**18**:881–892. DOI: 10.1038/s41592-021-01201-8

[24] De Simone M, Rossetti G, Pagani M. Single cell T cell receptor sequencing: Techniques and future challenges. Frontiers in Immunology. 2018;**9**:9. DOI: 10.3389/fimmu.2018.01638

[25] Han A, Glanville J, Hansmann L, Davis MM. Linking T-cell receptor sequence to functional phenotype at the single-cell level. Nature Biotechnology. 2014;**32**:684–692. DOI: 10.1038/nbt.2938

[26] Weng N. Numbers and odds: TCR repertoire size and its age changes impacting on T cell functions. Seminars in Immunology. 2023;**69**:101810. DOI: 10.1016/j.smim.2023.101810

[27] Murali-Krishna K, Altman JD, Suresh M, Sourdive DJD, Zajac AJ, Miller JD, et al. Counting antigen-specific CD8 T cells: A reevaluation of bystander activation during viral infection. Immunity. 1998;**8**:177–187

[28] Chao A. Nonparametric estimation of the number of classes in a population. Scandinavian Journal of Statistics.

Scandinavian Journal of Statistics. 1984;**11**:265–270

[29] Chao A, Lee S-M. Estimating the number of classes via sample coverage. Journal of the American Statistical Association. 1992;**87**:210–217. DOI: 10.1080/01621459.1992.10475194

[30] Liu X, Cui Y, Zhang Y, Liu Z, Zhang Q, Wu W, et al. A comprehensive study of immunology repertoires in both preoperative stage and postoperative stage in patients with colorectal cancer. Molecular Genetics & Genomic Medicine. 2019;7. DOI: 10.1002/mgg3.504

[31] Hosoi A, Takeda K, Nagaoka K, Iino T, Matsushita H, Ueha S, et al. Increased diversity with reduced "diversity evenness" of tumor infiltrating T-cells for the successful cancer immunotherapy. Scientific Reports. 2018;**8**:1058

[32] DeWitt WS, Emerson RO, Lindau P, Vignali M, Snyder TM, Desmarais C, et al. Dynamics of the cytotoxic T cell response to a model of acute viral infection. Journal of Virology. 2015;**89**:4517–4526

[33] Chiffelle J, Genolet R, Perez MA, Coukos G, Zoete V, Harari A. T-cell repertoire analysis and metrics of diversity and clonality. Current Opinion in Biotechnology. 2020;**65**:284–295. DOI: 10.1016/j.copbio.2020.07.010

[34] Stewart JJ, Lee CY, Ibrahim S, Watts P, Shlomchik M, Weigert M, et al. A Shannon entropy analysis of immunoglobulin and T cell receptor. Molecular Immunology. 1997;**34**: 1067–1082

[35] Sanz-Pamplona R, Melas M, Maoz A, Schmit SL, Rennert H, Lejbkowicz F, et al. Lymphocytic infiltration in stage II microsatellite stable colorectal tumors: A retrospective prognosis biomarker analysis. PLoS Medicine. 2020:17e1003292. DOI: 10.1371/journal.pmed.1003292

[36] Mika J, Polanska A, Blenman KR, Pusztai L, Polanska J, Candéias S, et al. A comprehensive evaluation of diversity measures for TCR repertoire profiling. BMC Biology. 2025;**23**:133

[37] Jaccard P. The distribution of the flora in the alpine zone. New Phytologist. 1912;**11**:37–50

[38] Horn H. Measurement of "Overlap" in comparative ecological studies. The American Naturalist. 1966;**100**:419–424

[39] Pogorelyy MV, Shugay M. A framework for annotation of antigen specificities in high-throughput T-cell repertoire sequencing studies. Frontiers in Immunology. 2019;**10**:10. DOI: 10.3389/fimmu.2019.02159

[40] Dash P, Fiore-Gartland AJ, Hertz T, Wang GC, Sharma S, Souquette A, et al. Quantifiable predictive features define epitope-specific T cell receptor repertoires. Nature. 2017;**547**:89–93

[41] Pogorelyy MV, Minervina AA, Shugay M, Chudakov DM, Lebedev YB, Mora T, et al. Detecting T cell receptors involved in immune responses from single repertoire snapshots. PLoS Biology. 2019:17e3000314. DOI: 10.1371/journal.pbio.3000314

[42] Zornikova KV, Sheetikov SA, Rusinov AY, Iskhakov RN, Bogolyubova AV. Architecture of the SARS-CoV-2-specific T cell repertoire. Frontiers in Immunology. 2023;14. DOI: 10.3389/fimmu.2023.1070077

[43] Zornikova K, Dianov D, Ivanova N, Davydova V, Nenasheva T, Fefelova E, et al. Features of highly homologous T-cell receptor repertoire in the immune response to mutations in immunogenic epitopes. International Journal of Molecular Sciences. 2024;**25**:12591

[44] Mayer-Blackwell K, Fiore-Gartland A, Thomas PG Flexible Distance-Based TCR Analysis in Python with Tcrdist3. Methods Mol Biol. 2022. 309–366 p. DOI: 10.1007/978-1-0716-2712-9_16

[45] Zhang H, Liu L, Zhang J, Chen J, Ye J, Shukla S, et al. Investigation of antigen-specific T-cell receptor clusters in human cancers. Clinical Cancer Research. 2020;**26**:1359–1371

[46] Ostmeyer J, Christley S, Toby IT, Cowell LG. Biophysicochemical motifs in T-cell receptor sequences distinguish repertoires from tumor-infiltrating lymphocyte and adjacent healthy tissue. Cancer Research. 2019;**79**:1671–1680. DOI: 10.1158/0008-5472.CAN-18-2292

[47] Vujović M, Marcatili P, Chain B, Kaplinsky J, Andresen TL. Signatures of T cell immunity revealed using sequence similarity with TCRDivER algorithm. Communications Biology. 2023;**6**:357. DOI: 10.1038/s42003-023-04702-8

[48] Hudson D, Lubbock A, Basham M, Koohy H. A comparison of clustering models for inference of T cell receptor antigen specificity. ImmunoInformatics. 2024;**13**:100033. DOI: 10.1016/j.immuno.2024.100033

[49] Britanova OV, Shugay M, Merzlyak EM, Staroverov DB, Putintseva EV, Turchaninova MA, et al. Dynamics of individual T cell repertoires: From cord blood to centenarians. The Journal of Immunology. 2016;**196**:5005–5013

[50] Fang M, Miao Y, Zhu L, Mei Y, Zeng H, Luo L, et al. Age-related dynamics and spectral characteristics of the TCRβ repertoire in healthy children: Implications for immune aging. Aging Cell. 2025;**24**. DOI: 10.1111/acel.14460

[51] Gaimann MU, Nguyen M, Desponds J, Mayer A. Early life imprints the hierarchy of T cell clone sizes. Elife. 2020;9. DOI: 10.7554/eLife.61639

[52] Britanova OV, Putintseva EV, Shugay M, Merzlyak EM, Turchaninova MA, Staroverov DB, et al. Age-related decrease in TCR repertoire diversity measured with deep and normalized sequence profiling. The Journal of Immunology. 2014;**192**:2689–2698

[53] Yoshida K, Cologne JB, Cordova K, Misumi M, Yamaoka M, Kyoizumi S, et al. Aging-related changes in human T-cell repertoire over 20 years delineated by deep sequencing of peripheral T-cell receptors. Experimental Gerontology. 2017;**96**:29–37

[54] Sun X, Nguyen T, Achour A, Ko A, Cifello J, Ling C, et al. Longitudinal analysis reveals age-related changes in the T cell receptor repertoire of human T cell subsets. Journal of Clinical Investigation. 2022:132. DOI: 10.1172/JCI158122

[55] Qi Q, Liu Y, Cheng Y, Glanville J, Zhang D, Lee J-Y, et al. Diversity and clonal selection in the human T-cell repertoire. Proceedings of the National Academy of Sciences. 2014;**111**:13139–13144

[56] Mittelbrunn M, Kroemer G. Hallmarks of T cell aging. Nature

Immunology. 2021;**22**:687–698. DOI: 10.1038/s41590-021-00927-z

[57] Palmer S, Albergante L, Blackburn CC, Newman TJ. Thymic involution and rising disease incidence with age. Proceedings of the National Academy of Sciences. 2018;**115**:1883–1888. DOI: 10.1073/pnas.1714478115

[58] Yager EJ, Ahmed M, Lanzer K, Randall TD, Woodland DL, Blackman MA. Age-associated decline in T cell repertoire diversity leads to holes in the repertoire and impaired immunity to influenza virus. Journal of Experimental Medicine. 2008;**205**: 711–723. DOI: 10.1084/jem.20071140

[59] Joseph M, Wu Y, Dannebaum R, Rubelt F, Zlatareva I, Lorenc A, et al. Global patterns of antigen receptor repertoire disruption across adaptive immune compartments in COVID-19. Proceedings of the National Academy of Sciences. 2022;**119**. DOI: 10.1073/pnas.2201541119

[60] Chang C-M, Feng P, Wu T-H, Alachkar H, Lee K-Y, Chang W-C. Profiling of T cell repertoire in SARS-CoV-2-infected COVID-19 patients between mild disease and pneumonia. Journal of Clinical Immunology. 2021;**41**:1131–1145. DOI: 10.1007/s10875-021-01045-z

[61] Wang GC, Dash P, McCullers JA, Doherty PC, Thomas PG. T cell receptor αβ diversity inversely correlates with pathogen-specific antibody levels in human cytomegalovirus infection. Science Translational Medicine. 2012;4. DOI: 10.1126/scitranslmed.3003647

[62] Baum PD, Young JJ, Schmidt D, Zhang Q, Hoh R, Busch M, et al. Blood T-cell receptor diversity decreases during the course of HIV infection, but the potential for a diverse repertoire persists. Blood. 2012;**119**:3469–3477

[63] Song R, Jia X, Zhao J, Du P, Zhang J. T cell receptor revision and immune repertoire changes in autoimmune diseases. International Reviews of Immunology. 2022;**41**:517–533. DOI: 10.1080/08830185.2021.1929954

[64] Simnica D, Akyüz N, Schliffke S, Mohme M, V. wenserski L, Mährle T, et al. T cell receptor next-generation sequencing reveals cancer-associated repertoire metrics and reconstitution after chemotherapy in patients with hematological and solid tumors. Oncoimmunology. 2019:8e1644110. DOI: 10.1080/2162402X.2019.1644110

[65] Cui J-H, Lin K-R, Yuan S-H, Jin Y-B, Chen X-P, Su X-K, et al. TCR repertoire as a novel indicator for immune monitoring and prognosis assessment of patients with cervical cancer. Frontiers in Immunology. 2018;**9**:9

[66] Pan Y, Gao J, Lin J, Ma Y, Hou Z, Lin Y, et al. High-dimensional single-cell analysis unveils distinct immune signatures of peripheral blood in patients with pancreatic ductal adenocarcinoma. Frontiers in Endocrinology (Lausanne). 2023:14. DOI: 10.3389/fendo.2023.1181538

[67] Jin Y, Luo W, Zhang G, Lin K, Cui J, Chen X, et al. TCR repertoire profiling of tumors, adjacent normal tissues, and peripheral blood predicts survival in nasopharyngeal carcinoma. Cancer Immunology, Immunotherapy. 2018;**67**:1719–1730

[68] Manna A, Pronzato P, Cordani S, Canessa P. CMV infection and pneumonia in hematological

malignancies. Journal of Infection and Chemotherapy. 2003;**9**:265–267. DOI: 10.1007/s10156-003-0251-9

[69] Marchesi F, Pimpinelli F, Ensoli F, Mengarelli A. Cytomegalovirus infection in hematologic malignancy settings other than the allogeneic transplant. Hematological Oncology. 2018;**36**:381–391. DOI: 10.1002/hon.2453

[70] Vilar-Compte D, Shah DP, Vanichanan J, Cornejo-Juarez P, Garcia-Horton A, Volkow P, et al. Influenza in patients with hematological malignancies: Experience at two comprehensive cancer centers. Journal of Medical Virology. 2018;**90**:50–60

[71] Atkins S, He F. Chemotherapy and beyond. Infectious Disease Clinics of North America. 2019;**33**:289–309. DOI: 10.1016/j.idc.2019.01.001

[72] Busca A. Viral infections in patients with hematological malignancies. Leukemia Supplements. 2012;**1**:S24–5. DOI: 10.1038/leusup.2012.15

[73] Sato K, Igarashi S, Tsukada N, Inamura J, Yamamoto M, Shindo M, et al. Cytomegalovirus infection in patients with malignant lymphomas who have not received hematopoietic stem cell transplantation. BMC Cancer. 2022;**22**:944

[74] Nguyen THO, Rowntree LC, Allen LF, Chua BY, Kedzierski L, Lim C, et al. Robust SARS-CoV-2 T cell responses with common TCRαβ motifs toward COVID-19 vaccines in patients with hematological malignancy impacting B cells. Cell Reports Medicine. 2023;**4**:101017

[75] Bange EM, Han NA, Wileyto P, Kim JY, Gouma S, Robinson J, et al. CD8+ T cells contribute to survival in patients with COVID-19 and hematologic cancer. Nature Medicine. 2021;**27**:1280–1289

[76] Keppler-Hafkemeyer A, Greil C, Wratil PR, Shoumariyeh K, Stern M, Hafkemeyer A, et al. Potent high-avidity neutralizing antibodies and T cell responses after COVID-19 vaccination in individuals with B cell lymphoma and multiple myeloma. Nature Cancer. 2022. DOI: 10.1038/s43018-022-00502-x

[77] Marasco V, Carniti C, Guidetti A, Farina L, Magni M, Miceli R, et al. T-cell immune response after mRNA SARS-CoV-2 vaccines is frequently detected also in the absence of seroconversion in patients with lymphoid malignancies. British Journal of Haematology. 2022;**196**:548–558

[78] Song Z, Chen X, Shi Y, Huang R, Wang W, Zhu K, et al. Evaluating the potential of T cell receptor repertoires in predicting the prognosis of resectable non-small cell lung cancers. Molecular Therapy - Methods & Clinical Development. 2020;**18**:73–83

[79] Liu Y, Yang Q, Yang J, Cao R, Liang J, Liu Y, et al. Characteristics and prognostic significance of profiling the peripheral blood T-cell receptor repertoire in patients with advanced lung cancer. International Journal of Cancer. 2019;**145**:1423–1431

[80] Guo L, Bi X, Li Y, Wen L, Zhang W, Jiang W, et al. Characteristics, dynamic changes, and prognostic significance of TCR repertoire profiling in patients with renal cell carcinoma. The Journal of Pathology. 2020;**251**:26–37

[81] Chiffelle J, Genolet R, Michielin O, Harari A. Harnessing TCR repertoires: Predictive insights and therapeutic monitoring in cancer immunotherapy. Immuno-Oncology and Technology. 2025;**28**:101076. DOI: 10.1016/j.iotech.2025.101076

[82] Huang A-L, He Y-Z, Yang Y, Pang M, Zheng G-P, Wang H-L. Exploring the potential of the TCR repertoire as a tumor biomarker (Review). Oncology Letters. 2024;**28**:413. DOI: 10.3892/ol.2024.14546

[83] Yuzhakova DV, Volchkova LN, Pogorelyy MV, Serebrovskaya EO, Shagina IA, Bryushkova EA, et al. Measuring intratumoral heterogeneity of immune repertoires. Frontiers in Oncology. 2020;**10**:10

[84] Wu B, Zhang B, Li B, Wu H, Jiang M. Cold and hot tumors: From molecular mechanisms to targeted therapy. Signal Transduction and Targeted Therapy. 2024;**9**:274. DOI: 10.1038/s41392-024-01979-x

[85] Bagaev A, Kotlov N, Nomie K, Svekolkin V, Gafurov A, Isaeva O, et al. Conserved pan-cancer microenvironment subtypes predict response to immunotherapy. Cancer Cell. 2021;**39**:845–865.e7

[86] Tsuji T, Eng KH, Matsuzaki J, Battaglia S, Szender JB, Miliotto A, et al. Clonality and antigen-specific responses shape the prognostic effects of tumor-infiltrating T cells in ovarian cancer. Oncotarget. 2020;**11**:2669–2683

[87] Zhang H, Chen L, Li L, Liu Y, Das B, Zhai S, et al. Prediction and analysis of tumor infiltrating lymphocytes across 28 cancers by TILScout using deep learning. NPJ Precision Oncology. 2025;**9**:76

[88] Scheper W, Kelderman S, Fanchi LF, Linnemann C, Bendle G, de Rooij MAJ, et al. Low and variable tumor reactivity of the intratumoral TCR repertoire in human cancers. Nature Medicine. 2019;**25**:89–94

[89] Joshi K, de Massy MR, Ismail M, Reading JL, Uddin I, Woolston A, et al. Spatial heterogeneity of the T cell receptor repertoire reflects the mutational landscape in lung cancer. Nature Medicine. 2019;**25**:1549–1559

[90] Lu Z, Zhang C, Sheng J, Shen J, Liu B. T cell receptor β-chain repertoire analysis reveals the association between neoantigens and tumour-infiltrating lymphocytes in multifocal papillary thyroid carcinoma. International Journal of Cancer. 2017;**141**:377–382. DOI: 10.1002/ijc.30743

[91] Reuben A, Gittelman R, Gao J, Zhang J, Yusko EC, Wu C-J, et al. TCR Repertoire Intratumor Heterogeneity in Localized Lung Adenocarcinomas: An Association with Predicted Neoantigen Heterogeneity and Postsurgical Recurrence. Cancer Discovery. 2017;**7**:1088–1097

[92] Pothuri VS, Hogg GD, Conant L, Borcherding N, James CA, Mudd J, et al. Intratumoral T-cell receptor repertoire composition predicts overall survival in patients with pancreatic ductal adenocarcinoma. Oncoimmunology. 2024:13. DOI: 10.1080/2162402X.2024.2320411

[93] Huisman W, Hageman L, Leboux DAT, Khmelevskaya A, Efimov GA, Roex MCJ, et al. Public T-Cell Receptors (TCRs) Revisited by Analysis of the Magnitude of Identical

and Highly-Similar TCRs in Virus-Specific T-Cell Repertoires of Healthy Individuals. Frontiers in Immunology. 2022:13. DOI: 10.3389/fimmu.2022.851868

[94] Price DA, Asher TE, Wilson NA, Nason MC, Brenchley JM, Metzler IS, et al. Public clonotype usage identifies protective Gag-specific CD8+ T cell responses in SIV infection. Journal of Experimental Medicine. 2009;**206**: 923–936

[95] Benati D, Galperin M, Lambotte O, Gras S, Lim A, Mukhopadhyay M, et al. Public T cell receptors confer high-avidity CD4 responses to HIV controllers. Journal of Clinical Investigation. 2016;**126**:2093–2108

[96] Schultheiß C, Paschold L, Simnica D, Mohme M, Willscher E, von Wenserski L, et al. Next-Generation Sequencing of T and B Cell Receptor Repertoires from COVID-19 Patients Showed Signatures Associated with Severity of Disease. Immunity. 2020;**53**:442–455.e4

[97] Emerson RO, DeWitt WS, Vignali M, Gravley J, Hu JK, Osborne EJ, et al. Immunosequencing identifies signatures of cytomegalovirus exposure history and HLA-mediated effects on the T cell repertoire. Nature Genetics. 2017;**49**:659–665

[98] Madi A, Shifrut E, Reich-Zeliger S, Gal H, Best K, Ndifon W, et al. T-cell receptor repertoires share a restricted set of public and abundant CDR3 sequences that are associated with self-related immunity. Genome Research. 2014;**24**:1603–1612

[99] Zornikova KV, Khmelevskaya A, Sheetikov SA, Kiryukhin DO, Shcherbakova OV, Titov A, et al. Clonal diversity predicts persistence of SARS-CoV-2 epitope-specific T-cell response. Communications Biology. 2022;**5**:1351

[100] Bilich T, Nelde A, Heitmann JS, Maringer Y, Roerden M, Bauer J, et al. T cell and antibody kinetics delineate SARS-CoV-2 peptides mediating long-term immune responses in COVID-19 convalescent individuals. Science Translational Medicine. 2021:13. DOI: 10.1126/scitranslmed.abf7517

[101] Floares AG, Zety AV, Floares C, Calin G, Kreutz Carvalho E, Radi K. i-Biomarker CaDx: A circulating miRNA-based multi-cancer detection tool with explainable AI for breast cancer. JCO Global Oncology. 2023;**9**: 5–5. DOI: 10.1200/GO.2023.9.Supplement_1.5

[102] Kim T, Lim H, Jun S, Park J, Lee D, Lee JH, et al. Globally shared TCR repertoires within the tumor-infiltrating lymphocytes of patients with metastatic gynecologic cancer. Scientific Reports. 2023;**13**:20485

[103] Yang M, He D, Sun Y, Guo Y, Ma Y, Feng L, et al. The intratumoral landscape of T cell receptor repertoire in esophageal squamous cell carcinoma. Journal of Translational Medicine. 2024;**22**:1069

[104] Bai X, Zhang Q, Wu S, Zhang X, Wang M, He F, et al. Characteristics of tumor infiltrating lymphocyte and circulating lymphocyte repertoires in pancreatic cancer by the sequencing of T cell receptors. Scientific Reports. 2015;**5**:13664

[105] Pan M, Li B. T cell receptor convergence is an indicator of antigen-specific T cell response in

cancer immunotherapies. Elife. 2022;11. DOI: 10.7554/eLife.81952

[106] Munson DJ, Egelston CA, Chiotti KE, Parra ZE, Bruno TC, Moore BL, et al. Identification of shared TCR sequences from T cells in human breast cancer using emulsion RT-PCR. Proceedings of the National Academy of Sciences. 2016;**113**:8272–8277

[107] Teng YHF, Quah HS, Suteja L, Dias JML, Mupo A, Bashford-Rogers RJM, et al. Analysis of T cell receptor clonotypes in tumor microenvironment identifies shared cancer-type-specific signatures. Cancer Immunology, Immunotherapy. 2022;**71**:989–998

[108] Thorsson V, Gibbs DL, Brown SD, Wolf D, Bortone DS, Ou Yang T-H, et al. The Immune Landscape of Cancer. Immunity. 2018;**48**:812–830.e14

[109] Li X, Zhang Y, Guo S, Wu Z, Wang H, Huang Y, et al. Global analysis of T-cell groups reveals immunological features and common antigen targets of digestive tract tumors. Journal of Cancer Research and Clinical Oncology. 2024;**150**:129

[110] Woolaver RA, Wang X, Krinsky AL, Waschke BC, Chen SMY, Popolizio V, et al. Differences in TCR repertoire and T cell activation underlie the divergent outcomes of antitumor immune responses in tumor-eradicating versus tumor-progressing hosts. Journal for ImmunoTherapy of Cancer. 2021;**9**: e001615

[111] Twyman-Saint Victor C, Rech AJ, Maity A, Rengan R, Pauken KE, Stelekati E, et al. Radiation and dual checkpoint blockade activate non-redundant immune mechanisms in cancer. Nature. 2015;**520**:373–377

[112] Ahmed H, Mahmud AR, Faijanur-Rob-Siddiquee M, Shahriar A, Biswas P, Shimul M, et al. Role of T cells in cancer immunotherapy: Opportunities and challenges. Cancer Pathogenesis and Therapy. 2023;**1**:116–126

[113] Chen Z, Zhang P, Xu Y, Yan J, Liu Z, Lau WB, et al. Surgical stress and cancer progression: The twisted tango. Molecular Cancer. 2019;**18**:132

[114] Zhang J, Ji Z, Caushi JX, El Asmar M, Anagnostou V, Cottrell TR, et al. Compartmental Analysis of T-cell Clonal Dynamics as a Function of Pathologic Response to Neoadjuvant PD-1 Blockade in Resectable Non–Small Cell Lung Cancer. Clinical Cancer Research. 2020;**26**:1327–1337

[115] Formenti SC, Rudqvist N-P, Golden E, Cooper B, Wennerberg E, Lhuillier C, et al. Radiotherapy induces responses of lung cancer to CTLA-4 blockade. Nature Medicine. 2018;**24**:1845–1851

[116] Sharma A, Bode B, Wenger RH, Lehmann K, Sartori AA, Moch H, et al. γ-Radiation Promotes Immunological Recognition of Cancer Cells through Increased Expression of Cancer-Testis Antigens In Vitro and In Vivo. PLoS One. 2011:6e28217. DOI: 10.1371/journal.pone.0028217

[117] Monjazeb AM, Schalper KA, Villarroel-Espindola F, Nguyen A, Shiao SL, Young K. Effects of Radiation on the Tumor Microenvironment. Seminars in Radiation Oncology. 2020;**30**:145–157. DOI: 10.1016/j.semradonc.2019.12.004

[118] Chow J, Hoffend NC, Abrams SI, Schwaab T, Singh AK, Muhitch JB. Radiation induces dynamic changes to the T cell repertoire in renal cell

carcinoma patients. Proceedings of the National Academy of Sciences. 2020;**117**:23721–23729. DOI: 10.1073/pnas.2001933117

[119] Wu L, Zhu J, Rudqvist N-P, Welsh J, Lee P, Liao Z, et al. T-Cell Receptor Profiling and Prognosis After Stereotactic Body Radiation Therapy For Stage I Non-Small-Cell Lung Cancer. Frontiers in Immunology. 2021;**12**. DOI: 10.3389/fimmu.2021.719285

[120] Öjlert ÅK, Nebdal D, Snapkov I, Olsen V, Kidman J, Greiff V, et al. Dynamic changes in the T cell receptor repertoire during treatment with radiotherapy combined with an immune checkpoint inhibitor. Molecular Oncology. 2021;**15**:2958–2968

[121] Gustafson CE, Jadhav R, Cao W, Qi Q, Pegram M, Tian L, et al. Immune cell repertoires in breast cancer patients after adjuvant chemotherapy. JCI Insight. 2020;**5**. DOI: 10.1172/jci.insight.134569

[122] Cai G, Guan Z, Jin Y, Su Z, Chen X, Liu Q, et al. Circulating T-Cell Repertoires Correlate With the Tumor Response in Patients With Breast Cancer Receiving Neoadjuvant Chemotherapy. JCO Precision Oncology. 2022. DOI: 10.1200/PO.21.00120

[123] Chen Y-T, Hsu H-C, Lee Y-S, Liu H, Tan BC-M, Chin C-Y, et al. Longitudinal High-Throughput Sequencing of the T-Cell Receptor Repertoire Reveals Dynamic Change and Prognostic Significance of Peripheral Blood TCR Diversity in Metastatic Colorectal Cancer During Chemotherapy. Frontiers in Immunology. 2022:12. DOI: 10.3389/fimmu.2021.743448

[124] Keane C, Gould C, Jones K, Hamm D, Talaulikar D, Ellis J, et al. The T-cell Receptor Repertoire Influences the Tumor Microenvironment and Is Associated with Survival in Aggressive B-cell Lymphoma. Clinical Cancer Research. 2017;**23**:1820–1828

[125] Manuel M, Tredan O, Bachelot T, Clapisson G, Courtier A, Parmentier G, et al. Lymphopenia combined with low TCR diversity (divpenia) predicts poor overall survival in metastatic breast cancer patients. Oncoimmunology. 2012;**1**:432–440

[126] Akiyoshi T, Gotoh O, Tanaka N, Kiyotani K, Yamamoto N, Ueno M, et al. T-cell complexity and density are associated with sensitivity to neoadjuvant chemoradiotherapy in patients with rectal cancer. Cancer Immunology, Immunotherapy. 2021;**70**:509–518

[127] Shiravand Y, Khodadadi F, Kashani SMA, Hosseini-Fard SR, Hosseini S, Sadeghirad H, et al. Immune Checkpoint Inhibitors in Cancer Therapy. Current Oncology. 2022;**29**:3044–3060

[128] Fan T, Zhang M, Yang J, Zhu Z, Cao W, Dong C. Therapeutic cancer vaccines: Advancements, challenges and prospects. Signal Transduction and Targeted Therapy. 2023;**8**:450. DOI: 10.1038/s41392-023-01674-3

[129] Qian J, Liu Y. Recent advances in adoptive cell therapy for cancer immunotherapy. Frontiers in Immunology. 2025;**16**. DOI: 10.3389/fimmu.2025.1665488

[130] Hodi FS, O'Day SJ, McDermott DF, Weber RW, Sosman JA, Haanen JB, et al. Improved Survival

with Ipilimumab in Patients with Metastatic Melanoma. New England Journal of Medicine. 2010;**363**:711–723

[131] Brahmer J, Reckamp KL, Baas P, Crinò L, Eberhardt WEE, Poddubskaya E, et al. Nivolumab versus Docetaxel in Advanced Squamous-Cell Non–Small-Cell Lung Cancer. New England Journal of Medicine. 2015;**373**:123–135

[132] Reck M, Rodríguez-Abreu D, Robinson AG, Hui R, Csőszi T, Fülöp A, et al. Pembrolizumab versus Chemotherapy for PD-L1–Positive Non–Small-Cell Lung Cancer. New England Journal of Medicine. 2016;**375**:1823–1833

[133] Ansell SM, Lesokhin AM, Borrello I, Halwani A, Scott EC, Gutierrez M, et al. PD-1 Blockade with Nivolumab in Relapsed or Refractory Hodgkin's Lymphoma. New England Journal of Medicine. 2015;**372**: 311–319

[134] Nghiem PT, Bhatia S, Lipson EJ, Kudchadkar RR, Miller NJ, Annamalai L, et al. PD-1 Blockade with Pembrolizumab in Advanced Merkel-Cell Carcinoma. New England Journal of Medicine. 2016;**374**:2542–2552

[135] Schmid P, Adams S, Rugo HS, Schneeweiss A, Barrios CH, Iwata H, et al. Atezolizumab and Nab-Paclitaxel in Advanced Triple-Negative Breast Cancer. New England Journal of Medicine. 2018;**379**:2108–2121

[136] Motzer RJ, Escudier B, McDermott DF, George S, Hammers HJ, Srinivas S, et al. Nivolumab versus Everolimus in Advanced Renal-Cell Carcinoma. New England Journal of Medicine. 2015;**373**:1803–1813

[137] Bellmunt J, de Wit R, Vaughn DJ, Fradet Y, Lee J-L, Fong L, et al. Pembrolizumab as Second-Line Therapy for Advanced Urothelial Carcinoma. New England Journal of Medicine. 2017;**376**:1015–1026

[138] Massard C, Gordon MS, Sharma S, Rafii S, Wainberg ZA, Luke J, et al. Safety and Efficacy of Durvalumab (MEDI4736), an Anti–Programmed Cell Death Ligand-1 Immune Checkpoint Inhibitor, in Patients With Advanced Urothelial Bladder Cancer. Journal of Clinical Oncology. 2016;**34**:3119–3125

[139] Ferris RL, Blumenschein G, Fayette J, Guigay J, Colevas AD, Licitra L, et al. Nivolumab for Recurrent Squamous-Cell Carcinoma of the Head and Neck. New England Journal of Medicine. 2016;**375**:1856–1867

[140] Robert L, Tsoi J, Wang X, Emerson R, Homet B, Chodon T, et al. CTLA4 Blockade Broadens the Peripheral T-Cell Receptor Repertoire. Clinical Cancer Research. 2014;**20**:2424–2432

[141] Cha E, Klinger M, Hou Y, Cummings C, Ribas A, Faham M, et al. Improved Survival with T Cell Clonotype Stability After Anti–CTLA-4 Treatment in Cancer Patients. Science Translational Medicine. 2014:6. DOI: 10.1126/scitranslmed.3008211

[142] Oh DY, Cham J, Zhang L, Fong G, Kwek SS, Klinger M, et al. Immune Toxicities Elicted by CTLA-4 Blockade in Cancer Patients Are Associated with Early Diversification of the T-cell Repertoire. Cancer Research. 2017;**77**:1322–1330

[143] Hopkins AC, Yarchoan M, Durham JN, Yusko EC, Rytlewski JA, Robins HS, et al. T cell receptor

repertoire features associated with survival in immunotherapy-treated pancreatic ductal adenocarcinoma. JCI Insight. 2018:3. DOI: 10.1172/jci.insight.122092

[144] Miller BC, Sen DR, Al Abosy R, Bi K, Virkud YV, LaFleur MW, et al. Subsets of exhausted CD8+ T cells differentially mediate tumor control and respond to checkpoint blockade. Nature Immunology. 2019;**20**:326–336

[145] Kvistborg P, Philips D, Kelderman S, Hageman L, Ottensmeier C, Joseph-Pietras D, et al. Anti–CTLA-4 therapy broadens the melanoma-reactive CD8 $^+$ T cell response. Science Translational Medicine. 2014:6. DOI: 10.1126/scitranslmed.3008918

[146] Postow MA, Manuel M, Wong P, Yuan J, Dong Z, Liu C, et al. Peripheral T cell receptor diversity is associated with clinical outcomes following ipilimumab treatment in metastatic melanoma. Journal for ImmunoTherapy of Cancer. 2015;**3**:23

[147] Hogan SA, Courtier A, Cheng PF, Jaberg-Bentele NF, Goldinger SM, Manuel M, et al. Peripheral Blood TCR Repertoire Profiling May Facilitate Patient Stratification for Immunotherapy against Melanoma. Cancer Immunology Research. 2019;7:77–85

[148] Subudhi SK, Aparicio A, Gao J, Zurita AJ, Araujo JC, Logothetis CJ, et al. Clonal expansion of CD8 T cells in the systemic circulation precedes development of ipilimumab-induced toxicities. Proceedings of the National Academy of Sciences. 2016;**113**: 11919–11924

[149] Akyüz N, Brandt A, Stein A, Schliffke S, Mährle T, Quidde J, et al. T-cell diversification reflects antigen selection in the blood of patients on immune checkpoint inhibition and may be exploited as liquid biopsy biomarker. International Journal of Cancer. 2017;**140**:2535–2544

[150] Tumeh PC, Harview CL, Yearley JH, Shintaku IP, Taylor EJM, Robert L, et al. PD-1 blockade induces responses by inhibiting adaptive immune resistance. Nature. 2014;**515**:568–571

[151] Roh W, Chen P-L, Reuben A, Spencer CN, Prieto PA, Miller JP, et al. Integrated molecular analysis of tumor biopsies on sequential CTLA-4 and PD-1 blockade reveals markers of response and resistance. Science Translational Medicine. 2017:9. DOI: 10.1126/scitranslmed.aah3560

[152] Amaria RN, Reddy SM, Tawbi HA, Davies MA, Ross MI, Glitza IC, et al. Neoadjuvant immune checkpoint blockade in high-risk resectable melanoma. Nature Medicine. 2018;**24**:1649–1654

[153] Gerlinger M, Rowan AJ, Horswell S, Larkin J, Endesfelder D, Gronroos E, et al. Intratumor Heterogeneity and Branched Evolution Revealed by Multiregion Sequencing. New England Journal of Medicine. 2012;**366**:883–892

[154] Miao D, Margolis CA, Vokes NI, Liu D, Taylor-Weiner A, Wankowicz SM, et al. Genomic correlates of response to immune checkpoint blockade in microsatellite-stable solid tumors. Nature Genetics. 2018;**50**:1271–1281

[155] Forde PM, Chaft JE, Smith KN, Anagnostou V, Cottrell TR, Hellmann MD, et al. Neoadjuvant PD-1

Blockade in Resectable Lung Cancer. New England Journal of Medicine. 2018;**378**:1976–1986

[156] Saxena M, van der Burg SH, Melief CJM, Bhardwaj N. Therapeutic cancer vaccines. Nature Reviews Cancer. 2021;**21**:360–378. DOI: 10.1038/s41568-021-00346-0

[157] Sheikh N, Cham J, Zhang L, DeVries T, Letarte S, Pufnock J, et al. Clonotypic Diversification of Intratumoral T Cells Following Sipuleucel-T Treatment in Prostate Cancer Subjects. Cancer Research. 2016;**76**:3711–3718

[158] Carreno BM, Magrini V, Becker-Hapak M, Kaabinejadian S, Hundal J, Petti AA, et al. A dendritic cell vaccine increases the breadth and diversity of melanoma neoantigen-specific T cells. Science. 2015;**348**:803–808

[159] Vroman H, Balzaretti G, Belderbos RA, Klarenbeek PL, van Nimwegen M, Bezemer K, et al. T cell receptor repertoire characteristics both before and following immunotherapy correlate with clinical response in mesothelioma. Journal for ImmunoTherapy of Cancer. 2020:8e000251. DOI: 10.1136/jitc-2019-000251

[160] Poran A, Scherer J, Bushway ME, Besada R, Balogh KN, Wanamaker A, et al. Combined TCR Repertoire Profiles and Blood Cell Phenotypes Predict Melanoma Patient Response to Personalized Neoantigen Therapy plus Anti-PD-1. Cell Reports Medicine. 2020;**1**:100141

[161] Hsu MS, Sedighim S, Wang T, Antonios JP, Everson RG, Tucker AM, et al. TCR Sequencing Can Identify and Track Glioma-Infiltrating T Cells after DC Vaccination. Cancer Immunology Research. 2016;**4**:412–418

[162] Escobar G, Berger TR, Maus MV. CAR-T cells in solid tumors: Challenges and breakthroughs. Cell Reports Medicine. 2025;**6**:102353. DOI: 10.1016/j.xcrm.2025.102353

[163] Hogquist KA, Jameson SC. The self-obsession of T cells: How TCR signaling thresholds affect fate "decisions" and effector function. Nature Immunology. 2014;**15**:815–823. DOI: 10.1038/ni.2938

[164] Davis MM, Boniface JJ, Reich Z, Lyons D, Hampl J, Arden B, et al. LIGAND RECOGNITION BY αβ T CELL RECEPTORS. Annual Review of Immunology. 1998;**16**:523–544

[165] Hudecek M, Lupo-Stanghellini M-T, Kosasih PL, Sommermeyer D, Jensen MC, Rader C, et al. Receptor Affinity and Extracellular Domain Modifications Affect Tumor Recognition by ROR1-Specific Chimeric Antigen Receptor T Cells. Clinical Cancer Research. 2013;**19**:3153–3164

[166] Valitutti S, Müller S, Cella M, Padovan E, Lanzavecchia A. Serial triggering of many T-cell receptors by a few peptide–MHC complexes. Nature. 1995;**375**:148–151. DOI: 10.1038/375148a0

[167] Harris DT, Kranz DM. Adoptive T Cell Therapies: A Comparison of T Cell Receptors and Chimeric Antigen Receptors. Trends in Pharmacological Sciences. 2016;**37**:220–230. DOI: 10.1016/j.tips.2015.11.004

[168] Kershaw MH, Westwood JA, Darcy PK. Gene-engineered T cells for cancer therapy. Nature Reviews Cancer. 2013;**13**:525–541. DOI: 10.1038/nrc3565

[169] Stone JD, Chervin AS, Kranz DM. T-cell receptor binding affinities and kinetics: Impact on T-cell activity and specificity. Immunology. 2009;**126**: 165–176. DOI: 10.1111/j.1365-2567.2008.03015.x

[170] Rees W, Bender J, Teague TK, Kedl RM, Crawford F, Marrack P, et al. An inverse relationship between T cell receptor affinity and antigen dose during CD4 + T cell responses in vivo and in vitro. Proceedings of the National Academy of Sciences. 1999;**96**: 9781–9786

[171] Johnson LA, Heemskerk B, Powell DJ, Cohen CJ, Morgan RA, Dudley ME, et al. Gene Transfer of Tumor-Reactive TCR Confers Both High Avidity and Tumor Reactivity to Nonreactive Peripheral Blood Mononuclear Cells and Tumor-Infiltrating Lymphocytes. The Journal of Immunology. 2006;**177**:6548–6559

[172] Roszkowski JJ, Yu DC, Rubinstein MP, McKee MD, Cole DJ, Nishimura MI. CD8-Independent Tumor Cell Recognition Is a Property of the T Cell Receptor and Not the T Cell. The Journal of Immunology. 2003;**170**:2582–2589. DOI: 10.4049/jimmunol.170.5.2582

[173] Tsuji T. Generation of tumor-specific, HLA class I-restricted human Th1 and Tc1 cells by cell engineering with tumor peptide-specific T-cell receptor genes. Blood. 2005;**106**:470–476. DOI: 10.1182/blood-2004-09-3663

[174] Itakura E, Huang -R-R, Wen D-R, Paul E, Wünsch PH, Cochran AJ. RT in situ PCR detection of MART-1 and TRP-2 mRNA in formalin-fixed, paraffin-embedded tissues of melanoma and nevi. Modern Pathology. 2008;**21**:326–333. DOI: 10.1038/modpathol.3801008

[175] Chodon T, Comin-Anduix B, Chmielowski B, Koya RC, Wu Z, Auerbach M, et al. Adoptive Transfer of MART-1 T-Cell Receptor Transgenic Lymphocytes and Dendritic Cell Vaccination in Patients with Metastatic Melanoma. Clinical Cancer Research. 2014;**20**:2457–2465

[176] Johnson LA, Morgan RA, Dudley ME, Cassard L, Yang JC, Hughes MS, et al. Gene therapy with human and mouse T-cell receptors mediates cancer regression and targets normal tissues expressing cognate antigen. Blood. 2009;**114**:535–546

[177] Rohaan MW, Gomez-Eerland R, van den Berg JH, Geukes Foppen MH, van Zon M, Raud B, et al. MART-1 TCR gene-modified peripheral blood T cells for the treatment of metastatic melanoma: A phase I/IIa clinical trial. Immuno-Oncology and Technology. 2022;**15**:100089

[178] Robbins PF, Morgan RA, Feldman SA, Yang JC, Sherry RM, Dudley ME, et al. Tumor Regression in Patients With Metastatic Synovial Cell Sarcoma and Melanoma Using Genetically Engineered Lymphocytes Reactive With NY-ESO-1. Journal of Clinical Oncology. 2011;**29**:917–924

[179] Robbins PF, Kassim SH, Tran TLN, Crystal JS, Morgan RA, Feldman SA, et al. A pilot trial using lymphocytes genetically engineered with an NY-ESO-1–reactive T-cell receptor: Long-term follow-up and correlates with response. Clinical Cancer Research. 2015;**21**:1019–1027

[180] D'Angelo SP, Melchiori L, Merchant MS, Bernstein D, Glod J,

Kaplan R, et al. Antitumor activity associated with prolonged persistence of adoptively transferred NY-ESO-1 c259T cells in synovial sarcoma. Cancer Discovery. 2018;**8**:944–957

[181] Rapoport AP, Stadtmauer EA, Binder-Scholl GK, Goloubeva O, Vogl DT, Lacey SF, et al. NY-ESO-1–specific TCR–engineered T cells mediate sustained antigen-specific antitumor effects in myeloma. Nature Medicine. 2015;**21**:914–921

[182] Parkhurst MR, Yang JC, Langan RC, Dudley ME, Nathan D-AN, Feldman SA, et al. T cells targeting carcinoembryonic antigen can mediate regression of metastatic colorectal cancer but induce severe transient colitis. Molecular Therapy. 2011;**19**: 620–626

[183] Telang G, Mishra S, Sureshbabu A, Kulkarni S, Joshi S, Singh R. MAGE-A3 as a target for cancer immunotherapy: A systematic review of clinical and preclinical evidence. Current Problems in Cancer. 2025;**58**:101237. DOI: 10.1016/j.currproblcancer. 2025.101237

[184] Nadal R, Barisic S, Scurti GM, Cherkasova E, Chen L, Wood K, et al. Final results of a phase I trial of HERV-E TCR transduced T cells for the treatment of HLA-A*11 patients with metastatic clear cell renal cell carcinoma (mccRCC). Journal of Clinical Oncology. 2024;**42**:435–435

[185] Kageyama S, Ikeda H, Miyahara Y, Imai N, Ishihara M, Saito K, et al. Adoptive transfer of MAGE-A4 T-cell receptor gene-transduced lymphocytes in patients with recurrent esophageal cancer. Clinical Cancer Research. 2015;**21**:2268–2277

[186] Blumenschein GR, Devarakonda S, Johnson M, Moreno V, Gainor J, Edelman MJ, et al. Phase I clinical trial evaluating the safety and efficacy of ADP-A2M10 SPEAR T cells in patients with MAGE-A10 + advanced non-small cell lung cancer. Journal for ImmunoTherapy of Cancer. 2022;**10**: e003581

[187] D'Angelo SP, Van Tine BA, Attia S, Blay J-Y, Strauss SJ, Valverde Morales CM, et al. SPEARHEAD-1: A phase 2 trial of afamitresgene autoleucel (Formerly ADP-A2M4) in patients with advanced synovial sarcoma or myxoid/round cell liposarcoma. Journal of Clinical Oncology. 2021;**39**:11504–11504

[188] Hong DS, Van Tine BA, Olszanski AJ, Johnson ML, Liebner DA, Trivedi T, et al. Phase I dose escalation and expansion trial to assess the safety and efficacy of ADP-A2M4 SPEAR T cells in advanced solid tumors. Journal of Clinical Oncology. 2020;**38**:102–102

[189] Mazziotta F, Martin LE, Egan DN, Bar M, Kinsella S, Paulson KG, et al. A phase I/II trial of WT1-specific TCR gene therapy for patients with acute myeloid leukemia and active disease post-allogeneic hematopoietic cell transplantation: Skewing towards NK-like phenotype impairs T cell function and persistence. Nature Communications. 2025;**16**:5214

[190] Chapuis AG, Egan DN, Bar M, Schmitt TM, McAfee MS, Paulson KG, et al. T cell receptor gene therapy targeting WT1 prevents acute myeloid leukemia relapse post-transplant. Nature Medicine. 2019;**25**:1064–1072

[191] Leko V, Rosenberg SA. Identifying and targeting human tumor antigens for T cell-based immunotherapy of solid

tumors. Cancer Cell. 2020;**38**:454–472. DOI: 10.1016/j.ccell.2020.07.013

[192] Kim SP, Vale NR, Zacharakis N, Krishna S, Yu Z, Gasmi B, et al. Adoptive cellular therapy with autologous tumor-infiltrating lymphocytes and T-cell receptor–engineered T cells targeting common p53 neoantigens in human solid tumors. Cancer Immunology Research. 2022;**10**:932–946

[193] Leidner R, Sanjuan Silva N, Huang H, Sprott D, Zheng C, Shih Y-P, et al. Neoantigen T-cell receptor gene therapy in pancreatic cancer. New England Journal of Medicine. 2022;**386**:2112–2119

[194] Hemmer B, Vergelli M, Gran B, Ling N, Conlon P, Pinilla C, et al Cutting edge: Predictable TCR antigen recognition based on peptide scans leads to the identification of agonist ligands with no sequence homology. The Journal of Immunology. 1998;**160**: 3631–3636

[195] Sewell AK. Why must T cells be cross-reactive? Nature Reviews Immunology. 2012;**12**:669–677. DOI: 10.1038/nri3279

[196] Wooldridge L, Ekeruche-Makinde J, van den Berg HA, Skowera A, Miles JJ, Tan MP, et al. A single autoimmune T cell receptor recognizes more than a million different peptides. Journal of Biological Chemistry. 2012;**287**:1168–1177

[197] Spear TT, Riley TP, Lyons GE, Callender GG, Roszkowski JJ, Wang Y, et al. Hepatitis C virus-cross-reactive TCR gene-modified T cells: A model for immunotherapy against diseases with genomic instability. Journal of Leukocyte Biology. 2016;**100**:545–557

[198] Hu C, Shen M, Han X, Chen Q, Li L, Chen S, et al. Identification of cross-reactive CD8+ T cell receptors with high functional avidity to a SARS-CoV-2 immunodominant epitope and its natural mutant variants. Genes & Diseases. 2022;**9**:216–229

[199] Lineburg KE, Grant EJ, Swaminathan S, Chatzileontiadou DSM, Szeto C, Sloane H, et al. CD8+ T cells specific for an immunodominant SARS-CoV-2 nucleocapsid epitope cross-react with selective seasonal coronaviruses. Immunity. 2021;**54**:1055–1065.e5

[200] Su LF, Davis MM. Antiviral memory phenotype T cells in unexposed adults. Immunological Reviews. 2013;**255**:95–109. DOI: 10.1111/imr.12095

[201] Straub A, Grassmann S, Jarosch S, Richter L, Hilgendorf P, Hammel M, et al. Recruitment of epitope-specific T cell clones with a low-avidity threshold supports efficacy against mutational escape upon re-infection. Immunity. 2023;**56**:1269–1284.e6

[202] Morgan RA, Chinnasamy N, Abate-Daga D, Gros A, Robbins PF, Zheng Z, et al. Cancer regression and neurological toxicity following anti-MAGE-A3 TCR gene therapy. Journal of Immunotherapy. 2013;**36**:133–151

[203] Linette GP, Stadtmauer EA, Maus MV, Rapoport AP, Levine BL, Emery L, et al. Cardiovascular toxicity and titin cross-reactivity of affinity-enhanced T cells in myeloma and melanoma. Blood. 2013;**122**:863–871

[204] Cameron BJ, Gerry AB, Dukes J, Harper JV, Kannan V, Bianchi FC, et al. Identification of a titin-derived HLA-A1–presented peptide as a cross-reactive

target for engineered MAGE A3–directed T cells. Science Translational Medicine. 2013;**5**. DOI: 10.1126/scitranslmed.3006034

[205] Chiou S-H, Tseng D, Reuben A, Mallajosyula V, Molina IS, Conley S, et al. Global analysis of shared T cell specificities in human non-small cell lung cancer enables HLA inference and antigen discovery. Immunity. 2021;**54**:586–602.e8

[206] Vujanovic L, Shi J, Kirkwood JM, Storkus WJ, Butterfield LH. Molecular mimicry of MAGE-A6 and Mycoplasma penetrans HF-2 epitopes in the induction of antitumor CD8 + T-cell responses. Oncoimmunology. 2014;3e954501. DOI: 10.4161/21624011.2014.954501

[207] Ottaiano A, Scala S, D'Alterio C, Trotta A, Bello A, Rea G, et al. Unexpected tumor reduction in metastatic colorectal cancer patients during SARS-Cov-2 infection. Therapeutic Advances in Medical Oncology. 2021;**13**. DOI: 10.1177/17588359211011455

[208] Filipazzi P, Pilla L, Mariani L, Patuzzo R, Castelli C, Camisaschi C, et al. Limited induction of tumor cross-reactive T cells without a measurable clinical benefit in early melanoma patients vaccinated with human leukocyte antigen class I–modified peptides. Clinical Cancer Research. 2012;**18**:6485–6496

[209] Speiser DE, Baumgaertner P, Voelter V, Devevre E, Barbey C, Rufer N, et al. Unmodified self antigen triggers human CD8 T cells with stronger tumor reactivity than altered antigen. Proceedings of the National Academy of Sciences. 2008;**105**: 3849–3854